ADVANCES IN CLINICAL CHEMISTRY

VOLUME 19

Advances in
CLINICAL
CHEMISTRY

Edited by
OSCAR BODANSKY
The Memorial Sloan-Kettering Cancer Center
New York, New York

A. L. LATNER
Department of Clinical Biochemistry, The University of
Newcastle upon Tyne, The Royal Victoria Infirmary,
Newcastle upon Tyne, England

VOLUME 19 • 1977

ACADEMIC PRESS
New York   San Francisco   London
A Subsidiary of Harcourt Brace Jovanovich, Publishers

ACADEMIC PRESS, INC.
111 Fifth Avenue, New York, New York 10003

United Kingdom Edition published by
ACADEMIC PRESS, INC. (LONDON) LTD.
24/28 Oval Road, London NW1

LIBRARY OF CONGRESS CATALOG CARD NUMBER: 58–12341

ISBN 0–12–010319–2

PRINTED IN THE UNITED STATES OF AMERICA

CONTENTS

Advances in Quality Control
T. P. WHITEHEAD

Biochemical Consequences of Intravenous Nutrition in the Newborn
GORDON DALE

LIST OF CONTRIBUTORS

Numbers in parentheses indicate the pages on which the authors' contributions begin.

GORDON DALE (207), *Department of Clinical Biochemistry, University of Newcastle upon Tyne and Royal Victoria Infirmary, Newcastle upon Tyne, England*

HECTOR F. DELUCA (125), *Department of Biochemistry, College of Agricultural and Life Sciences, University of Wisconsin-Madison, Madison, Wisconsin*

E. R. DESOMBRE (57), *Ben May Laboratory for Cancer Research, The University of Chicago, Chicago, Illinois*

E. V. JENSEN (57), *Ben May Laboratory for Cancer Research, The University of Chicago, Chicago, Illinois*

D. W. MOSS (1), *Department of Chemical Pathology, Royal Postgraduate Medical School, London, England*

BERNARD REES SMITH (91), *Departments of Clinical Biochemistry and Medicine, University of Newcastle upon Tyne, Newcastle upon Tyne, England*

T. P. WHITEHEAD (175), *Department of Clinical Chemistry, University of Birmingham, Queen Elizabeth Medical Center, Edgbaston, Birmingham, England*

PREFACE

As one would expect, clinical chemistry is encroaching more and more into the fields of medicine and surgery. This has enormously increased the load on the hospital clinical chemistry laboratory and called for automatic procedures required to handle it. At the same time greater attention has been given to quality control, so necessary to maintain the high standard of biochemical data required for the care of patients. This volume deals with important aspects of both automatic procedures and quality control. As always, in addition to the technical aspects of the discipline, the Editors have carefully chosen their contributors so as to provide up-to-date information related to the biochemical etiology of disease, as well as to the control of therapy. Furthermore, this volume contains an account of the important new radioreceptor assay technique which promises not only to provide diagnostic information but in itself has already shed light upon the etiology of Graves' disease.

In his review of automatic enzyme analyzers, Moss deals very thoroughly with the special requirements of enzyme analysis and the relative merits and applicability of continuous-monitoring and fixed-time enzyme assays. A full account is given of virtually all currently available automatic equipment. Guidance from so respected an authority always proves welcome.

In their article on the diagnostic implications of steroid binding in malignant tissues, Jensen and Desombre deal with the interaction of estrogenic hormones with target tissues in the uterus, mammary glands, and tumors. They give an account of hormone dependency of human breast cancer, including the need for predictive criteria for such dependency and the promising use of mastectomy specimens to predict a possible response to endocrine therapy should metastases appear at a later date. The hormone sensitivity of other neoplasms is also considered.

Radioreceptor assay is becoming increasingly important. In his review of membrane receptors for polypeptide hormones, Rees Smith discusses very fully the thermodynamic considerations involved in relation to methods of studying hormone receptor interaction. Not only does he discuss the receptors for assay of the polypeptide hormones, but goes fully into the subject of antibodies to these receptors. This is especially important in relation to the thyroid-stimulating antibody, which is now regarded as the agent for production of hyperthyroidism associated with Graves' disease.

In recent years, there has been a good deal of development in relation to the metabolism of vitamin D. No one has done more in this respect than DeLuca. In his chapter on the vitamin D endocrine system, he provides a full review of recent advances and the reasons for regarding the vitamin as a prohormone. A highly informative account is given of the absorption and transport of the vitamin, its hydroxylases, and the part played by 1,25-dihydroxycholecalciferol in both calcium homeostasis and phosphate mobilization. Analogs are fully discussed in relation to the biological significance of the hydroxyl groups. The review includes an account of diseases of calcium and phosphorus metabolism related to defects in vitamin D metabolism, and light is shed on the relationship of the vitamin to a variety of bone diseases including osteomalacia and osteoporosis.

As one would expect, Whitehead has written a very lucid account of advances in quality control in which he discusses appropriate quality control terminology and techniques, as well as necessary preventive measures. Good accounts are given of the various types of variance, the use of patients' results, developments in handling laboratory quality control data and the role of external quality control schemes.

Recent advances in neonatal surgery as well as experience with severe nutritional failure have made intravenous nutrition in the newborn a matter of the highest importance. In his chapter dealing with biochemical consequences of intravenous nutrition in the newborn, Dale has given a full account of the effects of individual nutrients and the disorders that might result from intravenous alimentation. These include disorders of hydrogen ion regulation, hypophosphatemia, essential fatty acid deficiency, and trace element deficiencies, as well as possible effects on the liver.

Once again, as is our custom, it is a great pleasure to thank our contributors and the publisher for making this volume possible by virtue of their excellent cooperation.

OSCAR BODANSKY
A. L. LATNER

AUTOMATIC ENZYME ANALYZERS

D. W. Moss

Department of Chemical Pathology, Royal Postgraduate Medical School,
London, England

1. Introduction

Mechanization of chemical analysis is widely accepted as the solution to the problems of rapidly rising work loads which have beset clinical chemistry laboratories throughout the past two decades. It would be impossible for all but a few laboratories to contemplate providing a diagnostic service on the scale that they now achieve without mechanical aids with which to increase the productivity of their limited resources of qualified analysts: however, the very success of mechanized analysis has itself fed the demand for analyses of blood specimens, through the more rapid provision of data of greater reliability which it has brought about. These mechanical aids to analysis are customarily referred to as "automatic" analyzers, although the element of feedback control of the process which is implied in the strict use of the term automation is not usually present in their operation.

1

Determinations of the activities of at least two enzymes in serum (alkaline phosphatase and aspartate transaminase) are among the most frequently requested analyses carried out in clinical chemistry laboratories. These estimations, together with those of a number of other enzymes, make up from 15 to 25% of the total analytical workload of the laboratory. Thus, during the phase of rapid expansion of diagnostic clinical chemistry, the growth of requests for determinations of enzyme activity has at least kept pace with, and probably has even exceeded, the growth of demand for other types of analyses.

This review discusses the extent to which the special requirements of enzymic analysis have been met in automatic analyzers that are currently available, as well as attempting to identify essential and desirable features in the design of such apparatus. Descriptions of some of these analyzers and their performance are also included.

1.1.   SPECIAL REQUIREMENTS OF ENZYME ANALYSIS

Under most circumstances the enzyme contents of different samples of serum, plasma, etc., can be compared quantitatively only in terms of their respective catalytic activities, i.e., by the relative effects which equal volumes of the different samples have on the rate of the specific chemical reaction catalyzed by the enzyme in question. Thus, in contrast to what is usually the case for other types of analysis, enzyme assays always imply the measurement of reaction rates; that is to say, the amount of chemical change produced in a defined interval of time in the presence of a known volume of the solution of the enzyme. Since the rates of enzyme-catalyzed reactions are markedly dependent upon several variables—notably pH and temperature—these must also be strictly controlled. The need to measure time intervals accurately and to control variables, such as temperature, introduces constraints into the design of automatic enzyme analyzers that do not apply with the same rigor to analyzers intended for nonenzymic determinations.

The initial rate of a reaction catalyzed by an enzyme is directly proportional to the number of active molecules present in the system: increasing the number of enzyme molecules results in a proportionate increase in rate, provided that no other factor becomes limiting. An example of such limitation is when the capacity of an indicator reaction (e.g., development of a color) is exceeded at high enzyme concentrations. However, the rate of an enzymic reaction eventually decreases during catalysis by a fixed, initial volume of enzyme solution (Fig. 1). This is the result of the operation of several factors: decrease in concentration of the substrate, increasing importance of the reverse reaction, accumulation of

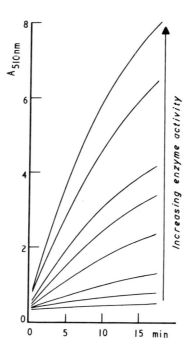

FIG. 1. Progress curves relating the amount of phenol released from phenyl phosphate at pH 10 by human liver alkaline phosphatase to the duration of the reaction. The amount of phenol released is expressed as the absorbance at 510 nm of its oxidized condensation product with 4-aminophenazone. The range of alkaline phosphatase activity is from 8 to 450 King–Armstrong units per 100 ml of sample.

reaction products which may be inhibitory, and inactivation of the enzyme itself. Consequently, the progress curve of the reaction ceases to be linear.

When the progress of reaction is continuously monitored, it is usual to calculate the amount of chemical change produced in unit time from the slope of a tangent drawn to the curve at its initial, or steepest, portion. In this method, no assumptions need to be made about the shapes of the curves for different samples of the enzyme. In the older two-point form of assay, the reaction is allowed to proceed for a fixed time and the relative amounts of chemical change produced in this period by different samples are taken as proportional to their respective enzyme contents. Fixed-time methods depend on the validity of the assumption that the progress curves of the reaction catalyzed by the different samples of enzyme are all linear, or if not linear, can all be described by the same function.

Typically, the nature of fixed-time enzyme assays does not permit any test of the linearity of the progress of reaction to be applied. However, some forms of automatic enzyme analyzers make use of a two-point calculation procedure to derive the value of enzyme activity, while retaining a chart recorder or other system to check linearity.

1.2. RELATIVE MERITS AND APPLICABILITY OF CONTINUOUS-MONITORING ("KINETIC") AND FIXED-TIME ENZYME ASSAYS (M6)

For any fixed-time procedure, an upper limit of enzyme activity exists beyond which the progress-curve of the reaction can no longer be assumed to remain linear during the incubation period. Samples of greater activity than this limit must receive special treatment: the assay must be repeated with a smaller sample, or with a shorter incubation period, or the enzyme sample must be diluted (a procedure which may result in a nonproportionate change in enzyme activity). In order to ensure a high degree of certainty that all samples with apparent activities below the upper limit can be assumed to have linear progress-curves the limit must be set conservatively, so that unnecessary repetition of an appreciable proportion of fixed-time enzyme assays is inevitable. Furthermore, individual variations from sample to sample (e.g., in enzyme stability) may result in undetected nonlinear progress curves in the case of some samples with activities below the limit accepted for the unmodified method.

Continuous-monitoring of the enzyme-catalyzed reaction allows the true initial rate to be derived from the appropriate phase of the reaction. In theory, the initial rate increases in proportion to increasing enzyme concentration, as long as saturation with substrate is maintained. In practice, the operations of initiating the reaction, mixing and commencing recording occupy a finite period of time which varies with the nature of the apparatus and analytical technique. Therefore, an upper limit of enzyme activity exists for continuous-monitoring assays, as well as for fixed-time procedures, above which samples require special treatment, although this limit is typically much higher in the former type of assay. Moreover, those samples which require special attention can be identified individually in continuous-monitoring assays, so that unnecessary repeat analyses or failures to detect unacceptable analyses occur less frequently than in fixed-incubation methods. As will be seen later, however, automated kinetic enzyme assays do not invariably have the same usable range of enzyme activity as their manual counterparts.

The assurance that the true initial rate is measured for each enzyme sample offered by the continuous-monitoring approach to enzyme assay gives it a decisive advantage over fixed-time procedures, making it unquestionably the method of choice for reference procedures in enzymology (B3). Present and future developments in automated enzyme assay are directed toward making this advantage available for routine assays on a large scale. However, fixed-incubation methods offer considerable practical convenience when large numbers of specimens have to be analyzed, and automated versions of them find extensive application.

2. Automation of Fixed-Time Enzyme Assays

2.1. THE AUTOANALYZER

The continuous-flow automatic analysis system invented by Skeggs (S1) and manufactured by the Technicon Instruments Corporation, Tarrytown, New York, as the several versions of the AutoAnalyzer has dominated laboratory automation for almost two decades, and has proved to be very suitable for application to fixed-time enzyme assays. Methods have been described for the automation of assays for virtually all the enzymes of clinical significance with the aid of this apparatus, e.g., alkaline phosphatase (M5), aspartate and alanine aminotransferases (A7, K2), lactate dehydrogenase (M4), and creatine kinase (A5).

An advantage of the AutoAnalyzer is that the introduction of a dialysis stage often removes much between-sample variation; e.g., that due to variations in bilirubin content in alkaline phosphatase assays with p-nitrophenyl phosphate as substrate. Thus, the need to provide a separate "blank" channel or duplicate blank run is avoided (A7). When the constituents of the sample which contribute to the blank are diffusible, dialysis is not effective in eliminating the need for blank correction. However, the sample stream can be split into two, one stream forming a substrateless blank channel. The readings in this channel are subtracted automatically from the corresponding readings obtained simultaneously in the stream in which the enzymic reaction takes place: this is the procedure adopted in the determination of aspartate transaminase at 340 nm in the Technicon SMA analyzers, for example. Alternatively, after division of the sample stream, one part is incubated with substrate for a longer time than the other. After the enzymic reaction has been stopped in both streams, the arrival of the two streams at a dual-differential colorimeter is synchronized by a delay coil in the shorter incubation stream. The difference between colorimeter readings in the two streams is a measure of reaction taking place during the period represented by the difference in incubation times (P4).

A disadvantage of the AutoAnalyzer in enzyme assays is the difficulty of estimating exactly the duration of incubation of the enzyme with its substrate, because of uncertainties about the precise moments at which the enzyme and substrate streams become mingled and at which the reaction effectively ceases. Moreover, flow rates vary over a period of time because of changes in the characteristics of the elastic pump tubing. Therefore, it is preferable to calibrate AutoAnalyzers with enzyme solutions of known activity, rather than with standard solutions of the reaction product (M7). The use of standard solutions of enzyme is itself subject to difficulties, however. The enzyme preparation in question must be of assured stability, unless its activity is to be redetermined regularly by the user with the aid of a reference method. Enzyme calibration standards are often supplied in the form of lyophilized preparations, and the time-dependent increase in activity of alkaline phosphatase which follows reconstitution of these preparations (B4) has been implicated as the cause of lack of agreement between redetermined and assigned values for the activity of this enzyme in AutoAnalyzer reference sera (T2).

When the sample volume (e.g., serum) forms an appreciable fraction of the total volume of the reaction mixture in a manual enzyme assay, a change in the ratio of these two volumes (e.g., by diluting the sample with water) may result in a nonproportionate change in enzyme activity. Therefore, it is preferable to reduce the incubation period in a fixed-time enzyme assay method, rather than to dilute the enzyme solution, when activities beyond the capacity of the method are to be measured. It is not usually convenient to reduce the incubation period in an enzyme assay with the AutoAnalyzer, so that dilution of high activity samples becomes obligatory. However, disproportionate changes in enzyme activity are more pronounced when the ratio of sample volume to total volume is high and, while some earlier AutoAnalyzer enzyme assays used high ratios with consequent anomalous effects of sample dilution, later, more sensitive AutoAnalyzer methods with lower ratios tend to be free from this particular drawback. For example, dilution of serum specimens for alkaline phosphatase assay up to 5-fold with 0.9% w/v saline has been shown in this laboratory to result in a strictly proportional change in activity, in an AutoAnalyzer method with p-nitrophenyl phosphate as the substrate.

Initial reaction velocities are more likely to be maintained in a fixed-time enzyme assay if the period of incubation is kept to the minimum necessary to produce a measurable chemical change. In this respect enzyme assays with the AutoAnalyzer are often better than the manual methods on which they are originally based, and thus the automated versions can be used over a greater range of enzyme activity. In the manual Kind–King alkaline phosphatase method with phenyl phosphate as substrate, for example, the fixed incubation period is 15 minutes, whereas in the corresponding AutoAnalyzer adaptation of the method it is less than half this; consequently, the range of enzyme activity which can be measured without recourse to dilution of samples is twice as great in the automated method as in the manual procedure (Fig. 2). Fluorometric detection of the reaction product, with its increased sensitivity, favors short incubation times and increases the range of linearity of enzyme assays, e.g., of creatine kinase (A5).

Certain criticisms of methods of enzyme assay with the AutoAnalyzer can be traced to the application to it of fixed-time methods which are themselves unsatisfactory, rather than to deficiencies in the apparatus itself. This is the case for the Reitman–Frankel method of aminotransferase assay (R1), for example, which has been criticized on the grounds of inadequate substrate concentration (A2). When well-designed fixed-time methods form the basis of AutoAnalyzer procedures, however, results are obtained which are at least as good as those obtained by hand, with the added advantage of the greater reproducibility characteristic of AutoAnalyzer methods. A coefficient of variation of $\pm 3\%$ was found for the AutoAnalyzer adaptation of the Kind–King alkaline phosphatase method in this laboratory, for example, a value slightly better than the $\pm 4\%$ obtained with the manual procedure.

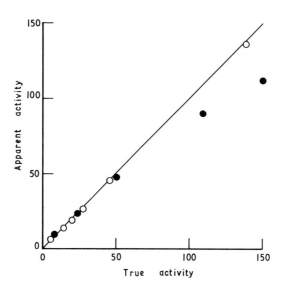

FIG. 2. Relationship of apparent alkaline phosphatase activity (King–Armstrong units per 100 ml) to "true" activity (determined from initial rates of reaction) for a manual procedure with a fixed incubation time of 15 minutes (●) and for an Auto-Analyzer method with about half this incubation period (○).

Good correlation is also obtained between results by suitable Auto-Analyzer methods of enzyme assay and those derived from continuous-monitoring methods, within the limits appropriate to the fixed-time procedures. This is true, for instance, when results of aspartate aminotransferase determinations with the AutoAnalyzer (using UV colorimetry) and with various manual or automated continuous-monitoring techniques are compared (Fig. 3). These data show not only good agreement between the two methods, but also that the standardization procedure with the

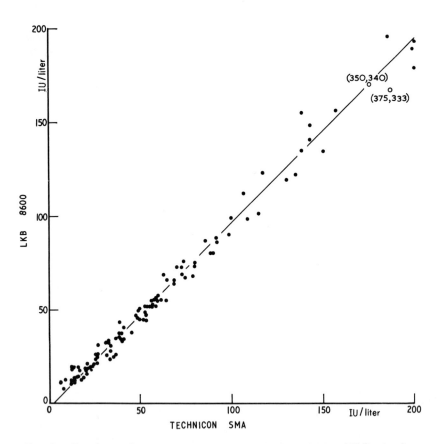

Fig. 3. Correlation between aspartate transaminase activities (IU/liter) of randomly selected serum samples obtained with a Technicon SMA apparatus (340 nm methodology) and with an LKB 8600 reaction-rate analyzer (SKI "Plus-Chem SGOT" reagents). Both sets of measurements were made at 37°C over a period of 3 months. The regression equation is $y = 0.99x - 2.9$ ($r = 0.993$; $n = 122$).

AutoAnalyzer is capable of giving consistent results over a period of some months.

2.2. DISCRETE AUTOMATIC ANALYZERS

Fixed-time enzyme assays have also been automated with the aid of the many types of discrete automatic analyzers that have been developed, although much less experience has been obtained with these analyzers than with the more widely used continuous-flow apparatus. As with the AutoAnalyzer, satisfactory manual fixed-time assays have been adapted to discrete analyzers with good results, provided that the automatic analyzer is free from defects in performance, such as the existence of excessive carry-over between samples, or inadequate control of incubation temperature. Deproteinization has proved to be an obstacle in the development of discrete analyzers, however, so that fixed-time enzyme assays which require this step are less adaptable to discrete analyzers than to the AutoAnalyzer, in which deproteinization by dialysis is available.

2.3. INCORPORATION OF FIXED-TIME ENZYME ASSAYS INTO MULTICHANNEL AUTOMATIC ANALYZERS

Developments in automated analysis have made available a series of instruments which can perform simultaneously a range of analyses on a single specimen of serum or plasma. Argument continues over the clinical value of unexpected abnormal results generated by the operation of these multichannel analyzers and, consequently, over whether programmable machines such as the Greiner Selective Analyzer GSAII (Greiner Electronic Ltd., Langenthal, Switzerland) are preferable to those with a fixed complement of analyses for each sample, of which the Technicon Sequential Multiple Analyzers (SMA) or the Vickers M300 analyzer (Vickers Medical Ltd., Basingstoke, England) are examples. Whatever the merits of the multichannel approach from the viewpoint of diagnostic information, most large clinical laboratories find greater efficiency in the use of multichannel analyzers to carry out a selected range of the most frequently requested tests on a large proportion of the samples submitted for analysis. When deciding which tests are to be included in such a multichannel chemical "screen" or "profile," at least two enzyme assays are invariably found to be among the analyses for which demand is greatest. Thus, enzyme assays have to be accommodated in multichannel analyzers within the constraints imposed by the configuration of the apparatus.

These constraints may include the need to complete each analysis within the cycle-time of the apparatus as a whole, the use of a sample-dilution ratio common to other analyses, and a shared-time system of reading or recording the colors produced in different analyses. This last restriction may prevent any recording or other intermediate check being made on the progress of the reaction in the enzyme channel, in cases where the nature of the reaction would otherwise allow this to be done. Although well-chosen fixed-time assay methods are capable of being automated with good results, as pointed out in the previous section, and perform well as part of multichannel systems, attempts have been made to incorporate continuous-monitoring analyzers into multichannel systems, or to make the fixed-time methods approach more closely to continuous-monitoring assays by introducing additional reading points into the course of the reaction.

A prototype reaction rate analyzer has been described (S4) which can be introduced into the Vickers M300 multichannel analyzer in place of one of the usual reaction modules. It consists of a scanning absorptiometer in which a beam of monochromatic light emerging radially from the center of the circular reaction rotor scans a series of 50 reaction cuvettes around the circumference. Absorbance measurements are made on each one at 100 msec intervals. The light beam is returned from a mirror behind the cuvettes to a photomultiplier below the central axis.

The Technicon Instruments Corporation computer-controlled multichannel analyzer (SMAC) makes three absorbance measurements during the course of each enzyme analysis. In the assay of aspartate aminotransferase, for example, these readings (at 340 nm) are taken 1.1, 2.8, and 4.5 minutes after the start of the reaction, during incubation at 37°C. Improved computer software allows interference by a number of factors which may confuse the interpretation of reaction progress curves (e.g., substrate depletion, presence of a lag phase, or high initial absorbance) to be identified with a high degree of certainty (K1). These improved programs have increased the measurable range of aminotransferase activities in this instrument, with day-to-day reproducibility of ±3-9 IU/liter, depending on sample activity.

3. Automation of Continuous-Monitoring Assays

A determination of enzyme activity by continuous monitoring can be divided into several stages (Fig. 4). A variety of apparatus is now available in which some or all of these stages are carried out automatically. Certain stages are common to all forms of automatic chemical analysis and therefore require no special comment in this review: they include sample measurement and dilution, and addition of reagents. However, the ways in which other functions are carried out, such as initiation of

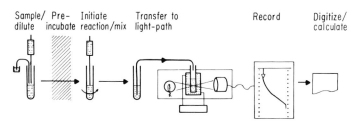

Sample/ Pre- Initiate   Transfer to   Record   Digitize/
dilute incubate reaction/mix light-path   calculate

FIG. 4. Diagrammatic representation of the stages in a typical continuous-monitoring ("kinetic") assay of enzymic activity.

the reaction and mixing, incubation and temperature control, and conversion of the analog signal (usually change in absorbance with time) into units of enzyme activity, can have a profound effect on the analytical performance of an automatic enzyme analyzer.

3.1. INITIATION OF THE REACTION

In the procedure usual in manual continuous-monitoring enzyme assay, the enzyme sample is added to the incomplete reaction mixture (i.e., minus substrate) and a period of incubation is allowed to ensure that side reactions which do not depend on the presence of substrate go to completion: this may be checked by registration of a constant absorbance. The enzymic reaction is then initiated by addition of the missing substrate and the substrate-dependent change is monitored. Although this change is due principally to the reaction catalyzed by the enzyme under study, substrate-dependent reactions of a different nature may also occur during the monitoring period, due, for example, to the presence in the sample of other enzymes which act on the initiating substrate. When complex, multisubstrate reactions are involved, or when coupled enzyme systems are used as indicator reactions, it may be possible to correct for all possible interfering reactions only by the use of one or more individual sample blanks, run either consecutively with the test or concurrently with it in a double-beam instrument.

Some automatic enzyme analyzers retain the preincubation period characteristic of manual enzyme assays, although it may not be possible to monitor absorbance changes during preincubation in these instruments. On the other hand, several automatic enzyme analyzers initiate the enzymic reaction by direct addition of a serum sample to the complete reaction mixture, thus avoiding the complication of having more than one reagent-dispensing module. In these instruments there is no possibility of allowing side reactions to reach completion as in a manual assay although their effect may be minimized by modification of the reaction chemistry (e.g., by including excess lactate dehydrogenase in assays of aspartate aminotransferase activity to promote rapid reduction of endogenous pyruvate). The effects of omission of preincubation may be overcome by the use of a substrateless blank in a two-channel analyzer (Fig. 5). Correction for the effects of unwanted reactions in aminotransferase assays has been studied by Rodgerson and Osberg (R2).

In instruments which retain preincubation as part of a fixed cycle of automatic operation, unavoidable prolonged exposure to elevated temperature (chosen to enhance the rate of reaction and to reduce measuring time) may have deleterious effects on some components of the reaction mixture which are not apparent in the equivalent manual procedure car-

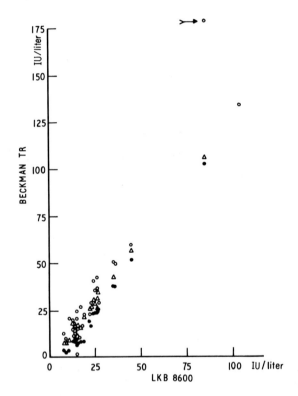

Fɪɢ. 5.   Relationship between aspartate transaminase activities in serum (IU/liter) determined by the Beckman System TR analyzer at 37°C and by the LKB 8600 analyzer at 35°C. The System TR was operated in the double-beam mode with various reference solutions: serum + water (○); serum + aspartateless reaction mixture (●); serum + 2-oxoglutarateless reaction mixture (△). One sample is included (arrowed), for which a serum + water blank fails to correct for spurious aspartate transaminase-like activity.

ried out at a lower temperature. Although thermal inactivation of measured enzymes seems not to be a serious problem in apparatus currently
in use, deterioration of substrates or cofactors during preincubation may
become significant.

Inefficient mixing delays the establishment of a steady rate of reaction
after initiation and may even prevent the true reaction rate being established during the measuring interval in automatic analyzers in which this
interval is short. Some analyzers rely on the mixing effect of expelling
one volume of liquid into a vessel which contains another liquid. Cook
(C2) has pointed out that, to obtain the kinetic energy necessary for efficient jet mixing, the volume of liquid added should be as large as possible
in relation to the volume already present in the vessel and not less than
50% of it. These relationships apply to aqueous solutions and a greater
relative volume of added liquid would be needed if the stationary liquid
were a viscous fluid such as serum. Serum-initiated enzymic reactions, in
which a small volume of serum is picked up by an automatic pipette and
ejected into a reaction vessel followed by a larger volume of buffer-
substrate solution, are examples of this kind of jet mixing. Overvigorous
mixing, whether by mechanical agitation or jet action, may also delay the
establishment of uniform conditions by promoting bubble formation.

As well as making mixing more difficult, the use of a high ratio of sample
volume to reaction-mixture volume can introduce problems of nonproportionate changes in activity when samples with high enzyme activity
have to be diluted before analysis. This effect may be due to interference
from side reactions at high sample to total volume ratios, which are incompletely compensated for in some analyzers.

3.2. Control of the Reaction Temperature

The need for close control of temperature during enzymic reactions is
sufficiently well known to require no further emphasis. However, the
choice of reaction temperature in automatic enzyme analyzers is subject
to considerations which are different from those that apply in manual
analysis.

In manual spectrophotometric assays, cuvette temperatures close to the
ambient temperature (e.g., 25°C or 30°C) provide better constancy of
temperature than temperatures such as 37°C, which are more remote
from room temperature, because of the fluctuations in cuvette temperature resulting from the inevitable repeated openings of the cuvette compartment (B1). This may not apply to some automatic analyzers, in which
samples may be drawn into the measuring position without disturbing
the environment of the measuring cuvette. Automatic analyzers fre-

quently aim to increase the throughput of samples by reducing the monitoring time to the minimum necessary to obtain a measurable absorbance difference, and therefore a higher temperature (usually 37°C) is chosen to accelerate the reaction. However, if the analyzer is of the type in which the reaction is serum-initiated, or if there is no period of preincubation at the measuring temperature, an appreciable fraction of the monitoring interval may be used up in attaining temperature equilibrium.

The use of higher temperatures in order to obtain greater rates of reaction is a more valid reason for their use than the frequently advanced argument that at, e.g., 37°C, a combination of heating cycles alternating with periods of cooling to the surroundings is adequate to ensure temperature stability. In such systems, the set-point of temperature is usually overshot after the heater switches off because of the residual heat of the element itself. While these fluctuations may be negligible over prolonged monitoring intervals, they become significant when monitoring time is shortened until it is of the same order of magnitude as the cyclical variations in temperature. Fluctuations in temperature are reduced if the control system cools as well as heats. Cooling no longer presents a major technical problem with the advent of small, inexpensive refrigeration units for use in water baths, and electrical cooling on the Peltier principle. Automatic enzyme analyzers are available which employ Peltier cooling to provide a controlled reaction temperature independent of the ambient temperature.

The Expert Panel on Enzymes of the International Federation of Clinical Chemistry has recently recommended 30°C as the preferred temperature for enzyme assays (B3). Although this recommendation applies in the first instance to reference methods, it is to be expected that it will influence routine practice also, including the specifications of automatic analyzers, and there seems to be no technological barrier to impede this trend.

The time required to achieve temperature equilibrium after initiation of the reaction is one of the factors determining the length of time which must elapse between initiation of the reaction and commencement of monitoring (see below). Rapid attainment of the set temperature is favored by the use of small volumes of reaction mixture, although the lower limit of volume is set by the dimensions of the cuvette and the sensitivity of the photometric system. Preincubation of the incomplete reaction mixture at the reaction temperature also facilitates rapid equilibration. In serum-initiated reactions, the buffer–substrate solution may be drawn from a thermostatted container, or through a heated tube. The accuracy and precision of temperature-controlling systems in automatic enzyme analyzers are usually not easily verified by the user. Some instruments operate with very small liquid volumes in the cuvette, while in others the cuvette is rotated or agitated mechanically to promote mixing, so that introduction of a temperature-sensing element into the cuvette is impracticable. The complete multiple cuvette assembly of centrifugal analyzers spins rapidly during measurement. In some analyzers, the output of a temperature sensor near the cuvette or in its wall is displayed as a temperature indication, but even in such instruments the operator usually has to rely on the initial and continuing accuracy of the calibration of the sensor.

In the LKB 8600 reaction-rate analyzer (Section 4.1.1), the reaction cuvettes progress sequentially through a heated tunnel in metal racks to bring them to the set temperature for measurement. Mixing is by a rapid alternate clockwise and anticlockwise rotation of each cuvette. The cuvettes are not usually accessible for measurement of temperature, therefore. However, a calibrated thermocouple was adapted to measure the temperatures reached in two of these analyzers in the author's laboratory. The preincubation period was found to be adequate to bring the reaction mixture to the set-point ($37\,^\circ$C) within the tolerance of $\pm 0.2\,^\circ$C claimed by the manufacturer, irrespective of whether the solution was initially at $0\,^\circ$C or at room temperature. A fall of 0.1–$0.2\,^\circ$C was produced by injection of 0.1 vol of cold starting reagent at the measurement position. The two analyzers could differ in their absolute operating temperature by nearly $0.2\,^\circ$C, however. (Data obtained by D. F. Carter, National Physical Laboratory, Teddington, England.)

An aqueous temperature-indicating system that is suitable for measuring the temperatures reached in the cuvettes of enzyme analyzers has been described by Bowie et al. (B3a). The system depends on the use of a buffer solution, Tris, which has a pronounced dependence of pH on temperature. The ionization of an indicator, cresol red, dissolved in the buffer changes in response to the temperature-induced shift in pH, with a corresponding change in absorbance of light. With suitable calibration, this system can be used as a sensitive and accurate indicator of intra-cuvette temperature. It has been used to measure cuvette temperatures in several enzyme analyzers (B3a).

3.3. Monitoring of the Reaction

As already indicated (Section 1.1), it is usual to compare the enzyme activities of different samples in terms of the respective initial rates of reaction that they produce under conditions in which the reaction is essentially zero-order with respect to substrate concentration. Therefore, it is necessary to identify in each assay that portion of the progress curve which follows zero-order kinetics and to derive its slope. Parts of the curve must be identified and rejected in which depletion of substrate has acted to reduce the rate, and the effects of such perturbations as mixing artifacts, instrumental noise, and temperature fluctuations must also be distinguished from changes in rate resulting from changes in enzyme activity. Besides the variations between samples in the period for which zero-order kinetics are followed that result from differences in their enzyme activities (Fig. 1), other sample-dependent effects on the shapes of progress curves may arise from variations in rates of enzyme activation or inactivation during the reaction. The program for monitoring the reaction in an automatic analyzer must be sufficiently flexible to accommodate these sample-to-sample variations, or, if a fixed sequence of reaction-initiation and monitoring is used, this must be timed so as to include the zero-order portion of the curve for the majority of samples.

Ingle and Crouch (I1) have pointed out that, in theory, measurements based on the variable time approach (in which the time required to produce a fixed change in concentration of a reactant is determined for each sample) are to be preferred to measurements of change occurring over a fixed period of time, in the assay of enzymatic activity. This is because, in the integrated form of the rate equation (I1), i.e.,

$$[E] = \frac{-K_m \ln ([S_2]/[S_1]) - \Delta[S]}{k\Delta t}$$

where $[E]$ is the initial concentration of enzyme, $[S_1]$ and $[S_2]$ are substrate concentrations at the beginning and end of time interval Δt, and k is the rate constant for the breakdown of ES to products, the numerator is the same for each concentration of enzyme, and $[E]$ is directly proportional to $1/\Delta t$. It is unnecessary, therefore, to ensure that zero-order kinetics with respect to $[S]$ are maintained throughout the measurement interval, and a wide range of activities can be measured. It is assumed, of course, that the rate equation describes the progress of reaction for each sample.

The variable-time approach has been little applied in automatic enzyme analyzers, however. Prolonged monitoring needed to reach the predetermined change in reactant concentration with samples of lower activities may introduce problems of enzyme inactivation, so that the essential condition of adherence to the rate equation is lost. Also, the rate of throughput of samples may be unacceptably low. A number of automatic analyzers now available do make provision for variation in monitoring intervals from sample to sample, but the purpose of this is to introduce flexibility in identifying the zero-order portion of the curve.

In manual kinetic enzyme assays the reaction is usually initiated with the reaction cuvette *in situ* in the beam of the spectrophotometer (or other measuring device), so that monitoring of the progress of reaction begins with a minimum of delay. Some automatic kinetic analyzers follow this principle. However, in other types of apparatus, the completed reaction mixture, or the cuvette containing it, has to be transported into the monitoring position. Thus, a delay may be introduced between the initiating of the enzymic reaction and the commencement of monitoring, which may be of the order of 30 sec or longer. A protracted interval between initiation and the start of monitoring may mean that the initial, zero-order phase of the reaction is lost for samples of high activity when this phase is brief in the reaction under study. Such a reaction is the conversion of pyruvate to lactate by lactate dehydrogenase in serum (Fig. 6). When the total interval for which the reaction is observed is short, any deviation of the progress curve from linearity may not be easy to detect.

The combination of a short interval between triggering of the reaction and the start of monitoring with a brief, fixed monitoring period is disadvantageous when the reaction being followed has an appreciable lag phase. The zero-order rate may then not be reached within the monitoring interval (G2).

Monitoring should ideally be continued until the zero-order portion of the curve has been identified and verified by a test of the constancy of the rate, and until a sufficient change in signal has taken place for the calculation of rate to be reliable. These requirements are modified in automatic enzyme analyzers by the needs to avoid undue complication and expense in computation and to process each sample as rapidly as possible to maintain an acceptable overall rate of analysis.

Enzymic reactions are almost invariably followed by observing changes in absorption of light. Enzyme analyzers thus are subject to the same errors and limitations as other photometric procedures. A brief recapitulation of these has been given by Ellis and Morrison (E2). In order to produce a signal which is linearly related to enzyme concentration, e.g., for display on a chart recorder, the photocurrent requires logarithmic amplification, since its magnitude is related to transmittance, not absorbance. The performance characteristics of the amplifier can have an important effect on the quality of the data. Some recent automatic enzyme analyzers employ small reaction volumes, to improve the speed and efficiency of temperature equilibration, and they combine these with measurement of small absorbance changes, to reduce the monitoring interval. High photometric sensitivity accompanied by low noise is needed in these instruments.

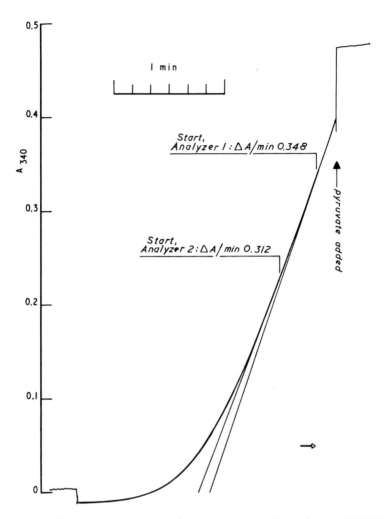

FIG. 6. Fall in absorbance at 340 nm accompanying the oxidation of NADH to NAD⁺ in the conversion of pyruvate to lactate by lactate dehydrogenase. Estimates of the reaction rate obtained from two automatic enzyme analyzers are shown. These differ because of the dissimilar fixed intervals between initiation of the reaction and the start of monitoring in the two instruments. The enzyme activity was equivalent to about 800 IU/liter at 25°C in this experiment.

It is usual to base calculations of enzyme activity on the known absorbance characteristics of some product of the catalyzed reaction. Therefore, the calibration of the photometer of an enzyme analyzer with respect to absorbance and wavelength must be stable, so that frequent checking and recalibration are unnecessary. Fluorometric detection of a reaction product is one or two orders of magnitude more sensitive than photometry in suitable cases and has been much used in manual enzyme assay (R3). Fluorescence intensity is linearly related to concentration of the fluorescent species in dilute solutions, so that logarithmic conversion of the signal is not necessary. However, there is no equivalent in fluorometry of the absorption coefficient, by which the fluorescence detector can be calibrated.

Electrometric methods of monitoring enzyme reactions have been applied in a few cases (C1, G3). A linear relationship exists between signal and concentration in the case of amperometric measurements, but not for potentiometry (I1).

3.4. Data Processing

The method adopted to convert the analog signal (usually generated as the change of absorbance with time) to a numerical value of catalytic concentration varies considerably from one automatic enzyme analyzer to another. The way in which this conversion is effected may have a profound influence on the quality of the results given by a particular analyzer, and on the agreement between them and corresponding values derived from an equivalent manual enzyme assay. The nature and complexity of the data-processing system can also account for an appreciable part of the capital cost of an automatic enzyme analyzer.

The progress of an enzymic reaction drawn on a recorder chart consists of an infinite number of points representing absorbance as a function of time, all of which are available to a human operator who assesses the record. Many automatic enzyme analyzers select only part of the available data in making their analog-to-digital conversion. Some examples of ways in which this selection may be made and the linearity of the progress curve tested are summarized in Fig. 7.

The simplest assessment of the data is to take three (or even only two) successive readings of absorbance on each reaction mixture, separated by fixed time intervals. Where three readings are taken, two rates over successive intervals can be calculated. These may be printed out for comparison by the operator, e.g., as in the Abbott Laboratories ABA 100 analyzer, or they may be compared by the instrument itself. Figure 8 shows diagrammatically the slope-assessment program in one analyzer with the latter type of data-processing, the Gilford Instrument Laboratories Inc. 3500 automatic enzyme analyzer.

The use of three-point assessment of enzymic reaction rates with computer evaluation of the linearity of the reaction in the Technicon SMAC multichannel analyzer has already been mentioned (Section 2.3). This

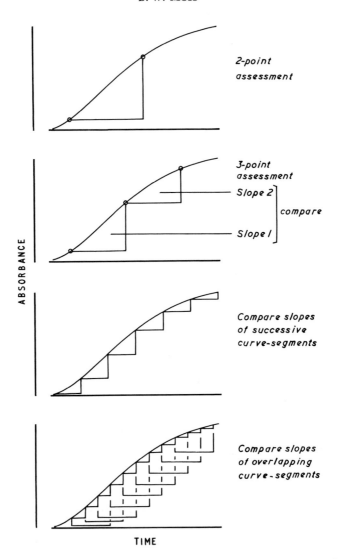

FIG. 7. Diagrammatic representation of various methods of converting the analog signal of change in absorbance with time to digital values of reaction rate used in automatic enzyme analyzers.

development represents a convergence between practice with regard to enzyme assays in this particular multichannel analyzer and in kinetic analyzers with three-point data processing.

More complicated assessments of the analog signal include comparison of the slopes of successive overlapping segments of the progress curve

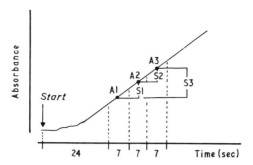

Fɪɢ. 8. Slope-assessment program used in the Gilford 3500 automatic enzyme analyzer. A1, A2, and A3 each indicate averages of 49 readings. [(S1 — S2)/S3] × 100 ⋫ ±5.

(Fig. 7). This method is applied in the LKB Produkter AB 8200 calculator available for use with the LKB 8600 reaction rate analyzer.

The parallel fast analyzers (A3) which employ centrifugation as a means of mixing sample and reagents and initiating the reaction provide examples of the collection of large numbers of readings of absorbance during enzymic reactions. In these instruments the individual reaction mixtures enter measurement cuvettes by centrifugal action. The cuvettes pass through the light beam of the photometer once in every revolution of the reaction rotor. For a rotation speed of 600 rpm, 10 readings are taken from each cuvette every second. Computer circuits are needed to record and analyze these large inputs of data.

The Beckman Instruments, Inc. System TR enzyme activity analyzer employs a different method of determining the slope and linearity of the progress curve. The first and second differentials of the analog signal are derived continuously (Fig. 9). When the second differential is zero, the rate of change of absorbance, represented by the first differential, is constant and its value is used in computing catalytic concentration.

Trayser and Seligson (T3) have described a method of data collection designed for use with automatic enzyme analyzers in which two absorbance readings, representing points on the progress curve of an enzymic reaction separated by a fixed time interval, are made in a double-beam photometer. This is achieved by initiating two identical enzyme reactions for each sample at a fixed time interval (Δt) apart. After a further interval (t_r) the absorbances in the two reactions are compared simultaneously in a double-beam photometer. The difference in absorbance (ΔA) represents the progress of reaction in the time Δt. Limits are set on the choice of the interval between the successive reaction-initiation processes, since this determines the magnitude of ΔA, by the sensitivity of the photometer.

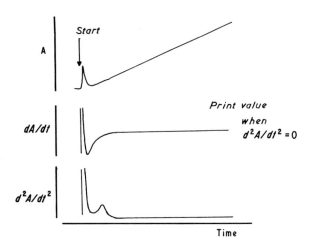

FIG. 9.   Determination of slope and linearity of the reaction progress curve in the Beckman System TR enzyme analyzer. Value of dA/dt is printed when $d^2A/dt^2 = 0$.

Similarly, t_r must be such that both reactions are still in the zero-order phase after this interval. A further condition of this method of data collection is that the twin reaction progress curves for each sample should have identical forms, i.e., that factors which affect the shape of the progress curve should not operate differentially.

In many automatic enzyme analyzers the rate-assessment programs operate with preset limits of maximum and minimum absorbance and of the periods of time for which individual reactions are monitored.

The degree of complexity necessary in data processing in automatic enzyme analyzers depends on whether the progress of reaction can be monitored separately and how the results obtained are to be used. If completely processed results are required, which are to be reported without further check, then they should carry the same degree of reliability as results obtained by a human operator. Therefore, complex calculation and validation programs are required. However, these programs may be part of the functions of a computer which monitors a wide range of activities and apparatus in the clinical chemistry laboratory as a whole, so that the enzyme analyzer itself is only required to digitize the analog signal with the appropriate frequency during the enzymic reaction to supply data to the computer.

Several automatic enzyme analyzers retain the conventional strip-chart recorder, or allow such a recorder to be fitted, on which the analog signal is displayed, in addition to incorporating calculation programs. If the operator is prepared to monitor each successive trace, the calculated result can be based simply on two readings separated by a fixed-time interval, assessment of linearity being entirely the operator's responsibility. This simplified approach loses some of the benefits of automation, however, and where an assessment of linearity based on at least 3 points on the progress curve is made by the instrument itself, the operator need only scrutinize the chart record in the case of those samples for which the criteria of linearity set by the calculation program have not been met. These criteria should be such that results which do satisfy them can be assumed to be reliable.

A comparison between results printed out by two automatic enzyme analyzers with results derived from a conventional assessment of the corresponding chart records was made in this laboratory. The automatic analyzers were the Gilford Instrument Laboratories 3500 analyzer and the Beckman System TR. In neither case was a printed result accompanied by an unacceptable chart record: the total number of analyses for various enzymes was of the order of 200 with each instrument. Thus, the criteria of acceptability of results programmed into these instruments appear to be appropriate.

Any program for dealing with the analog signal produced in an automatic enzyme analyzer is less flexible than assessment by a human operator. Therefore, a proportion of results will be printed with error messages of various kinds (e.g., indicating that the preset time limit has been exceeded or that linearity checks have not been satisfied) although inspection of the chart record reveals a usable trace. If the proportion of these unnecessarily rejected results is excessive, much of the advantage of automation may be lost. The proportion of unnecessarily rejected results in the case of the Gilford analyzer referred to earlier was only 12 out of a total of 851 analyses, however, indicating that it is possible to combine reliability of results printed out with a low rate of unjustified rejections.

Whatever the method of linearity-assessment and calculation that is adopted in an automatic enzyme analyzer, retention of a chart recorder by means of which individual reactions can be monitored is a highly desirable feature. When two-point calculations are employed, the use of a recorder to monitor the reactions is essential, since without it the operation of such an analyzer is indistinguishable from the use of fixed-time procedures.

4. Some Automatic Kinetic Analyzers

The earliest attempts to devise automatic continuous-monitoring enzyme analyzers incorporated AutoAnalyzer modules and made provision to interrupt the flow of reaction mixture so that the change in absorbance due to the enzymic reaction could be followed (B2, P3). However, the discrete system of automatic analysis has proved more adaptable to continuous-monitoring methods and forms the basis of most automatic enzyme analyzers in use at the present time.

Some automatic kinetic analyzers are described in this section. The analyzers have been broadly classified according to the extent to which the overall process of enzyme assay is mechanized, from dispensing of the sample to presentation of finished results. However, such a classification can only be approximate, since many partially mechanized analyzers offer the user the option of adding additional modules to mechanize stages not included in the functions of the basic instrument. Moreover, the list is not claimed to be complete.

4.1. PARTIALLY AUTOMATED ANALYZERS

Mechanization has been introduced into conventional manual kinetic enzyme assays by the use of automatic cuvette-positioners (Gilford Instrument Laboratories, Inc.; Pye Unicam, Ltd.). These devices permit time-sharing between several separate cuvettes in the light path of the photometer; thus several samples can be monitored in parallel. Considerable increases in productivity in the clinical laboratory have been reported as a result of incorporating cuvette-positioners in work-simplification schemes of enzyme assay (E1).

4.1.1. *The LKB 8600 Reaction-Rate Analyzer*

In its basic form, this instrument (LKB-Produkter AB, Bromma 1, Sweden) automates the stages of preincubation of incomplete reaction mixtures, initiation of the enzymic reaction, mixing, monitoring of the reaction, and recording of the analog signal of change in absorbance with time on a strip-chart recorder (Fig. 10). Measurement of serum or other samples into disposable plastic reaction cuvettes and addition of reagents other than the initiant is typically carried out off-line, although modules to perform this function mechanically are obtainable from the manufacturer and from Hook and Tucker Instruments Limited, New Addington, Croydon, England (Hook and Tucker K40 Sampler). Similarly, both LKB Produkter and other manufacturers supply calculators which can replace the need for assessment of the chart records by the operator (B6).

Enzyme samples diluted in the incomplete reaction mixture contained in cylindrical polystyrene cuvettes are loaded into metal racks. The racks are advanced mechanically through a thermostatted, electrically heated tunnel in which the racks fit closely, so that the first cuvette reaches the measuring position in 15 minutes. During passage through the tunnel the

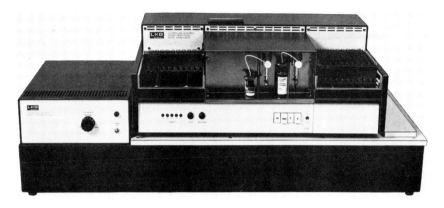

FIG. 10. The LKB reaction-rate analyzer. The analyzer is shown standing on a cooling stage which allows operation temperatures of 25°, 30°, 32°, 35°, or 37°C to be selected. The strip-chart recorder is not shown. (By courtesy of LKB Instruments Ltd., South Croydon, Surrey CR2 8YD, England.)

set temperature (35° or 37°C; ±0.2°C) is reached. Lower temperatures can be obtained by standing the apparatus on a cooling stage.

At the measuring position a pump (range 25–250 μl) adds a measured volume of initiating reagent. Mixing is effected by rotation of the cuvette alternately clockwise and anticlockwise 12 times during a period of 2.5 seconds. Internal vanes in the cuvette aid mixing. Absorbance is recorded for the preset interval (from 1 to 9 minutes) after a period of 1.5 seconds, during which the background absorbance is measured and the recorder is zeroed. Recording of absorbance changes begins within 10 seconds of initiation of the reaction. Rising or falling absorbance can be followed.

The photometer is a single-beam system with a stabilized tungsten-filament lamp and interference filters to select, e.g., wavelengths of 340 nm or 410 nm. The beam is focused in the center of the cylindrical cuvette. The photometer compensates automatically for background absorbance of the samples so that each reaction curve starts from zero on the chart. The total range of absorbance measurements is 0–1.8 A and background values of up to 1.1 A can be compensated for automatically over any part of this range. The minimum background absorbance likely to be met with for a range of samples in a given analysis is first backed off by an adjustable aperture. As each sample subsequently enters the light beam its absorbance is determined. This value is recorded as the background absorbance in the form of a peak on the chart. The output of the photocell adjusts the gain of the amplifier during background measurement and zeros the recorder. The measuring range is 0.05 A full-scale deflection, with automatic changeover to 0.2 A full-scale deflection if 0.05 A is reached during the measuring interval. Alternatively, the 0–0.2 A range can be selected initially.

The LKB reaction rate analyzer gives results that are well correlated with those by other methods (Fig. 11) with a precision as good or better than that of equivalent manual kinetic methods. In this laboratory the coefficient of variation of randomized duplicate lactate dehydrogenase assays was ±4.2% (mean value 233 IU/liter), compared with ±5.9% for the manual method, with the frequency distribution of agreement between duplicates showing more instances of closer agreement for the automated method (Fig. 12). Favorable evaluations have also been published from other laboratories (e.g., S3).

The analyzer also has a good record of reliability: during a 6-month period in this laboratory, only 4% of possible working time was lost due to breakdowns. The apparatus has been widely accepted into routine clinical laboratory practice. It is probable that a considerable part of this success has been due to its excellent photometry and efficient auto-zero mechanism.

4.1.2. *The Spectronic 400*

This modular spectrophotometric system (Bausch and Lomb, Rochester, New York 14625) aspirates reaction mixtures into the water-jacketed cuvette of the photometer, and an associated data-processer prints the corresponding absorbance values. Fixed-time or variable-time modes can be selected to give 10 readings at 6-second intervals or 12, 24, or 48 seconds apart. Samples are picked up and diluted by the hand-held probe of an automatic pipetting unit into tubes which are contained in the thermostatted sample presentation module. The enzymic reaction is initiated by automatic addition of substrate from the pipetting unit, with mixing by an air jet.

4.1.3. *The System Olli 3000*

The central feature of this semiautomatic system (Ollituote Oy, Kiven-lahti, Finland) is a photometer which contains an array of 24 individual detectors. Each detector is supplied with light from a single source by means of 24 parallel light paths, using quartz-fiber optics, and the signal from each channel is registered every 5 seconds. The first readings can be made within 30 seconds after initiation of the reaction. Reaction mixtures for enzyme assays (prepared and preincubated off-line in sample- and reagent-dispensing modules) are introduced into the photometer in racks of 24 containers. Temperature is maintained by heating circuits in the

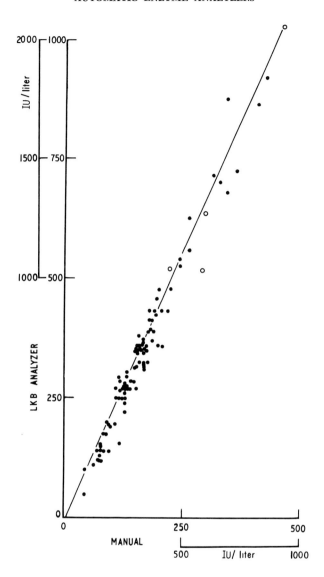

FIG. 11. Correlation between lactate dehydrogenase activities in serum (IU/liter) determined at 35°C with the LKB 8600 reaction-rate analyzer and at 25°C by manual spectrophotometry. The regression equation is: $y = 2.28x - 17.1$ ($r = 0.996$; $n = 101$). Points shown as ○ are referred to the outer pair of axes.

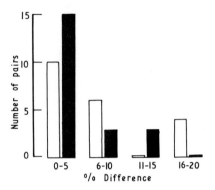

Fig. 12. Histogram of the agreement between duplicate estimations of lactate dehydrogenase activity in serum by a manual spectrophotometric method at 25°C (open bars) and by the LKB 8600 reaction-rate analyzer at 35°C (filled bars). Differences between duplicates are expressed as a percentage of the mean value for each pair.

aluminum block which contains the cuvettes during measurement, with an accuracy of ±0.1°C of the set temperature (from 25°–37°C) and with a between cuvette variation of ±0.05°C (A1).

The 24 readings collected from each of the 24 cuvettes within a 2-minute period are entered into the 16K memory of a Nova 1200 computer. The computer is programmed to search for the appropriate linear portion of the curve of absorbance change with time. This is achieved by fitting the data to a series of polynomial models of increasing degree from 0 to 3. The residual variance, representing the scatter of the data points about the model curve, is computed for each one, and the best-fit model is selected. The reaction rate is derived by differentiation of the selected model, taking the steepest slope within the measurement interval in more complex progress curves (due to lag phases, substrate exhaustion, etc.), for which models of higher degree are necessary to fit the data. Catalytic concentration values (IU/liter) obtained by multiplying the reaction rate by appropriate factors are printed out by an on-line typewriter.

The precision of the System Olli 3000 for duplicate assays of aspartate and alanine transaminases is of the order of ±6 to 7% and ±3% coefficient of variation at low and high activities, respectively, and correlation between results by this system and other manual and automatic analyses is good (A1). The values for precision are of the order to be expected in good, present-day practice in enzyme assay.

It has been reported that the Olli 3000 system is capable of high rates of analysis when appropriate dispensing and incubator modules are available, with 240 measurements completed in the first hour and 380 in each succeeding hour (A1). However, the process requires the continuous attention of the operator so that this rate of working must be regarded as a maximum one.

4.1.4. *Centrifugal Fast Analyzers*

Analyzers of this type have some similarities to the System Olli 3000 described above in that their construction allows a large number of readings to be taken in rapid succession from each of several reaction mixtures during the course of a single run. The reaction mixtures are prepared off-line, either manually or in an automatic sample- and reagent-dispensing module, and reaction-initiation and mixing are carried out in the analysis module.

It is the ability to collect large numbers of data points during a relatively brief period of any enzymic reaction, together with the facility for rapid initiation of the reaction and transfer of the reaction mixture to the measuring cuvette, that makes the centrifugal analyzer attractive from the point of view of enzyme assay. Against this is set the difficulty of close control of temperature in the spinning cuvette rotor, although it is claimed that this problem has been overcome in more recent versions of the apparatus.

Centrifugal analyzers are available from three manufacturers: the CentrifiChem (Union Carbide Corp., Rye, New York 10580), the Gemsaec (Electro-Nucleonics, Inc., Fairfield, New Jersey 07006) and the Rotochem II (American Instrument Co., Silver Spring, Maryland 20910). Although differing in detail, all three of these instruments are based on the original apparatus devised by Anderson (A3, A4).

A ring of radially arranged cuvettes is formed by sandwiching a slotted Teflon disk between stainless-steel plates. Glass or silica windows in the steel plates above and below each cuvette allow a beam of light to pass through the cuvettes from a source below the ring to a detector above it as the ring rotates in the horizontal plane. The center of the cuvette disk is filled by a removable, close-fitting transfer disk which contains sets of three interconnecting sample and reagent receptacles. Each set of three wells is aligned radially with a cuvette in the outer ring, the outermost well being connected to the adjacent cuvette by a narrow channel (Fig. 13).

The transfer disk is removed from the rotor and loaded with measured volumes of samples and reagents, either manually or in an automatic pipetting and dispensing module. After replacing the loaded transfer disk in the center of the cuvette ring the assembly is accelerated rapidly to a rotational speed of about 1000 rpm in a few seconds. The resulting centrif-

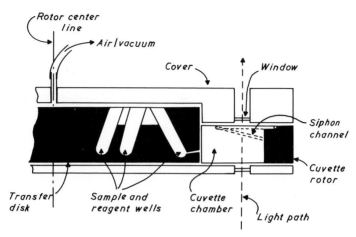

FIG. 13.   Diagrammatic cross section of the rotor of a parallel fast analyzer showing arrangement of sample and reagent wells and cuvettes.

ugal force transfers the samples and reagents rapidly and quantitatively
to the cuvettes. Some mixing takes place during transfer, but the effect of
centrifugal force also opposes mixing, so that later rotor designs incorporate siphons leading into the cuvettes through which air can be sucked
to promote mixing, by applying a vacuum to the center of the rotor for
2 seconds (A4). The cuvettes are drained of liquid at the end of analysis
through the siphons by applying air pressure at the rotor center and
washed by sucking water through them.

   The speed and efficiency of liquid transfer and mixing are of particular
importance in enzymic assays. Anderson (A4) has concluded that more
than 99% of the liquid volume is transferred during the 2–3 seconds
needed to reach 1000 rpm and that, with air suction, mixing is complete
within 1 second. Thus, these processes occupy only a negligible fraction
of the total analysis time of perhaps 1 minute or longer, but the time
needed for transfer and mixing could be reduced still further by a more
powerful drive giving greater acceleration.

   Readings of absorbance in each cuvette are taken at every passage of
the cuvette through the light beam: e.g., every 60 msec for a rotational
speed of 1000 rpm. The system is effectively double-beam if a reference
solution is placed in one of the cuvettes, to which the readings of the
other cuvettes are related at each revolution. Electronic collection and
processing of data are needed to deal with the large numbers of readings
which can be accumulated during even a brief analytical run. Data
processing is carried out in real time (i.e., during the run) so that results

can be scrutinized while the run is in progress, and the changing absorbances in each cuvette can be displayed on an oscilloscope for monitoring by the operator. The system is obviously well suited to the fitting of curves by a computer to the large number of data points obtained during the course of an enzymic reaction. However, simpler calculation programs have also been used, in which the computation of catalytic concentration of the enzyme is based on the difference in absorbance measured between two fixed times after the start of the reaction.

Control of temperature of the reaction mixtures within the cuvettes may be achieved by enclosing the rotor within an airtight chamber through which air at a controlled temperature is passed (e.g., as in the Union Carbide CentrifiChem) or by incorporating electrical heating elements into the cuvette ring (as in the Aminco Rotochem). The advantages gained by the rapid liquid transfer and mixing that are possible in centrifugal analyzers will be lost if an appreciably longer interval is then needed to reach equilibrium with respect to temperature. Starting with cold water in a cold transfer disk, one air-regulated system has been found to attain 37°C to within 0.1° in about 40 seconds: a longer time was needed to stabilize temperature at 30°C because this temperature was closer to the ambient temperature. Both set temperatures were reached within stated limits of accuracy (P. Henry and R. A. Saunders, personal communication, 1975). These intervals could perhaps be reduced by the use of prewarmed reagents.

Tiffany et al. (T1) have shown that the within-run and between-run variabilities for serum transaminase assays carried out with a CentrifiChem analyzer are of the same order as those obtained with other ultra-violet-spectrophotometric assays of these enzymes. They obtained within-run coefficients of variation of ±4.6% for activities within the normal range and ±1.6% for elevated activities. Corresponding values for between-run variations were ±7.7% and ±2.1%. Results obtained with the centrifugal analyzer were well correlated with those by other methods. Centrifugal analyzers have also been used in the determination of serum acid phosphatase activity (F1) and in the quantitation of tissue-specific forms of alkaline phosphatase in serum by differential inhibition with urea (S6). Statland et al. (S5) have used nonlinear regression analysis to determine lactate dehydrogenase in serum with data obtained with a Rotochem analyzer.

Maclin (M1) has analyzed the contribution made by different variables to the overall error of kinetic analyses in the Electro-Nucleonics Gemsaec analyzer and has concluded that feasible instrumental design parameters can be selected which will result in coefficients of variation of ±5% or less.

4.2. COMPLETELY AUTOMATED SYSTEMS

4.2.1. *The Abbott Bichromatic Analyzer*

The ABA-100 (Abbott Scientific Products Division, South Pasadena, California 91030) consists of a turntable around the periphery of which serum samples are placed (Fig. 14). The turntable rotates once every 5 minutes in the normal mode of operation. As each sample passes the dispensing position a measured volume of it is picked up by a syringe pump and transferred to the corresponding compartment of a 32-place disposable multiple cuvette followed by a measured volume of the complete reagent mixture. The cuvette rotates with the sample turntable. Mixing is by the jet effect of the additions, and the reaction is thus serum-initiated. The cuvette dips into a thermostatically controlled water bath

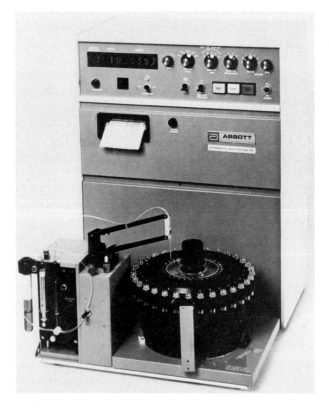

FIG. 14. The Abbott ABA-100 Bichromatic Analyzer. (By courtesy of Abbott Laboratories Diagnostics Division, South Pasadena, California 91030.)

through which the light beam of the photometer passes. The latter measures the difference in absorbance at two wavelengths, selected by interference filters, by a beam-chopping arrangement. For assays involving measurements of reduced NAD or NADP, for example, the difference in absorbance between 340 nm and 380 nm is measured. This approach removes between-cuvette variation and also much of the interference due to absorbing substances in the sample, but requires an accurate knowledge of the molar extinction of the substance being measured over the given wavelength interval: for NADH this represents about 80% of the value at 340 nm.

In the normal mode of operation the first absorbance reading is made 5 minutes after initiation of the reaction, with subsequent readings at further intervals of 5 minutes. The differences between successive pairs of readings, multiplied by a factor to give catalytic concentration, are printed out with sample-identification numbers and can be compared by the operator to check linearity. A "fast-kinetic" mode of operation can be selected in which readings on each sample are taken at 15-second or 30-second intervals after an initial delay of 2 minutes between the reaction-initiation and measurement positions.

The incubation bath of the ABA-100 is of relatively small volume and, being open, is prone to loss of liquid by evaporation or when the cuvette is removed. The inherent drawbacks of initiating enzyme reactions with serum are overcome by the choice of reaction chemistries and by the 5-minute incubation period before the first reading in the normal operational mode. Because of the rather long intervals between initiation and the first and subsequent absorbance measurements in the normal mode, the zero-order portion of the reaction may have been exceeded for some samples before the absorbance change over the second interval is measured, so that no check on linearity can be made. On the other hand, the fast-kinetic mode involves a rather long delay before the commencement of the more closely spaced readings that are possible in this mode.

In spite of these apparent disadvantages for enzyme assays, the ABA-100 has proved highly successful in practice. Good agreement with other methods of assay has been reported for several enzymes, with coefficients of variation fully comparable with those obtained by other manual and automatic equipment both on a within-batch and a day-to-day basis— e.g., by G. M. Widdowson, J. R. Penton and W. A. Hasson, at the 8th International Congress on Clinical Chemistry, Copenhagen, 1972.

4.2.2. The Beckman System TR

This analyzer (Beckman Instruments, Inc., Fullerton, California 92634; Fig. 15) uses the method of data processing already referred to in Section 3.4. The absorbance signal is electronically differentiated to obtain its rate

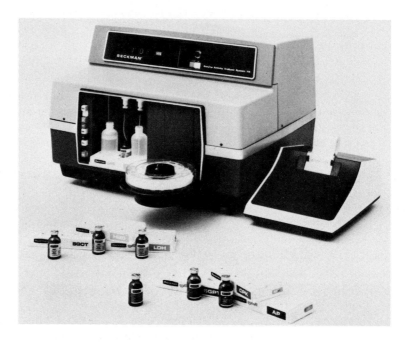

Fig. 15. The Beckman System TR enzyme activity analyzer. (By courtesy of Beckman-RIIC Ltd., Glenrothes, Fife KY7 4NG, Scotland.)

of change with time, and the variation of the first differential with time is monitored by a second differentiating circuit (Fig. 9). As long as the second derivative generated by this circuit is zero, the original absorbance change is linear with respect to time; i.e., the reaction is following zero-order kinetics. After the rapid fluctuations in absorbance due to reaction initiating and mixing have subsided, the second differential is monitored until a zero value lasting for 17 seconds is registered. The first differential corresponding to the period during which the second derivative is zero is then used to calculate catalytic concentration in IU/liter, and this result is printed out. If a linear rate is not maintained for 17 seconds during a maximum period which is programmed for each type of analysis, the rate derived from the final 17 seconds of monitoring is printed out with the symbol "T." The maximum monitoring period varies between 1.5 minutes, e.g. for lactate dehydrogenase determination, and 6 minutes for creatine kinase.

The basis of the calculation of enzyme activity is an absorbance change equivalent to 0.400 generated by pressing a "calibrate" push button. The rate given by samples is compared with this rate and converted to catalytic concentration by the appropriate factor, which is input at the start of each type of analysis and is a function of the sample-dilution factor, the molar extinction coefficient of the product of the reaction, and the temperature coefficient, if any.

Samples are loaded onto a 20-place turntable which plugs into the front of the instrument. Reagent and sample dispensing is by means of fixed-travel syringes set at 540 μl for the reagent and 50 μl for the sample. Part of the liquid picked up is used for washing the transfer tubing and cuvette so that the measured reaction mixture consists of 525 μl of reagent plus 35 μl of sample. The enzymic reaction is thus serum-initiated. Inserting the reagent carrier automatically primes the dispensing pump with reagent, and after measurement samples are automatically sucked out of the cuvette to waste. Replacement of the reagent by distilled water actuates a wash cycle.

Mixing within the cuvette is by a magnetic stirrer. The cuvette temperature is maintained to within $\pm 0.1°$C at $37°$C or, with external cooling, at $30°$C or $25°$C. Monitoring wavelengths of 405 ± 1 nm or 340 ± 1 nm (bandwidths < 5 nm) isolated by a diffraction grating are selected as appropriate by the push button which programs for each type of assay. The second, reference cuvette of the double-beam photometer normally contains air; however, a dual-probe sample pick up is provided so that a sample or reagent blank can be used to compensate for possible errors introduced into some assays by the use of serum initiation.

As already mentioned (Section 3.4), results printed out by the System TR were found in this laboratory to agree well with values calculated from a strip-chart recorder, thus establishing the validity of the computation system. Good correlation was also observed between results with the Beckman instrument and those by other methods for assays of alkaline phosphatase (Fig. 16), lactate dehydrogenase and creatine kinase. Coefficients of variation of less than $\pm 3\%$ were obtained for replicate analyses of pooled serum, and for agreement between randomized, duplicate estimations on serum specimens, in assays of these three enzymes (Table 1). Reports of good instrumental and analytical performance with the Beckman System TR have been published by Wolf (W1) and Passey et al. (P1).

4.2.3. The Coulter KEM-O-MAT Analyzer

This instrument (Coultronics Division Medicale, 95580 Andilly, France) consists of a turntable module which carries an outer ring of cups containing serum samples and an inner ring of disposable plastic cuvettes. The cups and cuvettes are held in a constant-temperature air bath. A measured volume of each sample is picked up and discharged into an adjacent cuvette with diluent by a syringe pump. The incomplete reaction

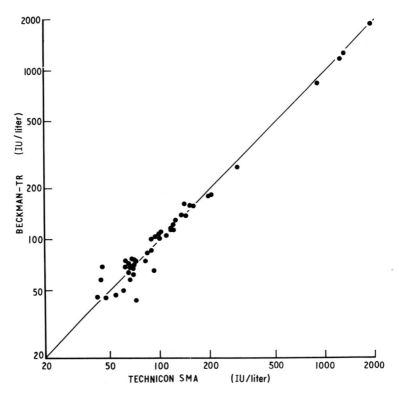

FIG. 16. Correlation between alkaline phosphatase activity in serum (IU/liter at 37°C) determined by the Beckman System TR analyzer and by the Technicon SMA multichannel analyzer. Both scales are logarithmic.

mixture is carried round to a second dispensing position by the movement of the turntable, and the reagent is added which initiates the reaction. Stirring is effected by a rotating rod. The cuvette progresses into the light beam of the photometer. The absorbance reading is stored in a programmable calculator, where it and subsequent readings on the same cuvette are used to compute catalytic concentration.

The calculator, which forms part of the apparatus, is programmed by magnetic-tape cassette according to the type of analysis being performed. A series of instructions to the operator are first printed, defining the necessary instrumental settings. The program also directs the operation of the turntable and of the dispensing and diluting pumps and calculates the results of the analyses.

No performance data are available yet for this recently announced analyzer.

TABLE 1

PRECISION ESTIMATES WITH THE BECKMAN SYSTEM TR ANALYZER[a]

Enzyme	No. of replicates or pairs of estimations	Mean value (IU/liter)	± Standard deviation	± Coefficient of variation (%)
Alkaline phosphatase	18 Pairs	153	1.7	1.1
	5 Replicates	183	2.5	1.4
Lactate dehydrogenase	7 Replicates	170	2.9	1.7
α-Hydroxybutyrate	7 Replicates	237	3.1	1.3
dehydrogenase	4 Replicates	246	7.4	3.0
Creatine kinase	5 Replicates	303	4.2	1.4
	7 Replicates	299	2.6	0.9
	5 Replicates	304	3.1	1.0
	6 Replicates	302	2.2	0.7
	Between above 4 batches	302	1.9	0.6
γ-Glutamyl	6 Replicates	64	0.9	1.3
transpeptidase	6 Replicates	29	1.5	5.2
	7 Replicates	18	0.9	5.0
	6 Replicates	113	1.4	1.2
Aspartate transaminase				
Serum + H₂O blank	6 Replicates	286	8.0	2.8
Aspartateless blank	6 Replicates	242	2.3	0.95
α-Oxoglutarateless blank	6 Replicates	249	1.5	0.6

[a] Values are based on replicate analyses at 37°C of a single specimen or on randomized duplicate estimations on different specimens, and refer to within-batch reproducibility unless otherwise stated.

4.2.4. The Eppendorf Automat 5010

The manufacturer of this instrument (Eppendorf Gerätbau Netheler & Hinz GmbH, 2000 Hamburg 63, W. Germany) makes a range of partially automated enzyme analysis equipment based on the addition of sample-presentation and data-processing modules to the company's mercury-lamp spectral-line photometer. However, the Automat 5010, while incorporating a similar photometer, is a fully automated two-channel enzyme analyzer.

Serum samples are loaded into a sample transport chain from which measured volumes of them are picked up by the probe of a dispensing and diluting pump and transferred to disposable cuvettes carried on a rotating turntable. Each serum is sampled twice, once into each of two cuvettes, with the diluent appropriate to each of the two different enzyme assays being carried out. The cuvettes dip into an incubator which maintains them at a temperature of 25° or 37° ± 0.2°C. The cuvette-turntable is automatically fed with empty cuvettes from a magazine.

The progression of the turntable in steps of 30 seconds brings each diluted serum sample after a 15-minute preincubation to a second reagent-addition station. Here the appropriate reagent is added to start the enzymic reaction. The cuvettes are then picked up in turn by a transporter and conveyed to a rotor in the thermoregulated cuvette compartment of the photometer.

The 6-place measuring rotor makes a complete revolution in 6 steps every 25.7 seconds, and the absorbance of each sample is measured 7 times in a period of 2.57 minutes (i.e., the readings are 25.7 seconds apart.) The time lapse between initiation of the reaction and the first measurement for a given sample is 46 seconds. When the set of 7 readings on any cuvette is complete, the cuvette is discarded automatically. The absorbance readings for each cuvette can be displayed on a chart recorder, and catalytic concentration values are computed from the linear regression of the readings by a calculation unit.

4.2.5. *The Gilford 3500 Analyzer*

Both the earlier Gilford 3400 analyzer and the later 3500 computer-directed analyzer are based on the manufacturer's 300-N spectrophotometer (Gilford Instrument Laboratories, Inc., Oberlin, Ohio 44074). The model 3400 provides for reaction-initiation and mixing, automatic spectrophotometry, and calculation of results (G1, M3), whereas the Model 3500 also incorporates the sample-dilution stage. It is thus fully automated.

The Gilford 3500 automatic enzyme analyzer (Fig. 17) dispenses fixed volumes (10–100 μl) of sample with up to 2.5 ml of a diluent. Sample and diluent volumes, as well as those of further reagent additions, are determined by interchangeable stops which limit the travel of the syringe pumps. Two further reagent volumes (0.25–2.5 ml) can be added after the initial sample dilution stage. No provision is made for mixing apart from that resulting from the forceful ejection of reagent into the reaction cup. The enzymic reaction is thus usually substrate-initiated, and the analyzer reproduces typical manual assay practice in allowing a preincubation period between sample-dilution and initiation of the enzymic reaction. When fully loaded, the sample transport system accommodates up to 56 sample cups, each with an adjacent reaction vessel, in 14 racks of 4 samples each. Adjustment of the position of the reagent-addition heads along a notched bar allows the lapse of time to be varied between sample dispensing and further reagent additions, or between these operations and introduction of the reaction mixture into the spectrophotometer cuvette.

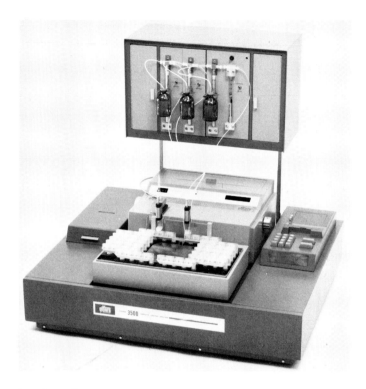

Fig. 17. The Gilford 3500 automatic enzyme analyzer. (By courtesy of Gilford Instruments Ltd., Teddington, Middlesex, England.)

The spectrophotometer is a single-beam diffraction-grating instrument with a wavelength range of 340–700 nm (bandwidth 8 nm), with direct readout of absorbance to 2 A. A resolution of 0.0001 A is claimed, but the fourth decimal place is not displayed. The cuvette (path length 10 mm) requires a minimum volume of 700 μl of solution. Its temperature is controlled by Peltier elements at nominal temperatures of 25°, 30°, 32°, or 37°C, which can be selected independently of ambient temperature by a switch. Depressing a push button displays the cuvette temperature to two places of decimals.

Results and other data are recorded by an alphanumeric printer. There is also provision for analog output to an optional strip-chart recorder. A keyboard on the printer module is used to input instructions (e.g., sample, purge, advance racks) or a dilution factor. Numerical data can also be input for calculation of means, standard deviations, and coefficients by the use of a separate "statistics program" card.

The operation of the analyzer is controlled by a digital computer programmed by the appropriate magnetically coded card for each test. Introduction of a card is first followed by the printing-out of a series of instructions to the operator: set temperature and wavelength, position diluter, select syringe volumes, set zero, and load the racks. A dilution factor can be entered at this stage if necessary for calculation. When the setting-up process is completed and the command to start is given, analysis of the samples proceeds automatically, the results (in IU/liter) appearing from the printer with identifying rack and cup numbers. The reagent blank is subtracted automatically from each result and error messages indicate samples for which the reaction progress curve does not meet the linearity criteria or for which initial absorbance is above or below programmed limits.

The method of monitoring the reaction in the Gilford 3500 analyzer has already been referred to (Section 3.4; Fig. 8). After addition of the reagent, which completes the reaction mixture and initiates the enzymic reaction, a minimum period of 24 seconds elapses before the progress of the reaction begins to be monitored. Forty-nine absorbance readings are then taken in each of three consecutive 7-second periods. The average reading in each period is calculated (A_1, A_2, A_3) and catalytic concentration is computed from $A_1 - A_3$, the absorbance change in 14 seconds. Linearity is considered acceptable if

$$\frac{(A_1 - A_2) - (A_2 - A_3)}{(A_1 - A_3)} \times 100$$

lies between -5 and $+5$. If these limits are exceeded, the result is printed with a message indicating an accelerating ("ACC") or decreasing ("DEC") rate. As has already been mentioned, no results printed without error messages were found to be accompanied by unacceptable traces when the performance of the analyzer was monitored by a chart recorder in this laboratory, and the incidence of results with error messages but with acceptable chart traces was very small.

Good correlation was found between results given by the 3500 analyzer and those by other methods for assays of aspartate transaminase, creatine kinase, and lactate dehydrogenase in serum (Fig. 18). Estimates of precision for these analyses, based on replicate determinations on single specimens and on randomized duplicate analyses, showed coefficients of variation which were generally comparable to those typical of these assays when performed manually or with other automatic analyzers (Table 2). These estimates of precision were obtained with an instrument with pneumatically operated reagent dispensing heads. These have now

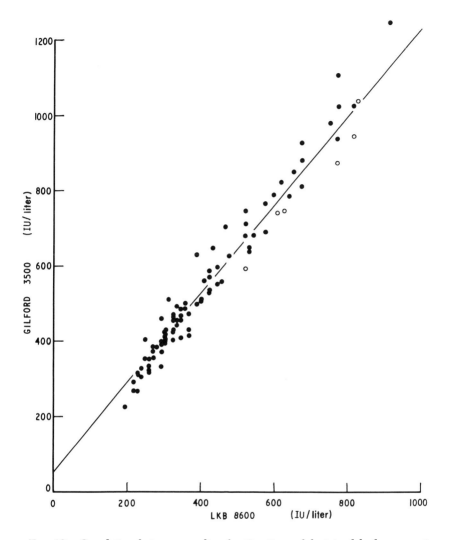

FIG. 18. Correlation between results of estimations of lactate dehydrogenase in serum (IU/liter) by the Gilford 3500 analyzer at 37°C and by the LKB 8600 reaction rate analyzer at 35°C. The regression equation is: $y = 1.18x + 55.5$ ($r = 0.991$; $n = 92$). Values shown by ○ have been divided by 2 for plotting.

been replaced by electrically actuated heads which, in our experience, give rather better precision as a result of reduced carry-over. Negligible carry-over, as well as excellent between-batch and within-batch reproducibility with the 3500 analyzer, have also been reported by Forrester *et al.* (F2).

TABLE 2

PRECISION ESTIMATES WITH THE GILFORD 3500 ENZYME ANALYZER[a]

Enzyme	Temperature (°C)	No. of replicates and pairs of estimations	Mean value (IU/liter)	± Standard deviation	± Coefficient of variation (%)
Lactate dehydrogenase	25	12 Pairs	238	8.4	3.5
		13 Pairs	390	24.9	6.4
		10 Replicates	187	3.8	2.0
		18 Replicates	198	11.5	5.8
		5 Replicates	187	4.7	2.5
		10 Replicates	197	4.2	2.2
		10 Replicates	200	4.7	2.3
		Between above 5 batches of replicates	194	6.3	3.3
	37	8 Pairs	532	19.1	3.6
		15 Pairs	780	19.7	2.5
		22 Pairs	659	14.6	2.2
		8 Replicates	415	14.9	3.6
		20 Replicates	418	28.7	6.9
		5 Replicates	391	10.2	2.6
		20 Replicates	440	12.1	2.7
		10 Replicates	420	12.1	2.9
		10 Replicates	431	9.6	2.2
		Between above 6 batches of replicates	419	16.6	4.0
Creatine kinase	25	9 Replicates	146	4.3	2.9
	37	15 Pairs	270	15.0	5.6
		14 Pairs	158	14.8	9.3
		19 Pairs	198	16.9	8.6
		8 Replicates	277	13.0	4.7
		15 Replicates	318	19.8	6.3
		10 Replicates	281	9.5	3.4
		Between above 3 batches of replicates	292	22.6	7.7
Aspartate transaminase	37	20 Pairs	89	5.8	6.6
		18 Pairs	39	3.6	9.1
		18 Pairs	50	3.6	7.3
		11 Replicates	205	3.6	1.8
		14 Replicates	256	4.1	1.6
		11 Replicates	258	4.3	1.7
		13 Replicates	267	4.3	1.6
		Between above 4 batches of replicates	247	28.1	11.4

[a] Values are based on replicate analyses of a single specimen or on randomized duplicate estimations on different specimens and refer to within-batch reproducibility unless otherwise stated.

A particularly impressive feature of the Gilford 3500 automatic enzyme analyzer is the rapid changeover that is possible from one temperature of measurement to another: a new indicated temperature is reached within seconds of changing from a different setting. Temperature accuracy to within $\pm0.1°C$ of the indicated temperature is claimed, with a precision of $\pm0.05°C$. It was not possible to check the accuracy of the temperature indication in this laboratory, but in order to test whether the instrument returned reproducibly to a particular temperature when reset from a different temperature, a series of replicate determinations of lactate dehydrogenase in pooled serum were made: 10 measurements were made at 37°C, the setting was changed to 25°C and 10 further measurements were made, followed by 10 replicates at 37°C and finally 10 at 25°C. The mean values (IU/liter) and coefficients of variance (CV) were:

Run No.:		1	2	3	4
Temperature (°C)	Nominal:	37	25	37	25
	Indicated:	37.02	24.98	37.00	24.98
Mean:		420	197	431	200
CV ($\pm$ %):		2.9	2.2	2.2	2.3

The differences between means at corresponding temperatures were significant only at the level of $p < 0.10$. It can be concluded therefore that the instrument returns essentially to the same temperature when the setting is changed and then reset to the original value.

4.2.6. The Perkin-Elmer Kinetic Analyzer KA-150

The KA-150 (Fig. 19) (Perkin-Elmer Corp., Norwalk, Connecticut 06856) bases its rapid rate of analysis of 150 samples per hour (S2) on the ability to detect absorbance changes of the order of 5×10^{-6} per second. The light-source of the photometer is a hollow cathode lamp, generating a narrow beam of high-energy monochromatic light at a wavelength of 340 nm, for reactions linked to oxidation or reduction of NAD or NADP. Emission lines at other wavelengths are blocked by interference filters. An alternative lamp and filter system allows reactions to be monitored at 404 nm. These light sources, which eliminate the errors due to wavelength inaccuracy and stray light associated with sources emitting continuous spectra, are combined with small silicon-diode detectors in a double-beam system. The temperature of the preamplifier is controlled to enhance its stability and to reduce noise.

The photometer cuvette is constructed of silver, to accelerate temperature equilibration, and has a path length of 1 cm. The volume of solution

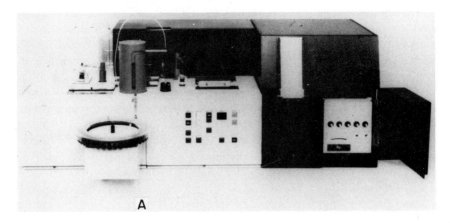

A

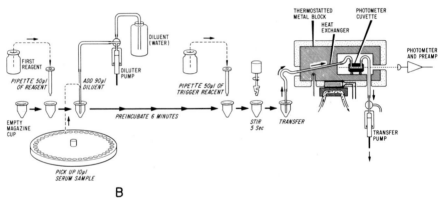

B

FIG. 19. (A) The Perkin-Elmer KA-150 Kinetic Analyzer. (B) Diagram of operational sequence. (By courtesy of Perkin-Elmer Corporation, Norwalk, Connecticut 06856, and the editors of *Clinical Chemistry*.)

required to fill it is 20 μl. Air-segmentation of the reaction mixture flowing through the cuvette is used to reduce carry-over from sample to sample. Control of the cuvette temperature is by Peltier-effect electrical regulation and gives an accuracy of ±0.2°C at 30°C, with a precision of ±0.05°C.

Reaction mixtures corresponding to each sample reach the photometer cell 25 seconds after the reaction has been triggered by substrate. (An additional 96-second delay can be introduced after the 7-second stirring period in assays of creatine kinase to allow for the lag phase of this reaction.) After initiation and stirring, transport to the cuvette occupies 18 seconds, and this period also provides for temperature equilibration as the solutions pass through a channel in the thermostatted metal block which encloses the cuvette. Measurement of the absorbance of each reaction mixture is made for 9 seconds, divided into four equal integrating periods. The curvature of the progress curve of the reaction is computed over these four intervals, and the rate of change of absorbance is calculated over the 9-second period. If the degree of curvature amounts to 5% of the rate, the result is printed with an accompanying error message. Error messages also draw attention to conditions such as excessively high initial absorbance, or low absorbance due to depletion of substrate.

The progress of samples (e.g., of serum) through the instrument begins at a 40-place turntable on which the samples are loaded. A measured volume (10 μl) of each sample is transferred to a transfer cup with 90 μl of water. The transfer cups, which are transported in racks of 10 cups, have already been charged with 50 μl of the first component of the reaction mixture. After a minimum of 6 minutes of preincubation to allow for the completion of side reactions, the cups reach the position of reaction initiation, which is effected by addition of 50 μl of substrate solution. The KA-150 analyzer thus follows the pattern of manual kinetic assays in providing for preincubation of incomplete reaction mixtures with triggering by substrate. After the measurement of each reaction mixture, the transfer path and photometer cell are purged by a wash liquid.

Results of an evaluation of the Perkin-Elmer KA-150 kinetic analyzer have been published by Hardin et al. (H1). Five enzymes were assayed: lactate dehydrogenase, creatine kinase, aspartate and alanine aminotransferases, and alkaline phosphatase. Rates of analysis were 122 samples per hour for creatine kinase and 125 per hour for the other four enzymes, and measured activities were linearly related to enzyme concentration up to at least 1500 IU/liter for all five enzymes. Within-run precision was of the order of ±3% CV or less for slightly or moderately elevated mean activities, the only value greater than this being recorded at low alanine transaminase activities. Between-run precision determined over a period of 30 days was also good, CV being ±11.5% at the upper limit of normal for alanine transaminase and less than ±10% for the other four enzymes. Carryover from high to low activity samples was negligible (4 IU/liter or less) and was less than the within-run standard deviation for most assays. Correlation of enzyme results by the KA-150 with those given by other assay methods was excellent for serum samples from patients. The analyzer incorporates error-detection devices designed to identify substrate-exhaustion and reaction progress-curves that deviate from linearity by more than 5% and these functioned satisfactorily. Less than 2% of possible operating time was lost during the trial.

An assessment of the use of the KA-150 for substrate determinations has been reported (A6).

4.2.7. *The Pye Unicam AC 30 Automatic Chemistry System*

For use in enzyme assays, this system (manufactured by Pye Unicam Ltd., Cambridge CB1 2PX, England) is made up of the AC 1 automatic chemistry unit, the SP 30 spectrophotometer, and the DR 16 digital printer (Fig. 20). A strip-chart recorder can also be added to monitor the reaction progress-curves.

The AC 1 unit performs the functions of sample dilution, reagent addition, mixing, preincubation, initiation of the enzymic reaction, and transfer of the completed reaction mixtures to the cuvette of the spectrophotometer. The serum or other samples are loaded in disposable cups into racks which also carry the disposable reaction tubes. The capacity of the unit is 10 loaded racks, although more can be added at any time as places become available. The racks carry machine- and human-readable identifying codes. The diluter depresses each reaction tube in turn to immerse it partially in the water bath which controls the preincubation temperature. The latter may be set over the wide range of 20°–70°C since the bath incorporates a cooling coil for use near ambient temperature. Measured volumes of sample and diluent are added to the reaction tube by the

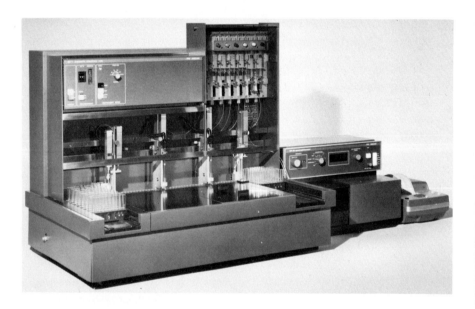

FIG. 20. The Pye Unicam AC 30 Automatic Chemistry System. The sample-processing and preincubation module is on the left. To the right are the spectrophotometer and printer. (By courtesy of Pye Unicam Ltd., Cambridge CB1 2PX, England.)

diluter. This and subsequent reagent-addition units (up to three in number) are pneumatically driven, and the reagent dispensers employ disposable plastic syringes for measurements of volumes. These syringes give excellent precision without the careful maintenance needed to prevent jamming with glass syringes. The volumes dispensed by all the syringes in a particular analysis are programmed by slotting in a single, shaped template ("VoluKey"), which sets all volumes simultaneously. Addition of a reagent is followed by stirring with a paddle.

The sequence of operations of the AC 30 system is timed by a reaction-rate accessory attached to the spectrophotometer. Either 30- or 60-second monitoring intervals can be selected. By placing the reagent dispenser which adds the initiating reagent next to the transfer unit, monitoring of enzymic reactions can begin within 12 seconds of initiation of the reaction. The dispenser can be moved away from the transfer unit to provide a delay before monitoring begins, for reactions which have an appreciable lag phase. The transfer unit is activated by a sensor which detects the presence of a reaction tube. One of the two syringes of the unit fills the photometer cuvette through a stainless-steel probe; the second syringe empties the cell after measurement. The volume required for absorbance measurement in the thermostatted cuvette is 80 μl, with a path length of 10 mm. However, a total volume of about 1.5 ml is necessary to ensure complete washing of the transfer tubing and the cuvette.

Arrival of a reaction vessel at the transfer station also triggers the auto-zero mechanism of the spectrophotometer. This offsets the initial absorbance of the reaction mixture and ensures that all traces begin from zero on the chart recorder, if this is in use. Computations of catalytic concentration are made by multiplying the absorbance change registered over 30 or 60 seconds by the appropriate factor, previously entered into the calculator. The results are printed out with sample identification numbers. The mode of calculation is thus two-point; however, the wide range of options with respect to preincubation times and intervals between reaction initiation and measurement makes it possible to select conditions for enzyme assays which ensure that the measuring interval will fall within the zero-order phase of the reaction for a majority of samples. The use of a chart recorder provides an additional safeguard, available for scrutiny by the operator to ensure that linearity has been maintained for samples with high enzyme activity.

A selective dispenser accessory can be fitted which allows each sample to be processed automatically with its own blank. This accessory can also be used for the measurement of two different enzyme activities (e.g., lactate and α-hydroxybutyrate dehydrogenases) on each sample loaded into the analyzer.

In the author's laboratory, good correlation between printed values based on two-point calculation and values computed from the chart recorder was found for about 100 apartate transaminase estimations (range, 10–200 IU/liter at 37°C). Successive 30-second printouts for each sample were in good agreement up to activities of nearly 700 IU/liter, showing that linearity was maintained for at least 60 seconds. Printed two-point values also agreed well with analog-derived values for creatine kinase with an appropriate choice of measuring interval.

Results obtained with the AC 30 agreed well with those given by other analyzers in the assay of aspartate transaminase, lactate dehydrogenase, and creatine kinase in serum. Within-run reproducibility was respectively better than ±5% CV and ±3% CV for normal and elevated activities of these three enzymes.

4.2.8. The Vitatron Automatic Kinetic Enzyme System (AKES)

The modular photometer system produced by this manufacturer (Vitatron Scientific BV, NL-6210, Diesen, Holland) is an example of the time-sharing systems that allow several reaction rates to be monitored simultaneously with the aid of an automatic cuvette-positioner. However, the AKES is a completely automatic enzyme analyzer (Fig. 21), based on the same photometric principles, but with the addition of an integral sample-processing unit.

Serum or other samples are loaded into a 100-place transport chain in disposable plastic vials, each with a capacity of up to 600 μl. The 10 sec-

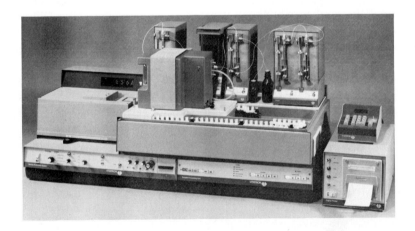

FIG. 21.   The Vitatron Automatic Kinetic Enzyme System (AKES). (By courtesy of MSE Scientific Instruments, Manor Royal, Crawley, Sussex, England.)

tions which make up the transport chain carry machine-readable identifying numbers. At the sample dispensing and diluting station, the needle of the adjustable sample syringe (100 μl capacity) pierces the plastic cap of the sample vial and removes the measured volume of sample. The pick-up probe rises and swings over a reaction cuvette in an adjacent 18-place reaction rotor where the sample is discharged with an appropriate volume of the incomplete reaction mixture. Sample and reagent pick-up and dispensing are effected by power-driven Hamilton syringes.

The 18 glass cuvettes carried in the reaction rotor are maintained at the selected temperature (25°, 32°, 35°, or 37°C) by Peltier elements to a claimed tolerance of ±0.05°C. The cuvettes are of 10 mm light path and accept reaction volumes of between 500 and 800 μl. The rotor advances one place every 20 seconds, and the 14 steps between the sample-addition and measurement positions thus introduce a minimum delay of 4 minutes 40 seconds before the enzymic reaction is initiated by a further reagent addition. Since the measurement interval is variable, depending on the activity of the samples, the preincubation time for samples other than the first is also variable. Measurement of absorbance changes begins about 10 seconds after addition of the triggering reagent and stirring. The light beam passes along a radius of the cuvette rotor from a mercury or quartz-iodine lamp to the centrally placed photocell. Wavelength selection is by interference filters. After measurement is completed, the cuvette is emptied to waste by suction and is refilled with 800 μl of water, which is again sucked away to waste. The maximum residual volume of liquid in the cuvette after each emptying is 8 μl, so that maximum cross-contamination of a 600-μl reaction mixture by its predecessor in the cuvette is 0.013%.

Data processing by the reaction-rate computer begins with an initial 5-second monitoring period to determine whether the initial absorbance of the mixture is acceptable. The sample is rejected if the value is above or below the programmed limits. Samples with acceptable initial absorbances are then monitored for a further 10 seconds and the area of the triangle (A_2) represented by the change in absorbance in this interval is computed. This is compared with the area corresponding to the first monitoring period (A_1). If $A_1 = 0.25 A_2$, within preset limits, the value of absorbance change per minute multiplied by an appropriate calibration factor is printed out as the catalytic concentration of the enzyme. If the expected relationship between A_1 and A_2 is not found, the reaction is followed for a further 20 seconds, then for 40 seconds more, and finally for 80 seconds. After each period linearity is assessed by comparing A_3 with A_2, etc., monitoring being terminated as soon as the required degree of linearity has been detected. If no two successive comparisons are satisfactory, a result based on the last monitoring period is printed together with a "nonlinear" warning message. The period for which the reaction is followed in the cuvette may vary between 20 seconds and 2 minutes 46 seconds.[1] The computer can be programmed by the operator to accept 1, 2, 5, or 10% deviations from linearity.

Several fault indicator lights are provided to draw attention to malfunctions of the sample transport system, the sample-identity reading head, and the waste system. The occurrence of the same error message from the reaction-rate computer on five consecutive samples is also signaled as a possible malfunction.

The results of two evaluations of the AKES in clinical chemistry laboratories have been published (M2, P2). Patel and O'Gorman (P2) found satisfactory within-run coefficients of variation at 25°C for assays of α-hydroxybutyrate dehydrogenase ($\pm 3.9\%$ at 150 IU/liter; $\pm 2.0\%$ at 830 IU/liter), alanine transaminase ($\pm 10\%$ at 11 IU/liter; $\pm 2.1\%$ at 56 IU/liter) and aspartate transaminase ($\pm 9.3\%$ at 11 IU/liter; $\pm 1.1\%$ at 99 IU/liter). McQueen and King (M2) found similar values for creatine kinase at 25°C ($\pm 9.4\%$ at 25 IU/liter; $\pm 3.3\%$ at 142 IU/liter) and 37°C ($\pm 5.6\%$ at 60 IU/liter; $\pm 1.9\%$ at 364 IU/liter). Reproducibility was satisfactory also for assays of lactate and α-hydroxybutyrate dehydrogenases, γ-glutamyl transpeptidase, and alkaline phosphatase. The results of McQueen and King (M2) were obtained with the 5% linearity setting. For the assay of creatine kinase, changing the setting from 2% to 10% increased the rate of analysis of samples from 71 per hour to 80 per hour, but the accompanying increase in coefficient of variation was only from $\pm 1.96\%$ to $\pm 2.12\%$ at a mean level of 330 IU/liter. Thus, the faster analysis rate did not result in an appreciable deterioration in reproducibility for this analysis. Patel and O'Gorman (P2) found between-run coefficients of variation that were of the same order of magnitude as the within-run values, with good correlation of the results of assays by the AKES and by other methods.

Both evaluations reported on the reliability of the AKES. In the laboratory of Patel and O'Gorman, only 1 day was lost during 7 months owing to breakdown, minor faults being corrected on the same day (P2). McQueen and King (M2) lost nearly 25% of possible working time owing to breakdowns, but these were due largely to failures of minor components, such as microswitches. Both studies comment on the general ease of use of the instrument, although McQueen and King (M2) note that the programmed maximum acceptable rate of 0.4 A per minute results in the need to repeat a substantial number of samples with high enzymic activity. The fixed position of substrate addition, immediately before the measurement

---

[1] The maximum period is reduced to 1 minute 47 seconds with a more recent model of the reaction rate computer.

position, reduces flexibility in dealing with reactions that have a lag phase (P2).

4.3. Multichannel Enzyme Analyzers

4.3.1. The Jeol Clinalyzer

The Clinalyzer (made by Jeol Ltd., 1418 Nakagani, Akishima, Tokyo 196, Japan) carries out six different enzyme assays simultaneously on each sample. Each assay is carried out in a separate, revolving reaction assembly, consisting of 12 reaction vessels, which also serve as measurement cuvettes. As the assembly rotates, the reaction vessels pass successively through stages of sample and reagent introduction, stirring by injected air bubbles, preincubation, addition of initiating reagent and stirring, photometric measurement, and discharge of the measured sample, after which the cuvette is washed twice with water. The whole rotor is enclosed in a thermoregulated air bath, which maintains the temperature to within ±0.1° of 37°C, with a variation of ±0.03°C.

Light from a tungsten lamp is directed outward radially through the measuring position to the photodetector. The path length of the reaction cuvettes is 12 mm. The photometric system is also enclosed in the thermostat to increase its stability. Wavelength selection is by filters.

Each sample is proportioned between the six parallel reaction modules by means of a rotating cutoff valve system. A sample picked up by a pump from the sample turntable, which is equipped with machine-readable sample identification, fills six interconnected channels in the valve rotor. When the rotor turns the sample is cut into six discrete, equal volumes, one connected to each of the appropriate reagent channels for the various analyses. Reagents are preheated to the reaction temperature before addition to the reaction vessels.

Absorbance changes in each reaction mixture are monitored for 44 seconds after initiation of the enzymic reaction. The changes over the two halves of this interval are compared by the calculation unit; if the difference between them is greater than ±12.5% of the total change, the final result is printed with a warning signal. A chart recorder is provided to monitor each channel as an additional check on linearity. Catalytic concentration values calculated by multiplying the observed absorbance difference (corrected for any blank reactions) by an appropriate factor are printed out with sample-identification numbers.

4.3.2. The Jobin-Yvon Multienzy

The Multienzy (Jobin-Yvon Instruments S.A., 91160 Longjumeau, France) carries out up to six preselected kinetic enzyme analyses on each sample. The reaction vessels for the several analyses move in parallel along the instrument and are washed and dried automatically. The reaction mixtures progress from the sample-measurement and dilution stage to successive stages of reagent addition and ultimate photometric measurement. Temperature is controlled throughout preincubation and in the cuvette at 25°, 30°, or 37°C to within 0.1°C. The last stage of reagent addition completes the reaction mixture and initiates the enzymic reaction. Transfer of the reaction mixture to the cuvette occupies 10 seconds and reading begins after a further 7 seconds. There is thus a minimum delay of 17 seconds between the start of the reaction and the commencement of monitoring. Three readings are taken on each reaction mixture, at intervals which can be varied between 2 seconds and 2 minutes.

5. Conclusions

This survey shows that a wide range of equipment exists with which the enzyme assays that form a major part of modern diagnostic clinical chemistry can be mechanized. Instruments are available which allow enzyme assays to be carried out alternatively with other forms of analysis, which can be used to incorporate enzyme assays into multichannel systems combining analyses for both enzymic and nonenzymic constituents, or which are designed exclusively for measurements of reaction rates. In selecting from this spectrum of equipment, therefore, a first consideration will be the needs of a particular laboratory with regard to the numbers of different enzymic and nonenzymic analyses performed, any requirement for instrumentation to fulfill more than one function, and policy toward the provision of multiparameter analysis of a majority of the specimens received.

When these criteria have been applied to identifying in general terms the category of automated equipment appropriate to the laboratory's requirements for enzyme analysis, further considerations become relevant. These include such factors as the amount of time and degree of skill which the operator will be able to devote to monitoring the performance of the chosen automatic enzyme analyzer, since this will affect, for example, the degree to which the validation of results will be a required function of the equipment itself. The rate at which samples are analyzed is a criterion which will differ in importance from one laboratory to another: the enzyme analyzers discussed in this review vary in this respect between rates of 20 or 30 specimens per hour to 150 or more per hour.

Indisputably the most important factors that influence the choice of any automatic laboratory equipment are its reliability in operation and the precision and accuracy of the analytical data it produces. It is undoubtedly true that discrete automatic analyzers, to which category many enzyme analyzers belong, have earned an unfavorable reputation in the opinion of many clinical chemists on the grounds of mechanical unreliability, while the long development times of some of these instruments attest to the complexity of the design of many of them. Nevertheless, a number of the enzyme analyzers described in this review have records of reliable service in the laboratory over long periods.

Now that the clinical chemist is faced with such a variety of choice in automatic enzyme analyzers, schemes for the evaluation of the performance of these and other analyzers have begun to attract attention. Several professional groups in various countries have inaugurated schemes for validating manufacturers' performance data or for assessing mechanical and analytical reliability (B5).

A further consideration in the design of automatic enzyme analyzers is the extent to which potential users of such apparatus should be prepared to advise manufacturers as to desirable specifications, and the form that such advice should take. At the Second International Symposium on Clinical Enzymology (Chicago, 1975), G. M. Widdowson considered different approaches to the formulation of specifications for automatic enzyme analyzers. First, detailed specifications might be prepared for each of the functions of the analyzer, e.g., reagent- and sample-dispensing, photometry, etc. Alternatively, an overall specification in terms of analytical reproducibility and accuracy might be set out, although "accuracy" in enzyme assay remains an ill-defined concept. A third approach might combine these two aspects, providing clearly defined specifications for functions such as temperature-control, photometry, and curve evaluation, with overall specifications based on analytical performance. At the present time, standards of overall analytical performance based on existing methods have largely guided the aims of manufacturers of new equipment.

It is possible that new methods of enzyme analysis, based on determination of the amount of enzyme protein present rather than on its catalytic activity, may ultimately render obsolete the methods and apparatus now in use. However, the widespread introduction of such methods seems remote: quantitative immunochemistry, for example, requires the availability of specific antisera, some of which at least may have to be raised against enzymes from human sources. Meanwhile, the automatic enzyme analyzers now available should ensure that the diagnostic applications of enzyme assays are not restricted by unsound or inadequate data.

Acknowledgments

I thank Mrs. K. B. Whitaker for assistance in obtaining the original data quoted in this review, and the companies named in the captions for the provision of illustrations.

REFERENCES

A1. Adlercreutz, H., Peltonen, V., and Volpio, T., Evaluation of the new "System Olli 3000" kinetic ultraviolet analyzer for measuring aspartate and alanine aminotransferase and lactate dehydrogenase activities in serum. *Clin. Chem.* **21**, 676–684 (1975).

A2. Amador, E., and Wacker, W. E. C., Serum glutamic-oxalacetic transaminase activity. A new modification and an analytical assessment of current assay techniques. *Clin. Chem.* **8**, 343–350 (1962).

A3. Anderson, N. G., Analytical techniques for cell fractions. XII. A multiple cuvet-rotor for a new microanalytical system. *Anal. Biochem.* **28**, 545–562 (1969).

A4. Anderson, N. G., Analytical techniques for cell fractions. XIV. Use of drainage syphons in a fast-analyzer cuvet rotor. *Anal. Biochem.* **32**, 59–69 (1969).

A5. Armstrong, J. B., Lowden, J. A., and Sherwin, A. L., Automated fluorometric creatine kinase assay. Measurement of 100-fold normal activity without serum dilution. *Clin. Chem.* **20**, 560–565 (1974).

A6. Atwood, J. G., and DiCesare, J. L., Making enzymatic methods optimum for measuring compounds with a kinetic analyzer. *Clin. Chem.* **21**, 1263–1269 (1975).

A7. Axelsson, H., Ekman, B., and Knutsson, D., Determination of SGOT, SGPT, and alkaline phosphatase, with a simplified AutoAnalyzer technique not requiring blank runs. *Automat. Anal. Chem. Technicon Symp., 1965* pp. 603–608 (1966).

B1. Bergmeyer, H. U., Standardization of the reaction temperature for the determination of enzyme activity. *Z. Klin. Chem. Klin. Biochem.* **11**, 39–45 (1973).

B2. Berry, M. N., and Walli, A. K., The automated assay of serum lactate dehydrogenase activity. *Automat. Anal. Chem. Technicon Symp., 1966* pp. 389–393 (1967).

B3. Bowers, G. N., Jr., Bergmeyer, H. U., and Moss, D. W., Provisional recommendation (1974) on IFCC methods for the measurement of catalytic concentration of enzymes. *Clin. Chim. Acta* **61**, F11-F24 (1975).

B3A. Bowie, L., Esters, F., Bolin, J., and Gochman, N., Development of an aqueous temperature-indicating technique and its application to clinical laboratory instrumentation. *Clin. Chem.* **22**, 449–455 (1976).

B4. Brojer, B., and Moss, D. W., Changes in the alkaline phosphatase activity of serum samples after thawing and after reconstitution from the lyophilized state. *Clin. Chim. Acta* **35**, 511–513 (1971).

B5. Broughton, P. M. G., Gowenlock, A. H., McCormack, J. J., and Neill, D. W., A revised scheme for the evaluation of automatic instruments for use in clinical chemistry. *Ann. Clin. Biochem.* **11**, 207–218 (1974).

B6. Brown, S. S., and Smith, A. F., Assessment of printing calculators for use with the LKB reaction rate analyzer. *Clin. Chim. Acta* **38**, 51–57 (1972).

C1. Castillo, J. del, Rodriguez, A., Romero, C. A., and Sanchez, V. Lipid films as transducers for detection of antigen-antibody and enzyme-substrate reactions. *Science* **153**, 185–188 (1966).

C2. Cook, J. G. H., Application of analytical methods to automatic analysers. *Ann. Clin. Biochem.* **12**, 163–168 (1975).

E1. Ellis, G., and Goldberg, D. M., Use of the Unicam SP 800 spectrophotometer with work simplification in routine aminotransferase determinations. *Spectrovision* **23**, 8–10 (1970).

E2. Ellis, K. J., and Morrison, J. F., Some sources of errors and artifacts in spectrophotometric measurements. *Clin. Chem.* **21**, 776–777 (1975).

F1. Fabiny-Byrd, D. L., and Erlingshausen, G., Kinetic method for determining acid phosphatase activity in serum with the use of the CentrifiChem. *Clin. Chem.* **18**, 841–844 (1972).

F2. Forrester, R. L., Collinge, W., Hashimoto, P., and Worrall, J., Evaluation of a discrete-sample computer directed clinical analyzer. *Clin. Chem.* **22**, 211–216 (1976).

G1. Goldberg, D. M., and Blomer, P. R., An evaluation of the Gilford 3400 automatic enzyme analyzer. *Z. Klin. Chem. Klin. Biochem.* **12**, 235 (1974).

G2. Goldberg, D. M., Ellis, G., and Wilcock, A. R., Problems in the automation of enzyme assays with lag, accelerated and blank reactions. *Ann. Clin. Biochem.* **8**, 189–194 (1971).

G3. Guibault, G. G., Kramer, D. N., and Cannon, P. L. Jr., A new, general electrochemical method of determining enzyme kinetics. Kinetics of the enzymic hydrolysis of thiocholine iodide esters. *Anal. Biochem.* **5**, 208–216 (1963).

H1. Hardin, E., Passey, R. B., Gillum, R. L., Fuller, J. B., and Lawrence, D., Clinical laboratory evaluation of the Perkin-Elmer KA-150 Enzyme Analyser. *Clin. Chem.* **22**, 434–438 (1976).

I1. Ingle, J. D., Jr., and Crouch, S. R., Theoretical and experimental factors influencing the accuracy of analytical rate measurements. *Anal. Chem.* **43**, 697–701 (1971).

K1. Kessler, G., Morgenstern, S., and Snyder, L., Possible errors in 3-point assays for ALT and AST in serum and how the Technicon SMAC high-speed biochemical analyzer computer flags such errors. *Clin. Chem.* **21**, 1005 (1975).

K2. Kessler, G., Rush, R. L., Leon, L., Delea, A., and Cupiola, R., Automated 340 nm measurement of SGOT, SGPT and LDH. *Clin. Chem.* **16**, 530–531 (1970).

M1. Maclin, E., A systems analysis of GEMSAEC precision used as a kinetic enzyme analyzer. *Clin. Chem.* **17**, 707–714 (1971).

M2. McQueen, M. J., and King, J., Evaluation of the Vitatron automatic kinetic enzyme system. *Clin. Chim. Acta* **64**, 155–164 (1975).

M3. Morell, S. A., Bach, D. A., and Ayers, V. E., Evaluation of a Gilford "Automatic Enzyme Analyzer" modified to assay 60 samples per hour. *Clin. Chem.* **20**, 1295–1304 (1974).

M4. Morgenstern, S., Flor, R., Kessler, G., and Klein, B., Automated determination of NAD-coupled enzymes. Determination of lactic dehydrogenase. *Anal. Biochem.* **13**, 149–161 (1965).

M5. Morgenstern, S., Kessler, G., Auerbach, J., Flor, R. V., and Klein, B., An automated *p*-nitrophenylphosphate serum alkaline phosphatase procedure for the AutoAnalyzer. *Clin. Chem.* **11**, 876–888 (1965).

M6. Moss, D. W., The relative merits and applicability of kinetic and fixed-incubation methods of enzyme assay in clinical enzymology. *Clin. Chem.* **18**, 1449–1454 (1972).

M7. Moss, D. W., Baron, D. N., Walker, P. G., and Wilkinson, J. H., Standardization of clinical enzyme assays. *J. Clin. Pathol.* **24**, 740–743 (1971).

P1. Passey, R., Gillum, R. L., Giles, M. L., and Fuller, J. B., Evaluation of the Beckman "System TR Enzyme Analyzer." *Clin. Chem.* **21**, 1107–1112 (1975).

P2. Patel, S., and O'Gorman, P., Assessment of a new enzyme reaction rate analyzer, the Vitatron AKES. *Clin. Chim. Acta* **60**, 249–258 (1975).

P3. Pitot, H. C., and Pries, N., The automated assay of complete enzyme reaction rates. 1. Methods and results. *Anal. Biochem.* **9**, 454–466 (1964).

P4. Pitot, H. C., Pries, N., Poirier, M., and Cutler, A., Rate analysis of enzyme reactions by continuous and interrupted flow procedures. *Automat. Anal. Chem. Technicon Symp., 1965* pp. 555–558 (1966).

R1. Reitman, S., and Frankel, S., A colorimetric method for the determination of serum glutamic oxaloacetic and glutamic pyruvic transaminases. *Am. J. Clin. Pathol.* **28**, 56–63 (1957).

R2. Rodgerson, D. O., and Osberg, I. M., Sources of error in spectrophotometric measurement of aspartate aminotransferase and alanine aminotransferase activities in serum. *Clin. Chem.* **20**, 43–50 (1974).

R3. Roth, M., Fluorimetric assay of enzymes. *Methods Biochem. Anal.* **17**, 189–285 (1969).

S1. Skeggs, L. T., Jr., An automated method for colorimetric analysis. *Am. J. Clin. Pathol.* **28**, 311–322 (1957).

S2. Slavin, W., Determining enzymes with the KA-150 kinetic analyzer. *Instrum. News* **24**, 7–9 (1975).

S3. Smith, A. F., Brown, S. S., and Taylor, R., Assessment of an automatic enzyme reaction rate monitor. *Clin. Chim. Acta* **30**, 105–113 (1970).

S4. Snook, M., Renshaw, A. E., and Rideout, J. M., A high capacity kinetic analyzer. *Z. Klin. Chem. Klin. Biochem.* **12**, 236 (1974).

S5. Statland, B. E., and Louderback, A. L., Non-linear regression analysis approach for determining "true" lactate dehydrogenase activity in serum with the centrifugal analyzer ("Rotochem"). *Clin. Chem.* **18**, 845–849 (1972).

S6. Statland, B. E., Nishi, H. H., and Young, D. S., Serum alkaline phosphatase: total activity and isoenzyme determinations made by use of the centrifugal fast analyzer. *Clin. Chem.* **18**, 1468–1474 (1972).

T1. Tiffany, T. O., Johnson, G. F., and Chilcote, M. E., Feasibility of multiple simultaneous enzyme assays, for diagnostic purposes, with the GeMSAEC fast analyzer. *Clin. Chem.* **17**, 715–720 (1971).

T2. Tracey, T. J., More on values for alkaline phosphatase activity in calibration sera. *Clin. Chem.* **21**, 787 (1975).

T3. Trayser, K. A., and Seligson, D., A new "kinetic" method for enzyme analysis suitable for automation. *Clin. Chem.* **15**, 452–459 (1969).

W1. Wolf, P. L., Evaluation and utilization of a kinetic enzyme direct measuring photometer. *J. Clin. Pathol.* **28**, 587–591 (1975).

THE DIAGNOSTIC IMPLICATIONS OF STEROID BINDING IN MALIGNANT TISSUES

E. V. Jensen and E. R. Desombre

Ben May Laboratory for Cancer Research, The University of Chicago,
Chicago, Illinois

1. Introduction

It has long been recognized that, during the course of differentiation, certain tissues acquire a need for continued exposure to minute amounts of steroid hormones for their optimal growth or function. Early studies of the physiologic fate of tritiated estradiol in immature rats (G6, J2, J7) and hexestrol in young goats and sheep (G2) demonstrated clearly that hormone-dependent tissues of the female reproductive tract are also characterized by the presence of an estrogen-binding component, called estrogen receptor, estrophile, or estrophilin, and that this substance is a protein (T6). Although it was later shown that most if not all tissues contain small amounts of estrogen receptor (J17), the presence of substantial amounts of estrophilin remains a feature of estrogen-dependent or target tissues. Subsequent studies by many investigators have shown that target tissues for all classes of steroid hormones contain analogous receptor proteins that interact with their respective hormones in a generally similar fashion (K4, R2).

Certain cancers likewise contain steroid hormone receptors. During neoplastic transformation some but not all tumors derived from hormone-dependent tissues retain the receptor systems characteristic of their cells

57

of origin. As discussed later, the presence of receptors appears to be a necessary but not sufficient indication of hormone dependency or sensitivity of such cancers.

The most extensive investigations of the relation between steroid hormone receptors and hormone response in malignant tissues have been carried out with estrogens in breast cancer. Because space does not permit a complete description of the many excellent investigations of receptors for all types of steroid hormones, this chapter will be limited to an overview of the principal features of the interaction pathway of the estrogens that has served as a prototype for the interaction of other classes of steroid hormones in their respective target tissues. After considering investigations of estrogen receptors in experimental mammary tumors, the clinical application of receptor studies in predicting hormone dependency in human breast cancer and in other endocrine-sensitive human neoplasms is discussed.

2.   Interaction of Estrogenic Hormones with Target Tissues

2.1.   INTERACTION OF ESTROGENS IN THE UTERUS

Using the immature rat (J8) or mouse (S17) uterus as a model, it was established that estrogen–receptor interaction and subsequent stimulation of uterine growth take place without chemical change of the estradiol molecule itself and that association of hormone with the receptor is an early if not the initial step in the uterotropic process (J4). As determined by either cell fractionation (J3, K3, N1) or autoradiographic (J14, S18) techniques, after administration of physiologic doses of tritiated estradiol, most (70–80%) of the radioactive hormone present in uteri of immature or castrate rats is found in the nucleus, from which it can be extracted as a steroid–protein complex by 0.3 M or 0.4 M potassium chloride (J22, P4). The remainder of the uterine hormone is extranuclear, bound to a macromolecular component of the high-speed supernatant or cytosol fraction of uterine homogenates (T1). The ratio of nuclear to extranuclear hormone remains relatively constant up to 6 hours after estradiol injection (J9).

The technique of sucrose gradient centrifugation (T6) provides a valuable method for detecting and measuring different forms of estradiol–receptor complexes. Although both the nuclear and extranuclear complexes sediment at about 8 S in low-salt sucrose gradients, they can be readily distinguished (J16) in the presence of 0.3 M KCl, which reversibly dissociates the complexes into steroid-binding subunits (E2, K10, R3). As shown in Fig. 1, in salt-containing sucrose gradients the cytosol complex sediments at 3.8 S and the nuclear complex at 5.2 S; for convenience these two complexes are usually designated 4 S and 5 S, respectively.

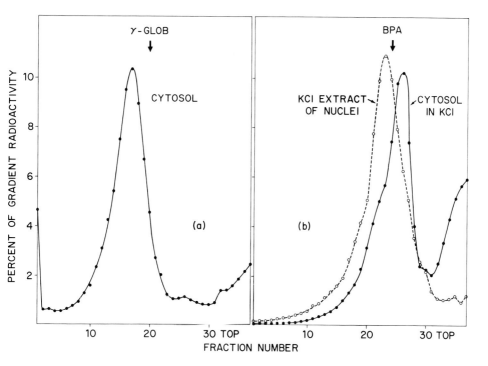

Fig. 1. Sedimentation patterns of radioactive estradiol–receptor complexes of cytosol of 20% homogenate in Tris–EDTA buffer (10 mM Tris, 1.5 mM EDTA, pH 7.4) and nuclear extract (0.4 M KCl in Tris-EDTA, pH 8.5) from uteri of immature rats 1 hour after subcutaneous injection of 0.1 μg (20.8 μCi) of [6,7-³H]estradiol. To saturate its receptor capacity, the cytosol fraction was made 5 nM with additional tritiated estradiol. Aliquots of 200 μl were layered on sucrose gradients; centrifugation was carried out at 2°C for 12 hours (a) at 308,000 g in 10–30% sucrose containing pH 7.4 Tris–EDTA, and (b) at 284,500 g in 5–20% sucrose containing 0.4 M KCl in Tris–EDTA, pH 8.5. Successive fractions (100 μl) were collected from the bottom of the gradient for determination of radioactivity. γ-Globulin (γ-GLOB) and bovine plasma albumin (BPA) indicate positions of bovine γ-globulin (7.0 S) and BPA (4.6 S) markers. Reproduced from Jensen and DeSombre (J6).

Incubation of excised uterine tissue with dilute solutions of tritiated estradiol at physiologic temperature *in vitro* gives rise to an intracellular distribution of hormone similar to that obtained *in vivo*, with formation of the same nuclear and extranuclear estradiol–receptor complexes (J9, J13). When uteri are exposed to estradiol at 2°C, most of the hormone is present as extranuclear 8 S complex, shifting to nuclear 5 S complex on subsequent warming of the tissues to 37°C (G4, J19). In contrast to the 8 S extranuclear complex, or its 4 S subunit, that forms directly when estradiol is added to uterine cytosol in the cold (J22, T7), little or no 5 S complex is produced by treatment of isolated uterine nuclei with estradiol unless uterine cytosol is also present, in which case warming of the mixture gives rise to a 5 S nuclear complex, indistinguishable from that obtained *in vivo* (J16, J19). The estradiol–receptor complex, present in uterine cytosol after the administration of a physiologic dose of estradiol *in vivo*, represents only a small fraction of its total estrogen-binding capacity, as can be demonstrated by the formation of additional amounts of 8 S complex by direct treatment of the cytosol with tritiated estradiol (G4, J19, J22, T7).

The foregoing observations, taken in conjunction with earlier experiments suggesting a relation between cytosol and nuclear binding (B5, J9, J13) and the fact that *in vivo* administration of estradiol causes a temporary depletion of extranuclear receptor protein levels (J16, J19, S7), provide a body of complementary experimental evidence for the concept of a two-step mechanism for the interaction of estradiol in uterine cells (G4, J16, J19, S11). In this mechanism, the predominant estradiol–receptor complex, found in the nucleus, is not derived from a nuclear receptor protein, but it arises from the temperature-dependent translocation of an initially formed extranuclear complex (Fig. 2). With the recent development of an exchange technique (A1) for measuring nonradioactive estrogen bound in the nucleus, it was shown that endogenous estrogen, like the

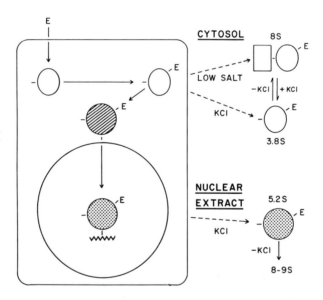

Fig. 2. Schematic representation of interaction pathway of estradiol (E) in uterine cell. Diagram at left indicates uterine cell with extranuclear estradiol–receptor complex undergoing transformation and entering nucleus to bind to chromatin. Diagrams at right indicate sedimentation properties of complexes extracted from the cell. Reproduced from Jensen and DeSombre (J6).

exogenous labeled hormone used in the previous experiments induces the translocation of extranuclear estrophilin to the uterine nucleus (C3).

The translocation of the extranuclear complex to its intranuclear binding or acceptor site, apparently in the chromatin (K7, M3, T2), is accompanied by conversion of the estrophilin from a 4 S to a 5 S form (J16). Contrary to original assumptions, this transformation of the receptor does not require the participation of the nucleus, but, as shown in Fig. 3, it can be effected by warming uterine cytosol to $25°-37°C$ in the presence of the estrogenic hormone (G5, J11). In addition to the change in sedimentation rate, the transformed estrogen–receptor complex shows two important properties not shared by the native (4 S) complex. Only the transformed complex binds strongly to isolated nuclei (J15) or to chromatin (M10), and only this form elicits a tissue-specific stimulation of RNA polymerase function in isolated nuclei of estrogen-dependent tissues (J15, M16). Thus, the temperature-dependent process associated with nuclear uptake in whole uterine tissue appears to be the estrogen-induced conversion of estrophilin from its native form to a transformed or active state that binds strongly to chromatin in the nucleus and in some way modulates RNA synthesis (J6).

2.2. Interaction of Estrogens with Mammary Tissue and Tumors

There have been relatively few investigations of the interaction of steroid hormones with normal breast tissue, probably because of difficulties in obtaining concentrated specimens of hormone-responsive cells. The observations that have been reported indicate the presence of estrogen receptors generally similar to those found in uterus. Specific uptake and binding of tritiated estrogens *in vivo* have been observed in mammary glands of the mouse (B6, B8, P3, P5), rat (S1, S5), and human (D1), using either biochemical or autoradiographic techniques; similar accumulation of hormone is seen with excised breast tissue exposed to tritiated estradiol *in vitro* (S2). With the mammary gland of the lactating mouse (S12) or rat (G1, K2), where the proportion of parenchymal cells is increased, the cytosol fraction is found to have a substantial content of estrogen-binding protein, reacting with tritiated estradiol to form an 8 S complex that dissociates into 4–5 S subunits in the presence of salt. Salt extraction of nuclei, obtained from mammary glands of either the lactating mouse (S12) or the lactating or pregnant rat (G1) injected with tritiated estradiol, yields a 5 S estrogen–receptor complex similar to that of uterine nuclei.

More extensive receptor studies have been carried out with tumors of the mammary gland, especially those arising in the Sprague-Dawley rat after the administration of 7,12-dimethylbenzanthracene (H9) as well as transplants of such DMBA-induced tumors. These cancers, the majority of

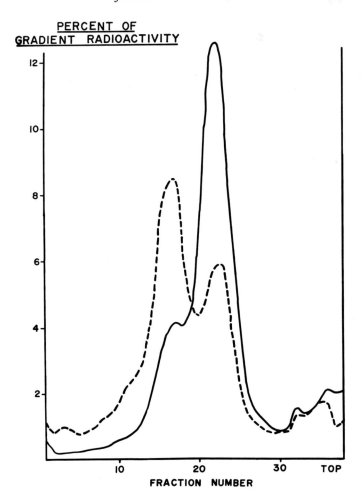

FIG. 3. Temperature-dependent transformation of the estradiol–receptor complex of rat uterine cytosol. Uterine horns from 22-day-old rats were homogenized in 9 volumes of 10 mM Tris buffer, pH 7.5. A 0.9 ml portion of the supernatant fraction was treated with 0.1 ml of buffer containing 20 nM [³H]estradiol to give a final hormone concentration of 2 nM and incubated for 30 minutes at either 26°C (---) or 0°C (——), after which 200-μl aliquots were layered on 5 to 20% sucrose gradients containing 400 mM KCl and centrifuged at 2°C for 15 hours at 308,000 g. As incubation at 26°C progresses, the 5 S component increases and the 4 S component disappears. Reproduced from Jensen et al. (J11).

which undergo regression after ovariectomy of the host, are found to accumulate radioactive steroid either after injection of the tritiated estradiol into tumor-bearing animals (J4, J10, J21, K5, K13, M8, M13, M14, S6) or on incubation of tumor slices with dilute solutions of the labeled hormone (J10, K13, S4, T3). Both *in vivo* (M13, S6) and *in vitro*, the mammary tumors that regress after oophorectomy show a greater incorporation of estradiol than do the autonomous tumors that continue to grow in the ovariectomized animal (Figs. 4 and 5). As in the case of uterus, administered estradiol is taken up and bound to receptors in mammary tumor without chemical change (J10, K5, K13), and this interaction is inhibited by estrogen antagonists such as nafoxidine (Upjohn 11,100A) or Parke-Davis CI-628 (J10, K13, S4). The difference in estradiol incorporation in the absence and in the presence of the inhibitor gives an indication of the specific binding in the specimen (Fig. 5).

After administration of tritiated estradiol to rats bearing DMBA-induced, hormone-dependent mammary tumors, most of the steroid in the tumor cells is present in the nucleus as determined both by cell-fractionation (B3, K5, K13) and by autoradiography (J10, S19). In comparison to uterus, where 70–80% of the incorporated estradiol is associated with the nucleus, the nuclear radioactivity in the tumor is usually 85–90% of the total. This nuclear estradiol can be solubilized as a macromolecular complex, either by extraction of the nuclei with 0.3 M–0.5 M KCl (B3, K6, K13, M8) or, to a lesser extent, with buffered 0.44 M sucrose (K13). The

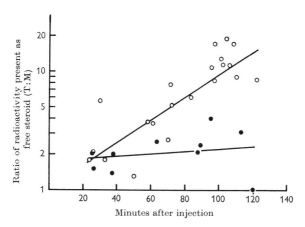

Fig. 4. Ratio of radioactivity present as free steroid in biopsy specimens of DMBA-induced rat mammary tumors (T) to that in muscle (M) after injection of 0.11 μg (16.7 μCi) of [6,7-³H]estradiol in 0.5 ml saline/100 g body weight. O——O, Responsive adenomata; ●——●, unresponsive adenomata. Reproduced with permission from Mobbs (M13).

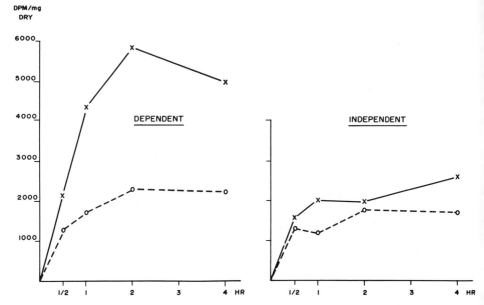

Fɪɢ. 5. Comparison of hormone-dependent and hormone-independent rat mammary tumor slices in uptake of radioactivity on exposure to 0.1 nM [6,7-³H]estradiol in the presence (○---○) and in the absence (×——×) of 10 μM nafoxidine (Upjohn 11,100). Each point is the median for 5 slices. Dependent tumors were taken from 42-week-old rats receiving dimethylbenzanthracene (3 × 2 mg, iv) at age 50–56 days and ovariectomized 24 hours before the experiment; nondependent tumors were those continuing to grow in similar rats ovariectomized 10 weeks before the experiment. Reproduced from Jensen et al. (J10).

extracted nuclear complex has been reported (K13, M8) to sediment at 5 S in sucrose gradients of either low or high ionic strength, although we find it to sediment closer to the 4.6 S bovine plasma albumin marker (Fig. 6).

After administration of a physiologic dose of tritiated estradiol, the amount of radioactivity found in the tumor cytosol is rather low. As shown in Fig. 6, it sediments as an 8 S complex, sometimes accompanied by a smaller unit sedimenting in the region of the bovine plasma albumin marker (B3, K6, K13). In salt-containing sucrose gradients, all the cytosol radioactivity present after hormone administration *in vivo* sediments near the BPA marker. As in the case of uterus, the complex formed *in vivo* represents only a small fraction of the total receptor capacity of the tumor. Addition of excess tritiated estradiol to tumor cytosol leads to the formation of a substantial amount of complex (Fig. 7), sedimenting in low-salt gradients as an 8 S entity (B3, K13, L1, M6, M8), sometimes accompanied by some 4 S complex (L1, M6, M8). In the presence of salt, the complex

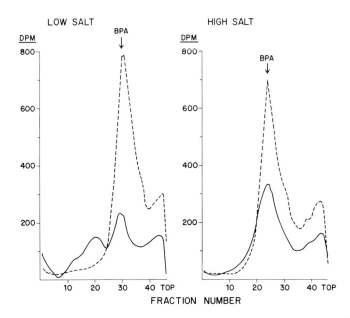

FIG. 6. Sedimentation patterns of radioactive estradiol–receptor complexes of cytosol (——) and nuclear extract (- - -) from hormone-dependent, dimethylbenzanthracene-induced rat mammary tumor excised from 90-day-old Sprague-Dawley rats 1 hour after the subcutaneous injection of 0.5 μg of [6,7-³H]estradiol in 0.5 ml of saline. Samples were prepared and centrifuged in low-salt and high-salt sucrose gradients as described in Fig. 1. BPA, bovine plasma albumin.

formed by adding estradiol to tumor cytosol sediments at about 4 S (K13, M6, M8).

It would appear that the receptor system of the hormone-dependent rat mammary tumor is generally similar to that of the uterus, involving the initial interaction of estradiol with the 4 S binding unit of an extranuclear 8 S receptor protein to form a complex that is translocated to the nucleus, from which it can be extracted as a 4.5–5 S entity. The translocation process with the formation of the nuclear complex seems to be temperature dependent (K13). However, there are certain differences between the receptor systems of mammary tumor and uterus. As mentioned earlier, the tumor contains a greater proportion of the incorporated estradiol in the cell nuclei, from which the hormone–receptor complex can be extracted somewhat more easily than from uterine nuclei. The 8 S complex of tumor cytosol appears to be more labile to warming or storage than that of uterine cytosol, and both the nuclear and cytosol complexes of mammary tumor are more sensitive to sulfhydryl reagents, such as p-chloromercuribenzoate (K13). Unlike the 5 S complex of uterine nuclei,

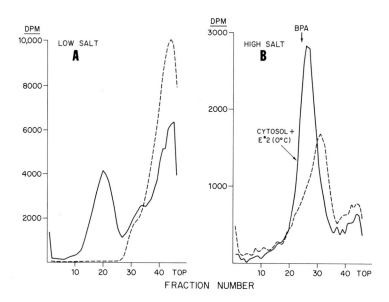

Fig. 7. Sedimentation patterns of radioactive estradiol–receptor complex in cytosol of first-generation transplant of hormone-dependent, dimethylbenzanthracene-induced rat mammary tumor. Cytosol, prepared as described in Fig. 1, was made 5 nM in tritiated estradiol and centrifuged: (A) in a low-salt 10–30% sucrose gradient in the absence (——) and in the presence (---) of 10 μM Parke-Davis CI628 and (B) in a 5–20% sucrose gradient containing 0.4 M KCl, after incubation with the hormone for 60 minutes at either 0°C (——) or 25°C (---). BPA, bovine plasma albumin.

which, when freshly prepared, aggregates to a 8–9 S form in low-salt sucrose gradients, the nuclear complex of mammary tumor does not aggregate, but sediments somewhat more slowly than 5 S in either high- or low-salt gradients. Of particular interest is the behavior of the receptor of tumor cytosol on warming with estradiol. Unlike the 4 S estradiol–receptor complex of uterine cytosol, which on warming is transformed to the 5 S nuclear form (Fig. 3), with most mammary tumors we have studied the cytosol complex that sediments at 4 S in salt-containing sucrose gradients is converted to a 3 S entity, different from the complex extracted from tumor nuclei (Fig. 7B). It has been reported previously (L1) that warming a mixture of estradiol and tumor cytosol to 18°C causes conversion of the extranuclear complex to a form that sediments at 3.5 S in low-salt sucrose gradients. This phenomenon is reminiscent of the change observed in the sedimentation of the androgen receptor when rat prostate cytosol is warmed with dihydrotestosterone, whereupon the 3.8 S complex is converted to a 3 S form, in this case similar to that extracted from prostate nuclei (L5).

Other experimental breast tumors have been observed to contain specific estrogen-binding components. One of the first experimental models to be studied was the spontaneous mammary tumor in the C3H mouse, some, but not all, of which bind estradiol specifically *in vivo* (B6). The estrogen-binding tumors were found to contain receptor proteins, and the low estrogen incorporation observed with other tumors was correlated with a reduction or absence of the estrogen-binding proteins originally present in the mammary gland (B7, P3). Pregnancy-dependent mammary tumors from the GR/A mouse were found to show greater incorporation of estradiol *in vitro* than autonomous tumors from the same host (T4). The R3230AC transplantable rat mammary tumor, a neoplasm that is estrogen-sensitive but not estrogen-dependent in that it does not regress on ovariectomy (H6), has been shown to have a low receptor content (M11) although it does incorporate some estradiol as rather poorly defined 8 S extranuclear and 4–5 S nuclear complexes (B2). The hormone-dependent subline of the transplantable MTW9 rat mammary tumor shows high estrogen affinity, giving rise to 8 S and 4 S extranuclear complexes on addition of tritiated estradiol to the cytosol fraction and to a 4 S nuclear complex after estradiol administration *in vivo* (C4). Estrogen-dependent kidney tumors of the hamster have been found to incorporate more estradiol *in vivo* than do corresponding autonomous renal tumors (S15) and to produce 8 S and 4 S cytosol complexes and 5 S nuclear complexes (S16).

Because of the many observations of greater estradiol uptake by hormone-dependent tumors as compared by their autonomous counterparts, and in view of the characteristic high levels of estrophilin in hormone-dependent normal tissues, it might be anticipated that the receptor content of a given tumor, determined as described in Section 3, would provide a measure of its hormone dependence. In general, mammary tumors that regress on ovariectomy contain significant receptor levels and most autonomous tumors show low receptor content, but there are examples of autonomous tumors with high receptor content, and there does not appear to be an absolute correlation between estrogen-binding capacity of a tumor and its growth response to oophorectomy.

With the DMBA-induced rat mammary tumor, it is rare to see regression of a tumor with low receptor content, but failure to regress after ovariectomy is relatively common among tumors with substantial estrophilin levels (B3, D2). Well established spontaneous mammary tumors in C3H mice all continue to grow after ovariectomy, whether or not they show estrogen uptake and contain receptor protein (B8). Virus-induced mammary tumors in GRS/A mice, all of which are autonomous, have been shown to contain substantial amounts of well defined 8 S extranuclear receptor, which seems to be unable to undergo translocation to the nucleus (S10). This interesting defect in nuclear translocation, however, does not appear to be a general property of receptor-containing autonomous tumors because formation of nuclear complex by translocation of extranuclear receptor has been observed both with autonomous DMBA-induced mammary tumors in the rat (B3) and kidney tumors in the hamster (S16).

Elucidation of the relation between tumor receptor content and hormone-dependence or autonomy will require further investigation, especially of the biochemical changes in the genome that accompany neoplastic transformation of a hormone-dependent cell. This, in turn, will require insight concerning the molecular biology of the original differentiation process that produces a hormone-dependent normal tissue. During normal differentiation, the acquisition of a need by the genome for exposure to estrogen-receptor complex is providentially accompanied by the development or activation of a system for synthesizing the receptor protein required for the hormone to act. During the "dedifferentiation" that accompanies neoplastic transformation, tumor nuclei may reacquire an ability to function optimally without need for hormonal stimulation, a change that may not always be accompanied by a shutdown of the receptor-synthesizing system. In some instances, the extranuclear receptor protein may continue to be produced and even undergo estrogen-induced translocation to the nucleus, even though its presence there is not required.

3. Hormone Dependency of Human Breast Cancer

3.1. NEED FOR PREDICTIVE CRITERIA OF DEPENDENCY

As was first established by experiments of Beatson (B1) and of Huggins and Bergenstal (H8), hormone deprivation, by surgically removing the organs responsible for sex hormone production, affords striking remission of disease in some but not all women with advanced breast cancer. Unfortunately, less than half the younger patients can expect benefit from ovariectomy, whereas an even smaller fraction (20–25%) of postmenopausal patients with breast cancer respond to adrenalectomy or hypophysectomy. Thus, there is need for a method to predict a priori which breast cancers are of the hormone-dependent type so that endocrine ablation can be restricted to those cases in which it has a reasonable chance of success, sparing the majority of patients the trauma of a major operation that cannot help them and that delays the inception of alternative methods of therapy. It now appears that this objective can be at least partially attained by determination of the estrogen receptor content of an excised specimen of the tumor.

The rationale of estrogen receptor determination derives from the previously discussed observations that the estrogen-responsive or target tissues of laboratory animals contain characteristic steroid-binding components, as indicated by their striking uptake and retention of hormone both *in vivo* and *in vitro*, and that hormone-dependent experimental mammary tumors usually incorporate more estrogen than do autonomous tumors. Early studies by Folca *et al.* (F4) indicated that, when injected with tritiated hexestrol, patients with breast cancer who responded favorably to adrenalectomy incorporated more radioactivity into their tumors than those who did not respond. With the subsequent development of techniques for measuring estrogen binding by mammary tumors *in vitro* (J10, S4, T3), and later the actual content of the receptor protein responsible for the binding, it became possible to examine excised specimens of breast cancers for correlation of their estrophilin levels with clinical response. Our early observations (J5, J12) that patients whose mammary tumors lack noteworthy amounts of estrophilin have little chance of responding to endocrine ablation or hormone administration, but that most but not all women with receptor-containing cancers receive benefit from such treatment, were soon confirmed by similar results from other laboratories (E1, L3, M1, S8). In July, 1974, the findings of fourteen research groups in regard to the relation between estrogen receptors and response of breast cancer patients to endocrine therapy were presented at a workshop sponsored by the Breast Cancer Task Force of the National Cancer Institute (M9). Despite the variety of experimental procedures used for the determination of estrophilin in breast cancer specimens, the overall conclusions were in remarkable agreement. Patients with tumors of low receptor content seldom received benefit from any kind of endocrine therapy, whereas from 50 to 75% of the patients with receptor-containing cancers showed objective remissions.

This section describes briefly some of the experimental procedures that are employed for the determination of estrophilin in human breast cancers and presents the correlations of estrogen receptor assays with clinical response that have been obtained in our laboratory.

3.2. EXPERIMENTAL PROCEDURES

The first method to be employed for the estimation of estrogen binding in excised tumor specimens was the incubation of tumor slices in dilute solutions of tritiated estradiol in the presence and in the absence of an inhibitor of specific binding (cf. Fig. 5). As carried out in our laboratory (J12), 0.5-mm slices of fresh tumor tissue are incubated at 37°C with 0.1 nM [6,7-^{3}H]estradiol in 300 ml of Krebs–Ringer–Henseleit glucose buffer, pH 7.3, in the presence and in the absence of an estrogen antagonist, either nafoxidine or Parke-Davis CI628, in 10 μM concentration. At appropriate intervals, usually 30 minutes, 5 or more slices are removed from each solution, blotted, dried from the frozen state, and weighed. The content of tritiated hormone is determined by combustion to yield tritiated water, which is counted in a liquid scintillation spectrometer. Results are expressed as disintegrations per minute per milligram of dry tissue, using the median of the individual values obtained for each time point. Figure 8 illustrates incorporation patterns for one receptor-poor and three receptor-rich breast cancers. It can be seen that the difference between the curves in the presence and in the absence of inhibitor is more significant than the actual magnitude of the uptake itself.

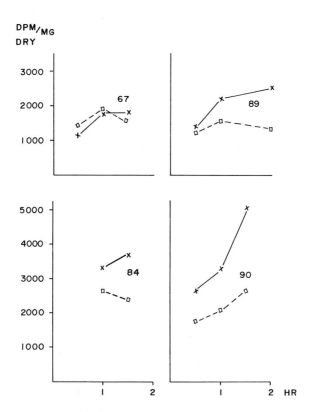

Fig. 8. Radioactivity uptake patterns in slices of typical human breast cancers incubated at 37°C in 0.1 nM [6,7-³H]estradiol in the absence (×——×) or in the presence (□---□) of 10 μM Parke-Davis CI628. Each point is median value for 5 slices. Specimen: No. 67, primary; No. 84, liver metastasis, No. 89, local breast mass; No. 90, primary. Receptor test: negative for No. 67, positive for Nos. 84, 89, 90.

Slice uptake procedures similar to this have been employed in other laboratories for determining estrogen binding in human breast cancer specimens (H3, J1, J20, S3) and for its correlation with clinical response to endocrine therapy (M1, T5). Compared to other techniques, slice uptake has the disadvantage that it is less sensitive, requires a larger tumor sample, and is restricted to fresh tumor specimens because cells that have been frozen lose their receptor protein to the medium during incubation with the hormone. The uptake technique has the advantage that it gives the total binding capacity of the specimen inasmuch as endogenous estrogen present in the tumor exchanges with radioactive hormone under the assay conditions.

After it was discovered (G4, J19) that the receptor protein of target cells is originally in the cytoplasm and moves to the nucleus only after combination with the hormone, it became possible to devise more sensitive and quantitative estimations of estrogen-binding capacity, applicable to frozen cancer specimens, simply by adding an excess of radioactive estradiol to a soluble extract of broken tumor cells and determining how much radioactivity is specifically bound to receptor protein. Separation of the estrogen–receptor complex from the unbound steroid may be effected in different ways, the principal methods employed being sucrose gradient ultracentrifugation, agar gel electrophoresis, dextran-coated charcoal, or gel filtration through Sephadex G-25.

Most of the studies of breast cancer patients carried out in our laboratory have employed sucrose gradient ultracentrifugation for measuring receptor content (D3, J12, J18). A number of other laboratories also have described the use of the sucrose gradient technique for the determination of estrophilin in human breast cancers (M4, M6, M7, S14, W3) and for the correlation of the results with clinical reponse to endocrine therapy (M12, P1, P2, S8, W2). In our procedure, as illustrated in Fig. 9 and described in more detail elsewhere (J18), the tumor specimen, after being pulverized in the frozen state, is homogenized in a buffer solution containing a small amount of dithiothreitol to protect the receptor protein against decomposition. The homogenate is centrifuged to precipitate nuclei and other particulate matter, and a portion of the cytosol fraction is treated with tritiated estradiol in a concentration (0.5 nM) sufficient to react with the amount of estrophilin usually found in hormone-dependent breast cancers. Because estradiol can also bind to certain serum proteins (albumin, α-fetoprotein) that are sometimes present in breast cancer specimens, a measure of this nonspecific binding is obtained by treating a second portion of the tumor cytosol with estradiol in the presence of Parke-Davis CI628, a compound that prevents the specific binding of hormone to estrophilin but has no effect on its interaction with serum

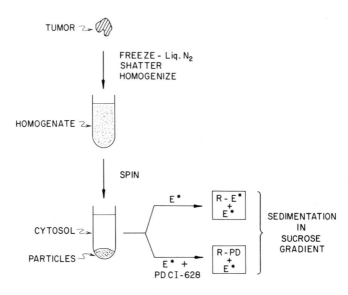

FIG. 9. Preparation of the specimen for determination of receptor content. E*
represents tritiated estradiol; R, the receptor protein; and PD, the inhibitor, Parke-
Davis CI628. Reproduced from DeSombre et al. (D3).

protein. An aliquot portion of each mixture is layered on a 10 to 30%
sucrose gradient and centrifuged at 2°C for 16 hours at 250,000 g. Successive 100-μl fractions are then collected from the bottom of the tube
and counted for radioactivity. Under the conditions of centrifugation,
estradiol bound to the large receptor protein molecule sediments into
the sucrose, whereas unbound estradiol remains at the top.

As illustrated in Fig. 10, some receptor-containing tumor specimens
exhibit only 8 S complex, whereas others show various amounts of specific
binding in the 4 S region as well. Radioactivity associated with the 8 S
form of estrophilin is estimated from the difference in the sedimentation
curves, with and without inhibitor, from fraction 1 to the minimum observed about fractions 18 to 22, depending on the conditions of ultracentrifugation. The 4 S radioactivity is similarly calculated by difference
of the curves between the minimum and the point where the curve with
inhibitor crosses the curve without inhibitor. For specimens with a large
amount of 8 S component, this procedure underestimates the 4 S complex,
because of the increased amount of unbound estradiol overlapping the
4 S region in the gradient with the inhibitor. This does not affect the
conclusion from the receptor test, inasmuch as specimens with large
amounts of 8 S complex are already considered to be receptor rich.

At the present time, DNA is being determined on the washed sediment

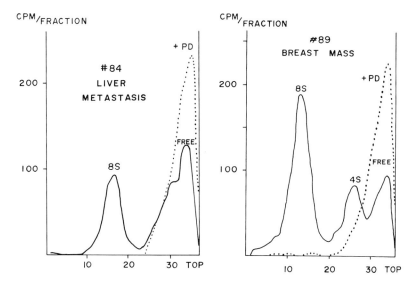

FIG. 10.   Typical sedimentation patterns in 10 to 30% sucrose gradients of receptor-rich human breast cancer cytosols containing 0.5 nM tritiated estradiol in the absence (———) or in the presence (....) of 0.2 μM Parke-Davis CI628 (PD). Some tumor cytosols show only 8 S complex in low-salt gradients: others show varying amounts of 4 S subunit as well.

from the original tumor homogenate, so that the assay results can be expressed in terms of femtomoles of estradiol bound per 100 μg of DNA. Because this procedure was not done with the earlier specimens, the results in this chapter are calculated in terms of femtomoles of estradiol binding capacity per gram of original tumor weight to permit comparison of all the patients. Expression of the results in terms of cytosol protein is not satisfactory, for the protein content of tumor cytosols varies widely, in part because of different amounts of serum proteins present. In our earlier experiments (D3, J12) cancers were classified as positive, borderline, or negative depending on whether or not there was a significant difference in the 8 S and 4 S regions between the curves with and without inhibitor. As discussed later, we now consider tumors to be receptor-rich or receptor-poor depending on whether their specific estradiol binding in the 8 S and 4 S regions is greater or less than an empirically determined critical level.

As an alternative to sedimentation, the estradiol–receptor complex of tumor cytosols can be estimated by electrophoresis in an agar gel (W1). This procedure, which has been employed for the correlation of receptor content with clinical response to endocrine therapy (K12, M1, M2), has the advantage of being simpler, faster, and less expensive than sucrose gradient centrifugation, but it has a minor disadvantage in that the cytosol complex does not separate from serum proteins that can bind estradiol, so that the specific binding often must be determined as a small difference between large numbers. A technique in which the estradiol–receptor complex is separated from excess unbound steroid by filtration of the estradiol–cytosol mixture through Sephadex G-25 (G3) has been employed both for correlation of clinical response with tumor receptor content (S13) and for demonstrating the presence of an estrogen receptor system in a stable line of human breast cancer cells maintained in culture (B9).

The method now most widely used for the determination of estrophilin in breast cancers is the dextran–charcoal procedure, first introduced by Korenman and Dukes (K9) and subjected to modification by various investigators (F1, H1, K11, L2, L3). This procedure, in which the unbound hormone is removed from an estradiol–cytosol mixture by adsorption on dextran-coated charcoal, is most accurate when aliquot portions of cytosol are incubated with different concentrations of hormone and, after addition of the charcoal and centrifuging, the amount of receptor-bound hormone remaining in solution is plotted against the ratio of bound to free steroid in the original mixture (Fig. 11). In such a Scatchard plot (S9) the total number of specific binding sites is calculated from the intercept on the abscissa of an extrapolation of a straight line through the experimental points, whereas the slope of the line gives a measure of the binding constant.

The charcoal technique is probably the simplest of the current methods for determining estrophilin in tumor cytosol and has been employed in a number of studies correlating tumor-receptor content with response to endocrine therapy (B4, C2, E1, H2, H5, K12, L3, L4, M12, W2). It gives values that are somewhat higher and probably more authentic than those obtained with the sucrose gradient procedure (C2, W2), although it suffers from the fact that artifacts of nonspecific binding may not be recognized as readily as with the sucrose gradient method. Moreover, it does not distinguish between the 8 S and 4 S forms of the receptor complex, a distinction that has been considered by some investigators to be important (W2). At the present time, the charcoal technique, properly employed, probably represents the method of choice for the routine assay of estrophilin in human breast cancers.

A recently described procedure for assay of estrophilin uses estradiol–albumin antibodies coupled to an insoluble matrix for the removal of unbound steroid from the estradiol–cytosol mixture (C1, F2). In preliminary studies this simple technique was found to compare favorably with

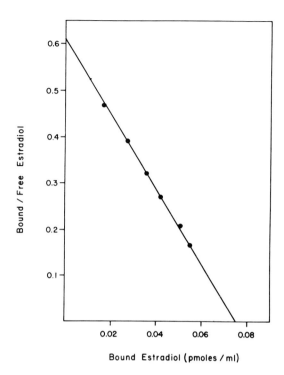

FIG. 11. Scatchard plot of the macromolecular binding of tritiated estradiol in cytosol of hormone-dependent, dimethylbenzanthracene-induced rat mammary tumor. $K_d = 1.2 \times 10^{-10}$ M. Reproduced with permission from McGuire and Julian (M8).

the charcoal procedure for the determination of estrogen receptors in human breast cancers (F3).

3.3. CLINICAL CORRELATIONS

So far our correlation of estrogen binding with response to endocrine therapy has been carried out for 133 women with advanced breast cancer. Ten of these were characterized by the slice uptake procedure only, and the remaining 123 by sucrose gradient ultracentrifugation, in some cases confirmed by uptake. Agreement between the two methods was good (Figs. 8 and 10).

As shown in Fig. 12, the 123 primary and metastatic cancers in patients undergoing therapy for advanced disease varied widely in estradiol binding capacity from undetectable levels to more than 3000 femtomoles per gram of tumor. With two exceptions, no patient without ovarian function whose tumor contained less than 750 femtomoles per gram, and no pre-

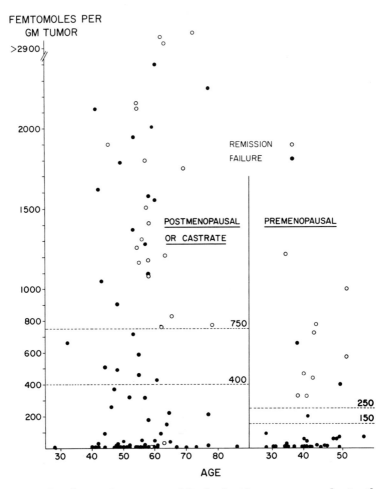

F_IG_. 12.   Correlation of tumor estrophilin level with response to endocrine therapy for 123 patients with advanced breast cancer.

menopausal patient with a level of less than 300 femtomoles per gram, responded to any type of endocrine therapy. Until results with larger numbers of patients permit a more precise assignment of values, we have defined the critical estrophilin level for a receptor-rich or positive test as >750 femtomoles per gram in the postmenopausal or castrate patient and >250 in the premenopausal patient. Tumors with estrophilin content below these values are classified as receptor-poor, divided into borderline (400–750 for postmenopausal, 150–250 for premenopausal patients) and negative (levels below these ranges). The fact that the estrophilin con-

centration required for response appears to be lower in tumors of premenopausal women presumably is due to the fact that these patients are
producing larger amounts of endogenous estrogen that not only masks
part of the receptor present in the cytosol, but also has caused some of it
to have moved into the tumor cell nuclei.

Of the 133 patients summarized in Table 1, 104 were treated with
ablative procedures and 29 received some type of hormone administration. Of the 87 women whose tumors gave negative or borderline tests,
only two showed objective responses to the endocrine therapy employed,
in marked contrast to remission in 29 of 46, or 63%, of the receptor-posi-
tive cases. In early 1974, the clinical records of 68 of these patients were
subjected to independent evaluation by an outside review team from the
Breast Cancer Task Force of the National Cancer Institute. As seen in
Table 2, the conclusions obtained from these reviewed patients are essentially the same as those from the total cases. It would appear that about
two-thirds of the patients whose cancers contain significant amounts of
estrophilin can expect benefit from some type of endocrine therapy. But
if the tumor estrophilin level is below a critical value, that patient has
little if any chance of response to endocrine therapy and probably is better
treated directly with chemotherapeutic agents. On the basis of the critical
estrophilin level as defined in Fig. 12, the more than 1200 women whose
primary and/or metastatic breast cancers have been assayed were found
to consist of about 70% classified as receptor poor and 30% receptor rich.

TABLE 1
OBJECTIVE REMISSIONS[a]—TOTAL CASES

	Receptor test		
	Positive	Borderline	Negative
Ablation—104			
Adrenalectomy	2/5	0/4	0/14
Adrenalectomy + oophorectomy	13/19	0/5	1/11
Hypophysectomy	2/4		0/9
Oophorectomy	6/8		0/25
Hormone—29			
Androgen	0/1		0/3
Estrogen	2/2	0/1	1/7
Antiestrogen	1/2		0/1
Estrogen + progestin	3/5		0/7
Total cases—133	29/46 (63%)	0/10	2/77

[a] Objective remissions were defined as responses of at least 6 months' duration, in
which at least 50% of the lesions regressed and no metastases showed progression.

TABLE 2

OBJECTIVE REMISSIONS—REVIEWED CASES[a]

	Positive	Borderline	Negative
Ablation—55			
Adrenalectomy	1/4	0/2	0/9
Adrenalectomy + oophorectomy	8/10	0/3	0/4
Hypophysectomy	1/2		0/7
Oophorectomy	3/4		0/10
Hormone—13			
Androgen	0/1		0/2
Estrogen	2/2		0/4
Antiestrogen	1/2		
Estrogen + progestin	1/1		0/1
Reviewed cases—68	17/26 (65%)	0/5	0/37

[a] The records of these patients, who are also included in Table 1, were reviewed by Drs. Mary Sears and George Escher according to the criteria of objective response established by the Breast Cancer Task Force.

Essentially none of the former group of patients and about two-thirds of the latter receive objective benefit from endocrine therapy; thus estrophilin determination can predict the optimal therapy for nearly 90% of the total patients (Fig. 13).

The reason why not all patients with receptor-rich tumors show objective remission to endocrine therapy is not entirely clear. In some instances it appears that the patient may have a mixture of estrophilin-rich and estrophilin-poor metastases or tumor regions, with a receptor-rich specimen being obtained for assay. The fact that many of these patients do experience subjective remissions of varying duration suggests that some but not all of their cancer is hormone-responsive. Alternatively, as suggested by the interesting recent findings by McGuire (M5), remission after endocrine ablation may require that breast cancers contain receptors for both estrogen and progestin, so that estrophilin-rich tumors lacking progestin receptor will be unresponsive. It is also possible that, during the course of neoplastic transformation, some mammary cells may retain their

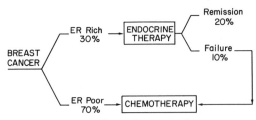

FIG. 13.   Receptor assay as a guide to therapy in breast cancer.

capacity for synthesizing estrophilin, even though they may escape from hormone dependency; examples of autonomous neoplasms with high estrophilin content have been found among experimental mammary tumors both in the mouse (B8, S10) and in the rat (A2, B3, D2).

3.4. USE OF MASTECTOMY SPECIMEN

Because samples of metastatic cancer are not always surgically accessible, it is of considerable interest whether the estrophilin level of a primary tumor, determined at the time of mastectomy, can predict subsequent response to endocrine therapy if metastases appear at a later time. Although only a limited number of such patients have been studied, the results so far appear promising. As indicated in Table 3, two patients with receptor-rich primary breast cancers showed objective remission to endocrine therapy 1–2 years later. Of eleven patients with receptor-poor tumors, all but one failed to respond to various endocrine treatments when metastases appeared from 4 months to more than five years later. Although many more patients must be studied before definitive conclusions can be drawn, these preliminary results suggest potential value in routinely characterizing primary breast cancers at the time of mastectomy

TABLE 3

USE OF MASTECTOMY SPECIMEN IN PREDICTING
SUBSEQUENT RESPONSE

Age	Test	$R_x{}^a$	Months	Response[b]
57	+	E	24	R
65	+	AdO	14	R
40	±	Ord	15	F
57	±	AdO	12	F
41	−	O	60	F
28	−	O	16	F
34	−	Ord	14	F
56	−	H	12	F
44	−	O	11	F
70	−	An	10	F
33	−	AdO	8	F
86	−	E	4	F
59	−	E	67	R

[a] AdO: adrenalectomy plus oophorectomy; An: Androgen; E: estrogen; H: hypophysectomy; O: oophorectomy; Ord: radiation castration.

[b] R: objective remission; F: failure

so that this information will be available as a guide to therapy in case of recurrence.

4.   Hormone Sensitivity of Other Neoplasms

It might be anticipated that different types of cancer, in which growth behavior is known to be influenced by endocrine manipulation, would have receptor proteins for the hormones to which they are sensitive. So far, relatively few investigations of neoplasms other than breast have been reported. In the case of prostatic carcinoma (M15), it has been reported that the capacity of the cytosol to bind dihydrotestosterone, as determined by the charcoal technique, varies widely among tumors of different individuals. Of a series of 12 patients undergoing treatment, no remissions to orchiectomy were observed when the androgen-binding capacity of the cytosol was low, whereas two patients with high binding levels experienced objective remissions. In endometrial carcinoma, which in some instances undergoes arrest when treated with progestational agents, it has been found by an equilibrium dialysis technique (H4), as well as by the charcoal method (R1), that some cancers show a high degree of progesterone binding and others very little affinity, with no relation to the degree of differentiation of the tumor. Correlation of progesterone-binding ability with response to therapy remains to be demonstrated.

The cytosol from cells of a glucocorticoid-sensitive line of the mouse lymphosarcoma P1798 has been shown to bind significantly more tritiated cortisol (H7) or triamcinolone acetonide (K1, K8) than cytosol from a resistant line and to form a hormone–receptor complex sedimenting at 8 S in low-salt sucrose gradients and 4–5 S in high-salt gradients (K1). However, cells of two human and one mouse leukemia lines that are steroid unresponsive also were found to have levels of cytoplasmic glucocorticoid-binding proteins comparable to those of steroid-responsive cells; these receptors participated in a temperature-dependent translocation of labeled dexamethasone to the nucleus (L6). Thus, as in the case of breast cancer, the presence of specific receptor proteins in the cytosol does not guarantee hormone responsiveness. In the case of human disease, it has been reported that the cytosol fraction of blast cells from six patients with acute lymphoblastic leukemia, who no longer responded to drug combinations including glucocorticoids, showed low or negligible binding of tritiated dexamethasone, as determined by the charcoal technique. In contrast, six patients whose cells showed the presence of glucocorticoid receptors responded to this therapy (L7).

The foregoing studies, although still preliminary, suggest that malignant neoplasms of various tissues that show sensitivity to some type of steroid hormone are characterized by the presence of specific receptors for the hormone. In some cases autonomous tumors may also contain such receptors. Further investigation is required to provide a better understanding of the relation of receptor content to hormone response in such malignancies.

5. Summary

Target tissues for steroid hormones have been found to contain receptor systems that interact with the hormone by a two-step mechanism. In the case of estrogens, the steroid first binds to an extranuclear receptor protein called estrophilin, inducing its conversion to an active form that can bind to chromatin. The transformed hormone–receptor complex is translocated to the nucleus, where it modulates RNA biosynthesis. Mammary gland and some but not all tumors derived from it also show hormone dependency and appear to contain a receptor system similar in most respects to that elucidated for the uterus. Some autonomous experimental mammary tumors also show a high level of estrophilin, even though hormonal stimulation through the receptor system apparently is not needed.

The determination of estrogen receptors in human breast cancers, both primary and metastatic, can furnish information useful to the clinician in his choice of the optimal therapy for the individual patient with advanced disease. Of patients with significant tumor estrophilin levels, most, but not all, will respond favorably to endocrine therapy. Women whose cancers lack sufficient amounts of estrophilin have little or no chance of benefit from endocrine ablation or hormone administration and probably should be treated directly by chemotherapy. On the basis of estrophilin assay, proper therapy can be selected in about 90% of the total cases.

Cancers derived from certain other hormone-responsive tissues appear to contain receptors for the particular steroid. The utility of receptor measurements in predicting hormone dependency in cancers of the prostate or endometrium, or hormone sensitivity of human leukemia, remains to be established.

REFERENCES

A1. Anderson, J. N., Clark, J. H., and Peck, E. J., Jr., Oestrogen and nuclear binding sites: Determination of specific sites by [³H]oestradiol exchange. *Biochem. J.* **126**, 561–567 (1972).

A2. Arbogast, L. Y., and DeSombre, E. R., Brief communication: Estrogen-dependent in vitro stimulation of RNA synthesis in hormone-dependent mammary tumors of the rat. *J. Natl. Cancer Inst.* **54**, 483–485 (1975).

B1. Beatson, G. T., On the treatment of inoperable cases of carcinoma of the mamma: Suggestions for a new method of treatment with illustrative cases. *Lancet* **2**, 104–107 (1896).

B2. Boylan, E. S., and Wittliff, J. L., Specific estrogen binding in vivo in the R3230AC mammary adrenocarcinoma of the rat. *Cancer Res.* **33**, 2903–2908 (1973).

B3. Boylan, E. S., and Wittliff, J. L., Specific estrogen binding in rat mammary tumors induced by 7,12-dimethylbenz[a]anthracene. *Cancer Res.* **35**, 506–511 (1975).

B4. Braunsberg, H., Carter, A. E., James, V. H. T., and Jamieson, C. W., Studies on the estimation and clinical significance of estrogen receptors in human malignant breast tumors. *In* "Estrogen Receptors in Human Breast Cancer" (W. L. McGuire, P. P. Carbone, and E. P. Vollmer, eds.), pp. 247–262. Raven, New York, 1975.

B5. Brecher, P. I., Vigersky, R., Wotiz, H. S., and Wotiz, H. H., An in vitro system for the binding of estradiol to rat uterine nuclei. *Steroids* **10**, 635–651 (1967).

B6. Bresciani, F., and Puca, G. A., Fissazione del 17β-estradiolo in ghiandola mammaria e in tumori mammari del topo C3H. *Atti Soc. Ital. Patol.* **9**, 661–664 (1965).

B7. Bresciani, F., Puca, G. A., and Maffettone, F., Riduzione del siti leganti l'estradiolo nella frazione citoplasmatica solubile dei tumori mammari del topo C3H. *Atti Soc. Ital. Patol.* **10**, 711–715 (1967).

B8. Bresciani, F., Puca, G. A., Nola, E., Salvatore, M., and Ardovino, I., Meccanismo dell'azione estrogena e trasformazione neoplastica. *Atti Soc. Ital Patol.* **11**, 203–224 (1969).

B9. Brooks, S. C., Locke, E. R., and Soule, H. D., Estrogen receptor in a human cell line (MCF-7) from breast carcinoma. *J. Biol. Chem.* **248**, 6251–6253 (1973).

C1. Castaneda, E., and Liao, S., The use of antisteroid antibodies in the characterization of steroid receptors. *J. Biol. Chem.* **250**, 883–888 (1975).

C2. Chester, Z., Feherty, P., Kellie, A. E., and Ralphs, D. L., Estrogen receptors in primary breast tumors in relation to the stage and progression of the disease. *In* "Estrogen Receptors in Human Breast Cancer" (W. L. McGuire, P. P. Carbone, and E. P. Vollmer, eds.), pp. 157–172. Raven, New York, 1975.

C3. Clark, J. H., Anderson, J. N., and Peck, E. J., Jr., Nuclear receptor-estrogen complexes of rat uteri: Concentration-time-response-parameters. *In* "Receptors for Hormones" (B. W. O'Malley and A. R. Means, eds.), pp. 15–59. Plenum, New York, 1973.

C4. Costlow, M. E., Buschow, R. A., Richert, N. J., and McGuire, W. L., Prolactin and estrogen binding in transplantable hormone-dependent and autonomous rat mammary carcinoma. *Cancer Res.* **35**, 970–974 (1975).

D1. Deshpande, N., Jensen, V., Bulbrook, R. D., Berne, T., and Ellis, F., Accumulation of tritiated oestradiol by human breast tissue. *Steroids* **10**, 219–232 (1967).

D2. DeSombre, E. R., Kledzik, G., Marshall, S., and Meites, J., Estrogen and prolactin receptor concentrations in rat mammary tumors and response to endocrine ablation. *Cancer Res.* **36**, 354–358 (1976).

D3. DeSombre, E. R., Smith, S., Block, G. E., Ferguson, D. J., and Jensen, E. V., Prediction of breast cancer response to endocrine therapy. *Cancer Chemother. Rep.* **58**, 513–519 (1974).

E1. Engelsman, E., Persijn, J. P., Korsten, C. B., and Cleton, F. J., Oestrogen receptor in human breast cancer tissue and response to endocrine therapy. *Br. Med. J.* **2**, 750–752 (1973).

E2. Erdos, T., Properties of a uterine oestradiol receptor. *Biochem. Biophys. Res. Commun.* **32**, 338–343 (1968).

F1. Feherty, P., Farrer-Brown, G., and Kellie, A. E., Oestradiol receptors in carcinoma and benign disease of the breast: An in vitro assay. *Br. J. Cancer* **25**, 697–710 (1971).

F2. Fishman, J., and Fishman, J. H., Competitive binding assay for estradiol receptor using immobilized antibody. *J. Clin. Endocrinol. Metab.* **39**, 603–606 (1974).

F3. Fishman, J., Fishman, J. H., Nisselbaum, J. S., Menendez-Botet, C., Schwartz, M. K., Martucci, C., and Hellman, L., Measurement of the estradiol receptor in human breast tissue by the immobilized antibody method. *J. Clin. Endocinol. Metab.* **40**, 724–727 (1975).

F4. Folca, P. J., Glascock, R. F., and Irvine, W. T., Studies with tritium-labeled hexoestrol in advanced breast cancer. Comparison of tissue accumulation of hexoestrol with response to bilateral adrenalectomy and oophorectomy. *Lancet* **2**, 796–798 (1961).

G1. Gardner, D. G., and Wittliff, J. L., Specific estrogen receptors in the lactating mammary gland of the rat. *Biochemistry* **12**, 3090–3096 (1973).

G2. Glascock, R. F., and Hoekstra, R. G., Selective accumulation of tritium labelled hexoestrol by the reproductive organs of immature female goats and sheep. *Biochem. J.* **72**, 673–682 (1959).

G3. Godefroi, V. C., and Brooks, S. C., Improved gel-filtration method for analysis of estrogen receptor binding. *Anal. Biochem.* **51**, 335–344 (1973).

G4. Gorski, J., Toft, D., Shyamala, G., Smith, D., and Notides, A., Hormone receptors: Studies on the interaction of estrogen with the uterus. *Recent Prog. Horm. Res.* **24**, 45–80 (1968).

G5. Gschwendt, M., and Hamilton, T. H., The transformation of the cytoplasmic oestradiol-receptor complex into the nuclear complex in a uterine cell-free system. *Biochem. J.* **128**, 611–616 (1972).

G6. Gupta, G. N., Tritium labelled estradiol-17β in rat tissues. Ph.D. Thesis, University of Chicago, Chicago, Illinois, 1960.

H1. Hähnel, R., and Twaddle, E., Estrogen receptors in human breast cancer. I. Methodology and characterization of receptors. *Steroids* **18**, 653–680 (1971).

H2. Hähnel, R., and Vivian, A. B., Biochemical and clinical experience with the estimation of estrogen receptors in human breast carcinoma. *In* "Estrogen Receptors in Human Breast Cancer" (W. L. McGuire, P. P. Carbone, and E. P. Vollmer, eds.), pp. 205–235. Raven, New York, 1975.

H3. Hähnel, R., Twaddle, E., and Vivian, A. B., Estrogen receptors in human breast cancer. 2. In vitro binding of estradiol by benign and malignant tumors. *Steroids* **18**, 681–708 (1971).

H4. Haukkamaa, M., Karjalainen, O., and Luukkainen, T., In vitro binding of progesterone by the human endometrium during the menstrual cycle and by hyperplastic, atrophic, and carcinomatous endometrium. *Am. J. Obstet. Gynecol.* **111**, 205–210 (1971).

H5. Heuson, J. C., Leclercq, G., Longeral, E., Deboel, C., Mattheim, W. H., and Heimann, R., Estrogen receptors: Prognostic significance in breast cancer. *In* "Estrogen Receptors in Human Breast Cancer" (W. L. McGuire, P. P. Carbone, and E. P. Vollmer, eds.), pp. 57–70. Raven, New York, 1975.

H6. Hilf, R., Michel, I., and Bell, C., Biochemical and morphological response of normal and neoplastic mammary tissue to hormonal treatment. *Recent Prog. Horm. Res.* **23**, 229–295 (1967).

H7. Hollander, N., and Chiu, Y. W., In vitro binding of cortisol-1,2-^{3}H by a substance in the supernatant fraction of P1798 mouse lymphosarcoma *Biochem. Biophys. Res. Commun.* **25**, 291–297 (1966).

H8. Huggins, C., and Bergenstal, D. M., Inhibition of mammary and prostatic cancer by adrenalectomy. *Cancer Res.* **12**, 134–141 (1952).

H9. Huggins, C., Grand, L. C., and Brillantes, F. P., Mammary cancer induced by a single feeding of polynuclear hydrocarbons, and its suppression. *Nature (London)* **189**, 204–207 (1961).

J1. James, F., James, V. H. T., Carter, A. E., and Irvine, W. T., A comparison of in vivo and in vitro uptake of estradiol by human breast tumors and the relationship to steroid excretion. *Cancer Res.* **31**, 1268–1272 (1971).

J2. Jensen, E. V., Studies of growth phenomena using tritium labelled steroids. *Proc. Int. Congr. Biochem., 4th, 1958* Vol. 15, p. 119 (1960).

J3. Jensen, E. V., Metabolic fate of sex hormones in target tissues with regard to tissue specificity. *Proc. Int. Congr. Endocrinol., 2nd, 1964* Int. Congr. Ser. No. 83, pp. 420–433 (1965).

J4. Jensen, E. V., Mechanism of estrogen action in relation to carcinogenesis. *Proc. Can. Cancer Conf.* **6**, 143–165 (1965).

J5. Jensen, E. V., The pattern of hormone-receptor interaction. *In* "Some Aspects of the Aetiology and Biochemistry of Prostatic Cancer" (K. Griffiths and C. G. Pierrepoint, eds.), pp. 151–169. Alpha Omega Alpha Publ., Cardiff, Wales, 1970.

J6. Jensen, E. V., and DeSombre, E. R., Estrogen-receptor interaction. *Science* **182**, 126–134 (1973).

J7. Jensen, E. V., and Jacobson, H. I., Fate of steroid estrogens in target tissues. *In* "Biological Activities of Steroids in Relation to Cancer" (G. Pincus and E. P. Vollmer, eds.), pp. 161–178. Academic Press, New York, 1960.

J8. Jensen, E. V., and Jacobson, H. I., Basic guides to the mechanism of estrogen action. *Recent Prog. Horm. Res.* **18**, 387–414 (1962).

J9. Jensen, E. V., DeSombre, E. R., and Jungblut, P. W., Interaction of estrogens with receptor sites in vivo and in vitro. *Proc. Int. Congr. Horm. Steroids, 2nd, 1966* Int. Congr. Ser. No. 132, pp. 492–500 (1967).

J10. Jensen, E. V., DeSombre, E. R., and Jungblut, P. W., Estrogen receptors in hormone-responsive tissues and tumors. *In* "Endogenous Factors Influencing Host Tumor Balance" (R. W. Wissler, T. L. Dao, and S. Wood, Jr., eds.), pp. 15–30 and 68. Univ. of Chicago Press, Chicago, Illinois, 1967.

J11. Jensen, E. V., Numata, M., Brecher, P. I., and DeSombre, E. R., Hormone receptor interaction as a guide to biochemical mechanism. *In* "The Biochemistry of Steroid Hormone Action" (R. M. S. Smellie, ed.), pp. 133–159. Academic Press, New York, 1971.

J12. Jensen, E. V., Block, G. E., Smith, S., Kyser, K., and DeSombre, E. R., Estrogen receptors and breast cancer response to adrenalectomy. *Natl. Cancer Inst., Monogr.* **34**, 55–70 (1971).

J13. Jensen, E. V., DeSombre, E. R., Hurst, D. J., Kawashima, T., and Jungblut, P. W., Estrogen-receptor interactions in target tissues. *Arch. Anat. Microsc. Morphol. Exp.* **56**, Suppl. 3–4, 547–569 (1967).

J14. Jensen, E. V., DeSombre, E. R., Jungblut, P. W., Stumpf, W. E., and Roth, L. J., Biochemical and autoradiographic studies of ^{3}H-estradiol localization. *In* "Autoradiography of Diffusible Substances" (L. J. Roth and W. E. Stumpf, eds.), pp. 81–97. Academic Press, New York, 1969.

J15. Jensen, E. V., Mohla, S., Gorell, T., Tanaka, S., and DeSombre, E. R., Estrophile to nucleophile in two easy steps. *J. Steroid Biochem.* **3**, 445–458 (1972).

J16. Jensen, E. V., Suzuki, T., Numata, M., Smith, S., and DeSombre, E. R., Estrogen-binding substances of target tissues. *Steroids* **13**, 417–427 (1969).

J17. Jensen, E. V., Numata, M., Smith, S., Suzuki, T., Brecher, P. I., and DeSombre, E. R., Estrogen-receptor interaction in target tissues. *Dev. Biol., Suppl.* **3**, 151–171 (1969).

J18. Jensen, E. V., Polley, T. Z., Smith, S., Block, G. E., Ferguson, D. J., and DeSombre, E. R., Prediction of hormone dependency in human breast cancer. In "Estrogen Receptors in Human Breast Cancer" (W. L. McGuire, P. P. Carbone, and E. P. Vollmer, eds.), pp. 37–55. Raven, New York, 1975.

J19. Jensen, E. V., Suzuki, T., Kawashima, T., Stumpf, W. E., Jungblut, P. W., and DeSombre, E. R., A two-step mechanism for the interaction of estradiol with rat uterus. *Proc. Natl. Acad. Sci. U.S.A.* **59**, 632–638 (1968).

J20. Johansson, H., Terenius, L., and Thorén, L., The binding of estradiol-17β to human breast cancers and other tissues in vitro. *Cancer Res.* **30**, 692–698 (1970).

J21. Jungblut, P. W., DeSombre, E. R., and Jensen, E. V., Estrogen receptor in induced rat mammary tumor. In "Hormone in Genese und Therapie des Mammacarcinoms" (H. Gummel, H. Kraatz, and G. Bacigalupo, eds.), pp. 109–123. Akademie-Verlag, Berlin, 1967.

J22. Jungblut, P. W., Hätzel, I., DeSombre, E. R., and Jensen, E. V., Über Hormon-Receptoren die oestrogenbindenden Prinzipien der Erfolgsorgane. *Colloq. Ges. Physiol. Chem.* **18**, 58–82 (1967).

K1. Kaiser, N., Milholland, R. J., and Rosen, F., Glucocorticoid receptors and mechanism of resistance in the cortisol-sensitive and -resistant lines of lymphosarcoma P1798. *Cancer Res.* **34**, 621–626 (1974).

K2. Keightley, D. O., and Okey, A. B., Effects of dimethylbenz[a]anthracene and dihydrotestosterone on estradiol-17β binding in rat mammary cytosol fraction. *Cancer Res.* **33**, 2637–2642 (1973).

K3. King, R. J. B., and Gordon, J., The localization of [6,7-³H]oestradiol-17β in the rat uterus. *J. Endocrinol.* **34**, 431–437 (1966).

K4. King, R. J. B., and Mainwaring, W. I. P., "Steroid-Cell Interactions." Univ. Park Press, Baltimore, Maryland, 1974.

K5. King, R. J. B., Cowan, D. M., and Inman, D. R., The uptake of [6,7-³H]oestradiol by dimethylbenzanthracene-induced rat mammary tumors. *J. Endocrinol.* **32**, 83–90 (1965).

K6. King, R. J. B., Gordon, J., and Steggles, A. W., The properties of a nuclear acidic protein that binds [6,7-³H]oestradiol-17β. *Biochem. J.* **114**, 649–657 (1969).

K7. King, R. J. B., Gordon, J., Cowan, D. M., and Inman, D. R., The intranuclear localization of [6,7-³H]oestradiol-17β in dimethylbenzanthracene-induced rat mammary adrenocarcinoma and other tissues. *J. Endocrinol.* **36**, 139–150 (1966).

K8. Kirkpatrick, A. F., Kaiser, N., Milholland, R. J., and Rosen, F., Glucocorticoid-binding macromolecules in normal tissues and tumors. *J. Biol. Chem.* **247**, 70–74 (1972).

K9. Korenman, S. G., and Dukes, B. A., Specific binding by the cytoplasm of human breast carcinoma. *J. Clin. Endocrinol. Metab.* **30**, 639–645 (1970).

K10. Korenman, S. G., and Rao, B. R., Reversible disaggregation of the cytosol-estrogen binding protein of uterine cytosol. *Proc. Natl. Acad. Sci. U.S.A.* **61**, 1028–1033 (1968).

K11. Korsten, C. B., and Persijn, J. P., A simple assay for specific estrogen binding capacity in human mammary tumors. *Z. Klin. Chem. Klin. Biochem.* **10**, 502–508 (1972).

K12. Korsten, C. B., Engelsman, E., and Persijn, J. P., Clinical value of estrogen receptors in advanced breast cancer. *In* "Estrogen Receptors in Human Breast Cancer" (W. L. McGuire, P. P. Carbone, and E. P. Vollmer, eds.), pp. 93–104. Raven, New York, 1975.

K13. Kyser, K. A., The tissue, subcellular and molecular binding of estradiol to dimethylbenzanthracene-induced rat mammary tumors. Ph.D. thesis, University of Chicago, Chicago, Illinois, 1970.

L1. Leclercq, G., and Heuson, J. C., Specific estrogen receptor of the DMBA-induced mammary carcinoma of the rat and its estrogen requiring molecular transformation. *Eur. J. Cancer* **9**, 675–680 (1973).

L2. Leclercq, G., Heuson, J. C., Schoenfeld, R., Mattheiem, W. H., and Tagnon, H. J., Estrogen receptors in human breast cancer. *Eur. J. Cancer* **9**, 665–673 (1973).

L3. Leung, B. S., Fletcher, W. S., Lindell, T. D., Wood, D. C., and Krippaehne, W. W., Predictability of response to endocrine ablation in advanced breast carcinoma. *Arch. Surg. (Chicago)* **106**, 515–519 (1973).

L4. Leung, B. S., Moseley, H. S., Davenport, C. E., Krippaehne, W. W., and Fletcher, W. S., Estrogen receptor in prediction of clinical responses to endocrine ablation. *In* "Estrogen Receptors in Human Breast Cancer" (W. L. McGuire, P. P. Carbone, and E. P. Vollmer, eds.), pp. 107–126. Raven, New York, 1975.

L5. Liao, S., Cellular receptors and mechanisms of action of steroid hormones. *Int. Rev. Cytol.* **41**, 87–172 (1975).

L6. Lippman M. E., Perry S., and Thompson E. B. Cytoplasmic glucocorticoid-binding proteins in glucocorticoid-unresponsive human and mouse leukemic cell lines. *Cancer Res.* **34**, 1572–1576 (1974).

L7. Lippman M. E., Halterman, R. H., Leventhal, B. G., Perry, S., and Thompson, E. B., Glucocorticoid-binding proteins in human acute lymphoblastic leukemic blast cells. *J. Clin. Invest.* **52**, 1715-1725 (1973).

M1. Maass, H., Engel, B., Hohmeister, H., Lehmann, F., and Trams, G., Estrogen receptors in human breast cancer tissue. *Am. J. Obstet. Gynecol.* **113**, 377–382 (1972).

M2. Maass, H., Engel, B., Nowakowski, H., Stolzenback, G., and Trams, G., Estrogen receptors in human breast cancer and clinical correlations. *In* "Estrogen Receptors in Human Breast Cancer" (W. L. McGuire, P. P. Carbone, and E. P. Vollmer, eds.), pp. 175–188. Raven, New York, 1975.

M3. Maurer, H. R., and Chalkley, R., Some properties of a nuclear binding site of estradiol. *J. Mol. Biol.* **27**, 431–441 (1967).

M4. McGuire, W. L., Estrogen receptors in human breast cancer. *J. Clin. Invest.* **52**, 73–77 (1973).

M5. McGuire, W. L., personal communication.

M6. McGuire, W. L., and Chamness, G. C., Studies on the estrogen receptor in breast cancer. *In* "Receptors for Reproductive Hormones" (B. W. O'Malley and A. R. Means, eds.), pp. 113–136. Plenum, New York, 1973.

M7. McGuire, W. L., and DeLaGarza, M., Similarity of estrogen receptor in human and rat mammary carcinoma. *J. Clin. Endocrinol. Metab.* **36**, 548–552 (1973).

M8. McGuire, W. L., and Julian, J. A., Comparison of macromolecular binding of estradiol in hormone-dependent and hormone-independent rat mammary carcinoma. *Cancer Res.* **31**, 1440-1445 (1971).

M9. McGuire, W. L., Carbone, P. P., and Vollmer, E. P., eds., "Estrogen Receptors in Human Breast Cancer." Raven, New York, 1975.

M10. McGuire, W. L., Huff, K., and Chamness, G. C., Temperature-independent binding of estrogen receptor to chromatin. *Biochemistry* 11, 4562–4565 (1972).

M11. McGuire, W. L., Julian, J. A., and Chamness, G. C., A dissociation between ovarian dependent growth and estrogen sensitivity in mammary carcinoma. *Endocrinology* 89, 969–973 (1971).

M12. McGuire, W. L., Pearson, O. H., and Segaloff, A., Predicting hormone responsiveness in human breast cancer. In "Estrogen Receptors in Human Breast Cancer" (W. L. McGuire, P. P. Carbone, and E. P. Vollmer, eds.), pp. 17–30. Raven, New York, 1975.

M13. Mobbs, B. G., The uptake of tritiated oestradiol by dimethylbenzanthracene-induced mammary tumours of the rat. *J. Endocrinol.* 36, 409–414 (1966).

M14. Mobbs, B. G., The uptake of simultaneously administered [^{3}H]oestradiol and [^{14}C]progesterone by dimethylbenzanthracene-induced rat mammary tumours. *J. Endocrinol.* 41, 339–344 (1968).

M15. Mobbs, B. G., Johnson, I. E., and Connolly, J. G., Hormonal responsiveness of prostatic carcinoma. In vitro technique for prediction. *Urology* 3, 105–106 (1974).

M16. Mohla, S., DeSombre, E. R., and Jensen, E. V., Tissue-specific stimulation of RNA synthesis by transformed estradiol-receptor complex. *Biochem. Biophys. Res. Commun.* 46, 661–667 (1972).

N1. Noteboom, W. D., and Gorski, J., Stereospecific binding of estrogens in rat uterus. *Arch. Biochem. Biophys.* 11, 559–568 (1965).

P1. Pearson, O. H., McGuire, W. L., Brodkey, J., and Marshall, J., Estrogen receptors and prediction of the response of metastatic breast cancer to hypophysectomy. In "Estrogen Receptors in Human Breast Cancer" (W. L. McGuire, P. P. Carbone, and E. P. Vollmer, eds.), pp. 31–35. Raven, New York, 1975.

P2. Pihl, A., Sander, S., Brennhovd, I., and Olsnes, S., Predictive value of estrogen receptors in human breast cancer. In "Estrogen Receptors in Human Breast Cancer" (W. L. McGuire, P. P. Carbone, and E. P. Vollmer, eds.), pp. 193–201. Raven, New York, 1975.

P3. Puca, G. A., and Bresciani, F., Decrease to loss of ability to bind estradiol by a soluble macromolecular fraction of C3H mammary tumors. *Eur. J. Cancer* 3, 475–479 (1968).

P4. Puca, G. A., and Bresciani, F., Receptor molecule for oestrogens from rat uterus. *Nature (London)* 218, 967–969 (1968).

P5. Puca, G. A., and Bresciani, F., Interactions of 6,7-^{3}H-17β-estradiol with mammary gland and other organs of the C3H mouse in vivo. *Endocrinology* 85, 1–10 (1969).

R1. Rao, B. R., and Wiest, W. G., Receptors for progesterone. *Gynecol. Oncol.* 2, 239–248 (1974).

R2. Raspé, G., ed., "Advances in the Biosciences," Vol. 7. Pergamon, Oxford, 1971.

R3. Rochefort, H., and Baulieu, E. E., Recepteurs hormonaux: Relations entre les récepteurs utérins de l'estradiol "8S" cytoplasmique et "4S" cytoplasmique et nucléaire. *C. R. Hebd. Seances Acad. Sci., Ser. D* 267, 662–665 (1968).

S1. Sander, S., The uptake of 17β-oestradiol in breast tissue of female rats. *Acta Endocrinol. (Copenhagen)* 58, 49–56 (1968).

S2. Sander, S., The capacity of breast tissue to accumulate oestradiol-17β in vitro. *Acta Pathol. Microbiol. Scand.* 73, 29–36 (1968).

S3. Sander, S., The in vitro uptake of oestradiol in biopsies from 25 breast cancer patients. *Acta Pathol. Microbiol. Scand.* **74**, 301–302 (1968).

S4. Sander, S., In vitro uptake of oestradiol in DMBA induced breast tumors of the rat. *Acta Pathol. Microbiol. Scand.* **75**, 520–526 (1969).

S5. Sander, S., and Attramadal, A., An autoradiographic study of oestradiol incorporation in the breast tissue of female rats. *Acta Endocrinol. (Copenhagen)* **58**, 235–242 (1968).

S6. Sander, S., and Attramadal, A., The in vivo uptake of oestradiol-17β by hormone responsive and unresponsive breast tumors of the rat. *Acta Pathol. Microbiol. Scand.* **74**, 169–178 (1968).

S7. Sarff, M., and Gorski, J., Control of estrogen binding protein concentration under basal conditions and after estrogen administration. *Biochemistry* **10**, 2557–2563 (1971).

S8. Savlov, E. D., Wittliff, J. L., Hilf, R., and Hall, T. C., Correlations between certain biochemical properties of breast cancer and response to therapy: A preliminary report. *Cancer* **33**, 303-309 (1974).

S9. Scatchard, G., The attraction of proteins for small molecules and ions. *Ann. N.Y. Acad. Sci.* **51**, 660–672 (1949).

S10. Shyamala, G., Estradiol receptors in mouse mammary tumors: Absence of the transfer of bound estradiol from the cytoplasm to the nucleus. *Biochem. Biophys. Res. Commun.* **46**, 1623–1629 (1972).

S11. Shyamala, G., and Gorski, J., Estrogen receptors in the rat uterus. *J. Biol. Chem.* **244**, 1097–1103 (1969).

S12. Shyamala, G., and Nandi, S., Interactions of 6,7-H³-17β-estradiol with the mouse lactating mammary tissue in vivo and in vitro. *Endocrinology* **91**, 861–867 (1972).

S13. Singhakowinta, A., Mohindra, R., Brooks, S. C., Vaitevicius, V. K., and Brennan, M. J., Clinical correlation of endocrine therapy and estrogen receptor. *In* "Estrogen Receptors in Human Breast Cancer" (W. L. McGuire, P. P. Carbone, and E. P. Vollmer, eds.), pp. 131–149. Raven, New York, 1975.

S14. Spaeren, U., Olsnes, S., Brennhovd, I., Efskind, J., and Pihl, A., Content of estrogen receptors in human breast cancers. *Eur. J. Cancer* **9**, 353–357 (1973).

S15. Steggles, A. W., and King, R. J. B., The uptake of [6,7-³H]oestradiol by oestrogen dependent and independent hamster kidney tumours. *Eur. J. Cancer* **4**, 395–401 (1968).

S16. Steggles, A. W., and King, R. J. B., Oestrogen receptors in hamster tumors. *Eur. J. Cancer* **8**, 323–334 (1972).

S17. Stone, G. M., The radioactive compounds in various tissues of ovariectomized mouse following systemic administration of tritiated oestradiol and oestrone. *Acta Endocrinol. (Copenhagen)* **47**, 433–443 (1964).

S18. Stumpf, W. E., Subcellular distribution of ³H-estradiol in rat uterus by quantitative autoradiography—a comparison between ³H-estradiol and ³H-norethynodrel. *Endocrinology* **83**, 777–782 (1968).

S19. Stumpf, W. E., Nuclear concentration of ³H-estradiol in target tissues. Drymount autoradiography of vagina, oviduct, ovary, testis, mammary tumor, liver and adrenal. *Endocrinology* **85**, 31–37 (1969).

T1. Talwar, G. P., Segal, S. J., Evans, A., and Davidson, O. W., The binding of estradiol in the uterus: A mechanism for derepression of RNA synthesis. *Proc. Natl. Acad. Sci. U.S.A.* **52**, 1059–1066 (1964).

T2. Teng, C. S., and Hamilton, T. H., The role of chromatin in estrogen action in the uterus. I. The control of template capacity and chemical composition and the binding of ^{3}H-estradiol-17β. *Proc. Natl. Acad. Sci. U.S.A.* **60**, 1410–1417 (1968).

T3. Terenius, L., Selective retention of estrogen isomers in estrogen dependent breast tumors of rats demonstrated by in vitro methods. *Cancer Res.* **28**, 328–337 (1968).

T4. Terenius, L., Parallelism between oestrogen binding capacity and hormone responsiveness of mammary tumours in GR/A mice. *Eur. J. Cancer* **8**, 55–58 (1972).

T5. Terenius, L., Rimsten, A., Thorén, L., and Lindgren, A., Estrogen receptors and prognosis in cancer of the breast. *In* "Estrogen Receptors in Human Breast Cancer" (W. L. McGuire, P. P. Carbone, and E. P. Vollmer, eds.), pp. 237–244. Raven, New York, 1975.

T6. Toft, D., and Gorski, J., A receptor molecule for estrogens: Isolation from the rat uterus and preliminary characterization. *Proc. Natl. Acad. Sci. U.S.A.* **55**, 1574–1581 (1966).

T7. Toft, D., Shyamala, G., and Gorski, J., A receptor molecule for estrogens: Studies using a cell-free system. *Proc. Natl. Acad. Sci. U.S.A.* **57**, 1740–1743 (1967).

W1. Wagner, R. K., Characterization and assay of steroid hormone receptors and steroid binding proteins by agar gel electrophoresis at low temperature. *Hoppe-Seyler's Z. Physiol. Chem.* **353**, 1235–1245 (1972).

W2. Wittliff, J. L., and Savlov, E. D., Estrogen-binding capacity for cytoplasmic forms of the estrogen receptors in human breast cancer. *In* "Estrogen Receptors in Human Breast Cancer" (W. L. McGuire, P. P. Carbone, and E. P. Vollmer, eds.), pp. 73–86. Raven, New York, 1975.

W3. Wittliff, J. L., Hilf, R., Brooks, W. F., Jr., Savlov, E. D., Hall, T. C., and Orlando, R. A., Specific estrogen-binding capacity of the cytoplasmic receptor in normal and neoplastic breast tissues of humans. *Cancer Res.* **32**, 1983–1992 (1972).

MEMBRANE RECEPTORS FOR POLYPEPTIDE HORMONES

Bernard Rees Smith

Departments of Clinical Biochemistry and Medicine,
University of Newcastle upon Tyne,
Newcastle upon Tyne, England

1. Introduction

The first stage in the mechanism of action of the large peptide hormones, which include growth hormone (GH), luteinizing hormone (LH), chorionic gonadotropin (CG), follicle-stimulating hormone (FSH), thyroid-stimulating hormone (TSH), prolactin (PRL), corticotropin (ACTH), insulin, glucagon, and parathyroid hormone (PTH) is contact with hormone-specific receptor sites on the target cell surface. The hormone receptor interaction appears to modify the cell in such a way as to activate the membrane-bound enzyme adenyl cyclase and possibly guanyl cyclase. This increased enzyme activity leads to increased intracellular levels of cyclic nucleotides which mediate the actions of the hormone.

There are now many studies of the binding of radioactively labeled hormones to various target cell preparations. The mechanism by which the hormone–receptor interaction activates adenyl cyclase is completely unknown at present, but the relationship between receptor binding and cyclic nucleotide production has been studied in several tissues. This review attempts to summarize current knowledge in these fields.

Recent work indicates that antibodies to hormone receptors play a major role in the pathogenesis of some diseases, and this area of research is also reviewed.

2. Labeling of Polypeptide Hormones with Radioisotopes

The isotope of choice for labeling peptide hormones is ^{125}I, which is usually supplied as $Na^{125}I$. The mixing of peptides with $Na^{125}I$ and an oxidizing system results in incorporation of the isotope into exposed tyrosine groups in the hormone. The two oxidizing systems that are currently widely used are the chloramine T method originally described by Hunter and Greenwood (H10) and the lactoperoxidase–hydrogen peroxide method originally described by Marchalonis (M7). Incorporation of one or two atoms of ^{125}I per molecule of hormone has generally been found not to influence the biological activity of peptide hormones greatly. However, some hormone denaturation usually occurs during iodination, and this is probably due to the effects of the oxidizing system on the labeled and unlabeled hormone. In the author's experience, there is considerable variation in the quality of $Na^{125}I$ supplied from the same manufacturers over a period of time, and trace contaminants in the $Na^{125}I$ may assist in hormone denaturation.

Different hormones have tyrosine groups that vary in their susceptibility to iodination. Also, different hormones show differences in their susceptibility to denaturation during labeling. Consequently, the conditions used for labeling different hormones vary considerably. Removal of denatured labeled hormone is usually necessary after labeling, and this can sometimes be effected by gel filtration or ion exchange chromatography. A method of general application in the preparation of labeled hormones suitable for studying receptor binding has been described by Manley et al. (M5) and Smith and Hall (S13, S14) for the purification of ^{125}I-labeled TSH. This technique, referred to as receptor purification was originally used to purify antibodies to the TSH receptor (S11, S15) and essentially involves adding the labeled hormone to particulate receptor preparations, washing, and eluting the bound hormone with a dissociating agent such as 2 M NaSCN or 2 M NaCl.

3. Methods of Studying the Hormone-Receptor Interaction

3.1. ANALYSIS OF EQUILIBRIUM BINDING

The study of labeled hormones interacting with their receptors clearly requires the separation of bound and free hormone. In the case of isolated cells or particulate receptor preparations, centrifugation or gel filtration can be used to separate bound and free hormone. In the case of soluble hormone receptors, bound and free hormone have been separated by gel filtration, precipitation with polyethylene glycol or ion exchange chromatography. The simplest and classical model of hormone-receptor binding at equilibrium can be represented as follows:

$$\text{Hormone (H)} + \text{receptor (R)} \rightleftharpoons \text{hormone--receptor complex (HR)}$$

The association constant of this system, K, is given by Eq. (1).

$$K = [HR]/([H] \times [R]) \tag{1}$$

Rearranging, we have $K \times [R] = [HR]/[H]$, and substituting $[R] = [R]_0 - [HR]$, where $[R]_0 = $ concentration of receptor sites before addition of any hormone, the equation gives:

$$K([R]_0 - [HR]) = [HR]/[H]$$

A plot of $[HR]$ vs $[HR]/[H]$ should be linear with a slope of $-K$. When $[HR] = [R]_0$, all the receptor sites are occupied and $[HR]/[H] = 0$. Consequently the intercept on the $[HR]$ axis gives the total binding capacity of the receptor preparation $[R]_0$. This is the classical Scatchard plot (S1).

Equation (1) can also be arranged to give

$$1/[HR] = 1/[R]_0 + 1/K[R]_0(1/[H])$$

A plot of $1/[HR]$ vs $1/[H]$ should be linear with a slope of $1/K[R]_0$; and when $1/[H] = 0$, $[HR] = [R]_0$. This plot, referred to as the reciprocal or Lineweaver–Burk plot (L17), gives the same information as the Scatchard analysis.

The Wilkinson plot (G1) is derived from yet another rearrangement of Eq. (1)

$$[H]/[HR] = 1/K[R]_0 + (1/[R]_0)[H]$$

A plot of $[H]/[HR]$ vs $[H]$ should therefore be linear with a slope of $1/[R]_0$ and intercept on the $[H]/[HR]$ axis of $1/K[R]_0$.

The choice between the various coordinate systems is arbitrary, depending on personal choice and experience. In the field of hormone–receptor interactions, the Scatchard plot is most widely used to analyze binding data.

The analysis consists of studying the effects of increasing amounts of cold hormone on the binding of labeled hormone to the receptor. The labeled hormone is assumed to have the same binding characteristics as the cold hormone, and the concentration of receptor-bound hormone equals: % label bound × (initial concentration of cold hormone + initial concentration of label). The concentration of free hormone equals (initial concentration − bound concentration).

Determinations of the amounts of bound and free hormone are susceptible to various errors that can lead to serious problems in analysis of binding data. Particularly troublesome is the problem of labeled hormone binding to reaction tubes. Also, labeled hormones are nonspecifically absorbed into particulate receptor preparations.

Correction for this nonreceptor binding is difficult. The amount of labeled hormone bound in the presence of large doses of cold hormone has been used as an indication of nonreceptor binding, but nonreceptor binding as well as receptor binding tends to be a function of hormone concentration, and this correction is in general erroneous. However, when the amount of labeled hormone bound to specific receptor sites is considerably greater than the nonreceptor binding, errors in estimating nonreceptor binding do not result in large errors in calculating [H] and [HR]. Further, the accurate estimation of [H] and [HR] by use of labeled hormone is possible only if the labeled hormone has the same receptor binding properties as the native hormone. Full biological activity of the labeled material is usually taken as an indication of identity between labeled and native material.

In addition to problems with nonreceptor binding, dissociation of the hormone–receptor complex can occur during separation of bound and free hormone. The extent of dissociation will depend on the method used to separate bound and free and the rate of complex dissociation. Procedures that depend on washing or dilution of the reaction mixture are most susceptible to problems of dissociation. A reduction in the rate of complex dissociation can usually be achieved by lowering the temperature during separation of the bound and free hormone.

If a hormone–receptor interaction can be represented by the simple model $H + R \rightleftharpoons HR$, then Scatchard-type analysis of the binding should lead to a linear plot and give the binding capacity of the receptor and the association constant of the system. Consideration of the difficulties in making accurate measurements of [H] and [HR] suggest that nonlinear Scatchard plots do not necessarily indicate that this model is incorrect. A linear Scatchard plot, however, probably indicates that the model is correct, and linear plots have been obtained in studies of many, but not all, polypeptide hormones interacting with their receptors.

It is of course possible for hormone–receptor interactions to be more complex than the simple $H + R \leftrightarrows HR$ model. Several different independent receptor sites could be involved, i.e.:

$$H + R_1 \rightleftharpoons HR_1$$
$$H + R_2 \rightleftharpoons HR_2$$
$$H + R_3 \rightleftharpoons HR_3$$
$$H + R_n \rightleftharpoons HR_n$$

and a plot of

$$[H] \Big/ \sum_{1}^{n} [HR_n] \text{ vs } \sum_{1}^{n} [HR_n]$$

would be expected to give an upwardly concave line. Graphical methods of analyzing this type of curve have been described by Rosenthal (R8) and Pennock (P4), but experimental results are rarely of sufficient precision to justify the introduction of more than three binding sites.

An alternative approach to the problem of multiple binding sites is analysis by use of the Hill or the Sips equation. Hill (H7) in 1910, studying the complex reaction between oxygen and hemoglobin, was able to fit his data to the equation:

$$\text{Fraction of oxygen bound} = Kc^a / (1 + Kc^a)$$

where c = concentration of free oxygen and K and a are constants.

Much later, a similar equation derived by Sips (S9) was used by Nisonoff and Pressman (N1) to analyze the binding of haptens to antibodies. Application of the Sips equation to the analysis of a hormone binding to several different receptor sites gives

$$\text{Fraction of sites occupied} = [HR]/[R]_0 = (K[H])^a / \{1 + (K[H])^a\}$$

where K is the average association constant and a (a constant) is the index of site heterogeneity.

Inversion of both sides of the equation gives

$$[R]_0/[HR] = 1/(K[H])^a + 1 \qquad (2)$$

A value for a can be obtained by plotting $1/[HR]$ vs $1/[H]^a$ for different values of a until a straight line is obtained. When $[HR] = [R]_0/2$, i.e., when half the total number of receptor sites are occupied, it is evident from Eq. (2) that $K = 1/[H]$.

The parameter a is a quantitative representation of the variation in apparent association constant with changes in hormone concentration. When $a = 1$, the Sips equation reduces to the simple mass action law, indicating that a homogeneous population of receptors is involved in hormone binding.

Values of a less than 1 indicate decreases in apparent association constant with increasing hormone concentration. This could be due to the hormone binding to sites with lower affinity as the higher affinity sites become occupied. Consequently, values of a less than 1 could be an indication of receptor site heterogeneity. An alternative explanation, however, is that the association constant is reduced by a cooperative effect in which the binding of hormone to one site reduces the association constant of adjacent sites.

Values of a greater than 1 would indicate increases in apparent association constant with increasing hormone concentration and would suggest the existence of a cooperative effect in which the binding of hormone to a receptor increases the association constant of adjacent receptor sites.

3.2. Kinetic Analysis

The Scatchard and Sips–Hill-type analyses apply only to reactions at equilibrium, and the first step in studying any hormone–receptor system must be to follow the time dependence of association and dissociation.

For the simple model $H + R \rightleftharpoons HR$

$$-\frac{d[H]}{dt} = k_1[H][R] - k_2[HR]$$

where k_1 and k_2 are the association and dissociation rate constants, respectively, and at equilibrium $d[H]/dt = 0$, giving

$$k_1[H][R] = k_2[HR]$$

and

$$k_1/k_2 = [HR]/[H][R] = K$$

and, from a knowledge of any two of the parameters k_1, k_2, and K (the association constant), it is possible to calculate the third.

Direct determination of k_1 should be possible by observing the variation in hormone concentration with time, and $d[H]/dt$ will be given by the slope of the $[H]$ vs time (t) plot and at $t = 0$ $[HR] = 0$ and $d[H]/dt = k_1[H]_0[R]_0$. In practice, however, this type of analysis is difficult for many hormone–receptor systems. The method uses only data obtained close to zero time, when $[HR]$ is small, and the problems frequently associated with accurate determination of small amounts of $[HR]$ have already been discussed. Further, the methods used to separate bound and free hormone, e.g., centrifugation, often take considerable time, and this clearly adds to the inaccuracy of the method. In addition to problems of determining the amount of hormone bound, it is necessary to determine the initial concentration of receptor $[R]_0$ by analysis of equilibrium binding.

In general, determination of the dissociation rate constant k_2 is easier than determination of k_1. Hormone and receptor are allowed to interact to form a complex, and then dissociation is studied under conditions where reassociation is prevented, preferably by dilution. For the simple model $HR = H + R$,

$$- d[HR]/dt = k_2[HR]$$

giving the integrated rate expression

$$\ln [HR] = \ln [HR]_0 - k_2 t$$

and a plot of $\ln[HR]$ vs t should be linear with a slope of $-k_2$.

In the case of n independent binding sites, the expression can simply be extended to

$$\ln [HR_n] = \ln [HR_n]_0 - k_{2_n} t$$

and when receptor site heterogeneity is suspected, attempts should be made to make a best-fit analysis of the dissociation data for a few selected values of n.

The rate constants of most chemical reactions increase with temperature (T), and it is usually found that a plot of $\log k$ vs $1/T$ (where k is the rate constant) is nearly linear with negative slope. This is equivalent to the Arrhenius equation:

$$(d \ln k)/dT = E_a/RT^2$$

where E_a is the Arrhenius or empirical activation energy.

A curved or "broken" Arrhenius plot can indicate the existence of reactions with different activation energies. In the case of hormone–receptor interactions, changes in activation energy could result from alterations in membrane lipid mobility. A recent report by Bashford et al. (B1) indicates that TSH and ACTH receptor binding show temperature variations that are consistent with changes in activation energy due to increased membrane lipid fluidity.

Observation of the dissociation of hormone–receptor complexes can be particularly useful when hormone-dependent receptor site–receptor site interaction is suspected. Such an approach has recently been used by De Meyts and his colleagues in their studies of the insulin receptor (D2, D3). Scatchard-type analysis of the insulin–insulin receptor reaction (using

cultured human lymphocytes as a source of insulin receptor) gives upwardly concave plots; i.e., as the amount of hormone bound increases, the
apparent association constant of the binding reaction decreases. This phenomenon could clearly be due to the presence of multiple binding sites or
to some interaction between insulin and the insulin receptor that results in
a decrease in the association constant K as the amount of insulin bound
increases. Now, as K is given by $K = k_1/k_2$, a hormone concentration-
dependent reduction in K could clearly result from an increase in k_2, the
dissociation rate constant. In order to investigate this possibility, the effect
of hormone concentration on the dissociation rate constant of the insulin–
insulin receptor interaction was studied by De Meyts et al. (D3).

Labeled insulin–insulin receptor complex was diluted 100-fold so that
only dissociation of labeled insulin could occur, and the effect of cold
insulin on the rate of dissociation was studied.

The dissociation rate contant k_2 was increased dramatically by addition
of cold insulin. This indicated that the insulin–insulin receptor interaction
influenced other insulin receptors in such a way as to increase the dissociation rate constant and consequently reduce the association constant K.

De Meyts and Roth have used a modification of the classical Scatchard
analysis to graph this effect, which they have termed negative cooperativity (D2). Binding data are plotted as [HR]/[H] vs [HR], giving an
upwardly concave plot. When [HR] = 0, all the sites are in the high-
affinity conformation and, in the absence of any negative cooperativity,
[HR]/[H] would fall along a straight line joining [HR]/[H] at[HR]= 0
with the intercept on [HR] axis $[R]_o$. The negative slope of this line,
shown as $\bar{k}_1$ in Fig. 1, is the association constant of the empty sites. When
site occupancy increases, the average affinity of all the receptor sites decreases owing to site–site interactions, and this changing affinity is repre-

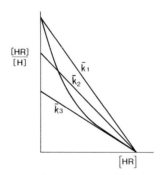

FIG. 1. Scatchard-type analysis of a hormone–receptor interaction which shows
variation in association constant with amount of hormone bound.

sented by successive lines of decreasing slope joining each point of the curve to the intercept on the [HR] axis, e.g., $\bar{k}_2$ in Fig. 1. When [HR] approaches $[R]_o$, $\bar{k}$ reaches a limiting low value shown as $\bar{k}_3$ in Fig. 1.

This situation is graphed by plotting $\bar{k}$ vs log $[HR]/[R]_o$, as shown in Fig. 2. The main characteristics of this curve are (a) the limiting high association constant $\bar{k}_1$ for the empty site conformation of the receptor; (b) the threshold occupancy (shown as x) at which $\bar{k}$ starts to fall with increasing site occupancy; (c) the limiting low association constant $\bar{k}_3$.

3.3. THERMODYNAMIC ANALYSIS

The mechanism by which the binding of a hormone to the surface of a cell is able to induce changes in the cell surface which lead to activation of adenyl, and possibly guanyl, cyclase is unknown. An understanding of this system will probably come from a study of the interaction between various combinations of the isolated constituents, i.e., hormone, receptor, membrane, and enzyme. Some insight into the nature of these interactions is obtainable from a knowledge of the thermodynamic parameters ΔF (the free energy change), ΔH (the enthalpy change), and ΔS (the entropy change) involved in the various reactions. Karush (K3) has elegantly analyzed the antibody–antigen interaction in terms of these thermodynamic parameters. The interaction between antigen and antibody has many characteristics that are similar to hormone receptor interactions, and, in the case of thyroid-stimulating antibodies (see Section 5.1), the interaction between antibody and antigen (the thyrotropin receptor) has a virtually identical effect to the interaction between hormone (TSH) and

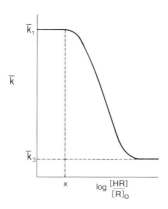

FIG. 2. Plot for the average association constant for a hormone–receptor interaction against the fraction of receptor sites occupied.

receptor (see Section 5.1, on thyrotropin receptors and thyroid-stimulating antibodies).

The free-energy change involved in the simple hormone–receptor interaction $H + R \rightleftharpoons HR$ is given by the equation:

$$\Delta F = -RT \ln K$$

When K (the association constant) is calculated using molar concentrations, the value deduced from this equation is the standard free-energy change, $\Delta F°$. It represents the change in free energy of the system resulting from the formation of 1 mole of the complex HR in an infinite volume of a hypothetical solution in which the concentration of H, R, and HR are each 1 molal and the temperature pH, ionic strength, and concentrations of other components are the same as they were in the experiment. The concentrations of H and R are usually sufficiently small to make activity corrections unnecessary.

The hormone receptor site and the binding site on the hormone will usually be surrounded by water molecules prior to formation of the hormone–receptor complex. Consequently, water will have to be removed during the reaction between hormone (H) and receptor (R), and the binding process is probably more accurately represented:

$$H_{(x+a)H_2O} + R_{(y+b)H_2O} = H_{aH_2O}R_{bH_2O} + (x + y)H_2O$$

The free-energy change resulting from this release of bound water is likely to make a considerable contribution to the overall ΔF. Contributions from hydrogen bonds and interactions between oppositely charged groups are probably also important, as evidenced by the increased rate of dissociation of many hormone–receptor complexes at high ionic strength.

The free-energy change for the combination of hormone and receptor is composed of an enthalpic term (ΔH) and an entropic term (ΔS) according to the equation

$$\Delta F = \Delta H - T \Delta S \tag{3}$$

The value of ΔH can be determined by observing the temperature dependence of the association constant and use of the integrated form of the van't Hoff equation

$$\ln (K_2/K_1) = \Delta H/R[(1/T_1) - (1/T_2)]$$

where K_1 and K_2 are the association constants at temperatures T_1 and T_2, and R is the gas constant.

Since very dilute solutions are always used in the study of hormone–receptor interactions, the experimental value of ΔH corresponds to that for an infinitely dilute solution and can be equated to $\Delta H°$, the standard enthalpy change. From a knowledge of ΔF and ΔH, ΔS, the entropy change, can clearly be determined from Eq. (3)

4. Receptors for Polypeptide Hormones

4.1. LUTEINIZING HORMONE (LH) AND CHORIONIC GONADOTROPIN (CG)

In the female, luteinizing hormone is involved in the development of Graafian follicles and the control of follicular secretion of estrogens and progesterone. In the male, LH is responsible for stimulating androgen production by the interstitial cells (Leydig cells) of the testis and stimulating Leydig cell development. Chorionic gonadotropin is structurally and functionally closely related to LH and is important in maintaining the corpus luteum and ensuring implantation of the fertilized ovum.

4.1.1. Receptors for LH and CG in the Testis

Receptors for LH and CG have been demonstrated in homogenates of rat testis (C1, C2), and the binding system has been used to develop a receptor assay for LH and CG (C2, C3, L8). Scatchard analysis of the adult rat testis–human chorionic gonadotropin (hCG) binding system has indicated an association constant of $2.4 \times 10^{10}\ M^{-1}$ at 24°C and a binding capacity of 10^{-12} mole per gram of testis (C4). Studies of the variation in rat Leydig cell binding capacities with age have shown that the binding capacity correlates with the cell number and secretory activity (P1).

There is evidence to suggest that cyclic AMP (cAMP) functions as an intermediate in the action of LH and CG on the rat testis (C5, D11). However, recently Mendelson et al. (M11) used dispersed rat interstitial cells to study the relationship between CG binding, cAMP production, and testosterone synthesis. Analysis of the data showed a marked dissociation between steroidogenesis and cAMP production, and Mendelson et al. have concluded that membrane responses other than activation of adenyl cyclase may be important in gonadotropin-induced steroidogenesis.

Gonadotropin receptors have been extracted from homogenates of the rat testis in soluble form using the detergent Triton X-100 (D10). The activity of the soluble receptors was monitored by mixing with labeled hCG followed by addition of polyethylene glycol to precipitate the hormone–receptor complex (D9). Purification of the soluble receptors has been achieved using affinity chromatography and analysis of the purified material by sodium dodecyl sulfate (SDS) gel electrophoresis indicated a molecular weight of about 100,000 (D10).

The binding of labeled LH or CG to receptors in the rat testis is not inhibited by pituitary hormones other than LH or CG (C2, L8). Isolated

subunits of hCG do not in themselves influence intact hormone binding
(R2), indicating that the receptor-binding activity of hCG is formed by
combination of the two subunits. Studies with LH and CG from different
species indicate that the affinity of the hormones for the rat testis receptor
shows phylogenetic variation (C2, C3, L8).

4.1.2. Ovarian Receptors for LH and CG

Luteinizing hormone labeled with ^{125}I has been shown to bind to slices
of ovary from rats made pseudopregnant with pregnant mare's serum
gonadotropin and hCG (L3). Danzo (D1) has studied the binding of
^{125}I-labeled hCG to sedimentable compounds of pseudopregnant rat
ovaries and found an association constant of $2 \times 10^9 \ M^{-1}$ at $37°$. Isolated
porcine granulosa cells have also been used to study the ovarian gonadotropin receptor (K1, K2). The LH-hCG binding properties of the rat ovary
have been shown to depend on the functional state of the ovary (L4). The
number, but not the affinity, of ovarian gonadotropin receptors is increased
by administration of gonadotropin (L4). This increase is followed by a
rapid decrease in receptor numbers during luteolysis. The pattern of
ovarian binding corresponds with changes in ovarian progesterone levels
suggesting that binding activity is closely associated with the formation
and luteolysis of corpora lutea. This suggestion is supported by the observation of Lee and Ryan (L3) that estrogen treatment, which prevents
luteolysis, as evidenced by sustained high levels of progesterone in both
blood and ovary, also prevents the decline in ovarian binding of ^{125}I-la-
beled hCG.

Studies with porcine granulosa cells (K2) have shown that the number
of gonadotropin receptors per cell increases as the follicle enlarges. There
was, however, no appreciable change in association constant (about
$2 \times 10^9 \ M^{-1}$ for hCG at 37°C). Mature follicle cells are sensitive to LH
and hCG as measured by stimulation of cAMP production, progesterone
secretion, and morphological luteinization whereas small follicle cells are
unresponsive (C6, C7). This difference between mature and immature
cells corresponds with the number of gonadotropin receptors per cell, and
the increased responsiveness of the large follicle cell may well be due to
the increased number of receptors (K2).

The binding of labeled LH to the ovary shows a similar specificity to
the LH– or CG–testis interaction (D1, K2, L2), and the ovarian receptor
binding activity of LH and CG is formed by combination of the hormone
subunits. Studies with gonadotropins from different species indicate phylogenetic variations in the affinity of hormones for the ovarian LH and CG
receptor (P2).

Gonadotropin receptors in bovine corpora lutea have been studied by

Gospodarowicz (G11) and Haour and Saxena (H3). Purified membranes from the corpora lutea were found to have an association constant of about 10^9 M^{-1} at 37°C. Comparison of the hormone-binding properties of the membranes with those of intact luteal cells has indicated that they have similar receptor characteristics (P2). Solubilization of the bovine membranes with detergents has indicated that the receptor activity is principally associated with a protein fraction molecular weight 30,000–70,000 (H3).

4.2. FOLLICLE-STIMULATING HORMONE (FSH)

Follicle-stimulating hormone controls the development of the primary ovarian follicle and stimulates granulosa cell proliferation. In the male, FSH increases spermatogenesis and seminiferous tubule development.

Studies of the effects of FSH and LH on cAMP production in various cell types from the rat testis (D6, D7) indicate that FSH acts only on the Sertoli cells of the seminiferous tubule and that LH acts only on the interstitial cells.

This independence of the effects of FSH and LH has been confirmed by studies of the binding of ^{125}I-labeled FSH, CG, and LH to homogenates of rat testis tubule (R1), which showed that only FSH bound to the tubule homogenate.

Radioreceptor assays based on the ^{125}I-labeled FSH–testis interaction have been described for measuring FSH in human serum (C10, R3). Studies with ^{125}I-labeled human FSH and membranes prepared from homogenates of bovine testis (C9) have shown that the bovine membranes contain a single population of binding sites with an association constant of about 10^{10} M^{-1} at 25°C.

4.3. THYROTROPIN (TSH)

The overall effect of thyrotropin on the thyroid is to increase the production and secretion of thyroid hormones and almost all metabolic processes in the thyroid can be stimulated by TSH. There is good evidence that many of these effects of TSH are mediated by cAMP. The increased levels of cAMP then lead to activation of protein kinases, which, by phosphorylating key enzymes and other proteins, are able to induce the effects of the hormone.

Specific binding sites for radioactively-labeled TSH have been described in a variety of thyroid extracts. Lissitzky et al. (L18) and Verrier et al. (V1) have used isolated porcine thyroid cells to study the TSH–TSH receptor interaction. Scatchard analysis of the binding data indicated the

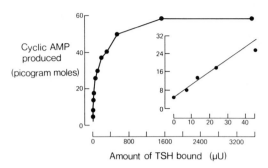

FIG. 3. Comparison of the amount of thyroid-stimulating hormone (TSH) bound to human thyroid membranes with the amount of cyclic adenosine monophosphate produced.

existence of a single population of binding sites with an association constant of about 10^9 M^{-1} at 35°C. Comparison of hormone binding to intact cells and plasma membranes isolated from the cells showed that the TSH receptors in the two preparations were similar.

Manley (M5) and Smith and Hall (S14) used a crude preparation of guinea pig thyroid membranes to study TSH binding. This guinea pig thyroid preparation contained a single population of binding sites with an association constant of about 10^{10} M^{-1} at 37°C.

The binding of labeled TSH to bovine plasma membranes has been described by Moore and Wolff (M12) and Kotani (K10), and these workers reported an association constant of about 10^8 M^{-1} at 22°C. The human thyroid membrane preparations used to study hormone binding contain TSH-sensitive adenyl cyclase. A plot of the amount of hormone bound versus amount of cAMP produced by the membranes is shown in Fig. 3. The curve is linear for small amounts of TSH bound, and from the slope of this part of the curve it is possible to calculate that, in the membrane system, 1 molecule of hormone bound results in the production of 400 molecules of cAMP. This is an interesting example of the amplifying effect of the hormone-receptor–adenyl cyclase–cAMP system.

The studies with porcine, guinea pig, and bovine thyroid membranes have also demonstrated a close relationship between TSH receptor binding and activation of adenyl cyclase (M5, M12, V1).

The effects of thyrotropin appear to be principally restricted to the thyroid. The tissue and hormone specificity of the TSH–TSH receptor interaction has been established by studies using hormones structurally closely related to TSH (K10, L18, S13) and different tissues (K10, T3). However, TSH has been shown to stimulate lipolysis in isolated fat cells from several species (G10, H4, K6), and recently thyrotropin binding sites have been described in crude guinea pig fat cell membrane preparations (T3). In the guinea pig, TSH receptors in fat and thyroid tissue appear to have identical hormone-binding properties. The function of TSH receptors in guinea pig fat is not clear at present but clearly warrants investigation. In contrast to the guinea pig, human fat does not contain readily detectable specific TSH binding sites (C. S. Teng and B. Rees Smith, unpublished observations).

4.4. PARATHYROID HORMONE (PTH)

The main function of PTH is to regulate the concentration of ionized calcium in body fluids by its actions on bone, the small intestine, and the kidneys. The effects of PTH on bone and kidney appear to be mediated by cAMP (C8, G8, M9, S20).

The binding of ^{125}I-labeled PTH to receptors in renal cortex membranes has been described by Sutcliffe et al. (S20), Malbon and Zull (M3), and Di Bella et al. (D4). The binding reaction is not influenced by vasopressin, growth hormone, epinephrine, glucagon, ACTH, angiotensin, or calcitonin (S20).

Sutcliffe et al. (S20) have reported that insulin inhibits the binding of labeled PTH to kidney membranes and inhibits PTH stimulation of cAMP formation in the membrane preparations. Di Bella et al. (D4), however, were unable to demonstrate these effects of insulin in a similar membrane system.

Parathyroid hormone consists of a single chain of 84 amino acids, and the structural requirements for virtually full biological activity are present in residues 1 through 34 for porcine and human PTH and 2 through 27 for bovine PTH (K7).

The binding of labeled intact hormone or labeled 1–34 peptide to renal membranes has been shown to be inhibited competitively by unlabeled 1–34 peptide over the same concentration range that activates membrane adenyl cyclase (D4), emphasizing the close link between PTH-receptor binding and adenyl cyclase activation.

Studies of the effects of various synthetic peptide fragments of bovine PTH on parathyroid hormone stimulation of cAMP production in bovine kidney membranes have indicated that the complete sequence from residue 3 to 27 is required for receptor binding (G8). A dichotomy between receptor binding and adenyl cyclase activation was demonstrated only by sequence alterations or deletions involving the first two N-terminal residues. This implies considerable importance for these two amino acids in providing a structure capable of interacting with the receptor in such a way as to activate adenyl cyclase.

An interesting approach to studying PTH binding to renal membranes has recently been described by McIntosh and Hesch (M2). These workers mixed renal membranes with cold PTH and then estimated the amount of hormone bound by adding ^{125}I-labeled anti-PTH antibody.

4.5. PROLACTIN

One of the principal target tissues for prolactin is the mammary gland where the hormone is involved in growth, differentiation, and milk secretion.

Turkington (T5) has shown that prolactin coupled to agarose beads can stimulate RNA synthesis in dispersed mammary epithelial cells, indicating that the effects of the hormone are mediated by a cell surface receptor. The binding of ^{125}I-labeled prolactin to membranes prepared from mid-pregnant mice (T6) and rabbits (S7) has been described and the binding system used to develop an assay for prolactin in serum (S7).

Membranes prepared from rabbit mammary tissue contain a single population of prolactin binding sites with an association constant of $3 \times 10^9 \ M^{-1}$ (S5). Solubilization of the receptor with Triton X-100 and purification of the soluble extract by affinity chromatography indicates that the molecular weight of the receptor is about 200,000 (S6). The soluble receptor was found to have an association constant five times greater than the membrane-bound receptor.

The labeled prolactin–mammary tissue membrane interaction is specific insofar as the gonadotropins, insulin, glucagon, TSH, and ACTH do not influence hormone binding (S7).

However, human growth hormone and human placental lactogen are capable of competing with ^{125}I-labeled prolactin for mammary tissue receptors (S7). Growth hormones from other species that are not lactogenic in the rabbit are unable to compete with labeled prolactin for its receptor (S5, S7). These observations emphasize the close relationship between receptor binding and mammary cell stimulation.

The effects of prolactin are not restricted to the mammary gland and the hormone has many metabolic effects on different tissues similar to those of growth hormone. Consistent with these observations is the report by Shiu and Friesen (S6) of prolactin receptors in membranes prepared from rabbit adrenal, ovary, liver, and kidney. Gelato et al. (G6) have studied prolactin binding sites in rat liver membranes and showed that ovariectomy or thyroidectomy reduced the number of prolactin binding sites in the liver. They conclude that the thyroid and ovaries are important regulators of liver prolactin binding activity.

4.6. CORTICOTROPIN (ACTH)

Binding sites for ^{125}I-labeled ACTH have been described in soluble extracts of mouse adrenal tumors (L7), particulate fractions of beef adrenal cortex (H8), isolated rat adrenocortical cells (M1), and crude particulate preparations of ovine, rat, and rabbit adrenal (W1). The interaction of ^{125}I-labeled ACTH with soluble or particulate adrenal preparations has been used to develop assays for the measurement of ACTH in serum (L1, L6, W1).

Studies of the effects of ACTH and cAMP on isolated rat adrenal cells (R4) and adrenal homogenates (G12) suggests that the effects of ACTH are mediated by cAMP, and corticotropin-stimulated production of cAMP formation in isolated adrenal cells has been reported to precede stimulation of steroidogenesis (B2). However, Sharma et al. (S4) have reported that small doses of ACTH that stimulate corticosterone production in isolated rat adrenal cells do not stimulate dectectable increases in cAMP production, and their studies showed that the effects of low doses of ACTH corresponded with increases in cGMP. The cGMP-producing systems did not appear to operate at high doses of ACTH, and Sharma et al. have proposed that the effects of ACTH on the adrenal are mediated by cGMP at low hormone concentrations and by cAMP at high hormone concentrations.

Corticotropin 1–24 coupled to agarose (L5) and corticotropin coupled to polyacrylamide (R4) has been shown to stimulate steroidogenesis in isolated adrenal cells. The relatively large size of the agarose or polyacrylamide beads used restricts the effects of the hormone to the adrenal cell surface, and these studies, together with the studies of ^{125}I-labeled ACTH binding to adrenal membrane fractions, indicate that the ACTH receptor is localized on the cell surface.

Studies on the binding of fragments, derivatives, and analogs of ACTH to the hormone receptor have been described by Lefkowitz et al. (L7), Hofmann et al. (H8), and Finn et al. (F1). In general, receptor-binding activity correlates with the biological activity, but Finn et al. (F1) have reported that the biologically inactive corticotropin 11–26 amide binds to adrenal cell membranes.

4.7. INSULIN

The major physiological effect of insulin is to increase tissue utilization of glucose by stimulating glucose transport across the cell membrane. Insulin acts principally on tissues such as muscle, fat, the lens, and leukocytes, where there is a high resistance to glucose penetration and entry of glucose is the rate-limiting step in carbohydrate metabolism.

Cuatrecasas (C12) was able to show that insulin covalently attached to Sepharose beads could increase glucose utilization and suppress GH- and ACTH-stimulated lipolysis in isolated fat cells. His results indicated that the interaction of insulin with superficial membrane structures alone suffices to initiate at least some of the actions of the hormone.

Specific binding sites for ^{125}I-labeled insulin were first described in isolated fat cells by Cuatrecasas (C13) and Kono and Barham (K9) and in liver cell membranes by House and Weidemann (H9), Freychet *et al.* (F3), and Cuatrecasas *et al.* (C16). More recently, insulin receptors have been described on the surface of leukocytes (G5). Later studies by Schwartz *et al.* (S2) indicated that the insulin-binding properties of the leukocytes were associated with monocytes rather than lymphocytes. Insulin receptors have also been demonstrated in plasma membranes prepared from the human placenta (H2, M8).

Gavin *et al.* (G2) have developed a radioreceptor assay for insulin based on the interaction of ^{125}I-labeled insulin with insulin receptors in rat liver membranes and cultured human lymphocytes. Studies with plasma and pancreatic insulins and proinsulins indicate that receptor-binding activity parallels biological activity.

The role of cAMP in the effects of insulin on fat cells was first studied by Butcher *et al.* (B5). These workers were able to demonstrate that epinephrine-induced increases in cAMP were reversed by insulin suggesting that insulin may act by reducing cAMP levels. More recent studies indicate that this effect of insulin is due at least in part, to a hormone-induced increase in membrane phosphodiesterase activity (L19, M4, S3, S18).

The relationship between insulin receptor-binding and insulin-induced lipogenesis in isolated rat fat cells has recently been studied by Gliemann *et al.* (G7). They reported that at low concentrations of hormone, the rate of increase in lipogenesis was proportional to the receptor occupancy (receptor association constant about $3 \times 10^8 \ M^{-1}$). Further when insulin was removed, the decrease in lipogenesis followed the decrease in receptor occupancy. At high concentrations of insulin, however, maximum lipogenesis was obtained before complete receptor occupancy and did not decrease as rapidly as dissociation of the hormone–receptor complex. Gliemann *et al.* conclude that insulin receptor binding is rate limiting at low concentrations of hormone, but at high insulin concentrations some other step becomes rate determining.

Solubilization of insulin receptors from rat liver or fat cell membranes with the nonionic detergent Triton X-100 has been described by Cuatrecasas (C14, C15). The receptors derived from both tissues appear to have identical properties and, on the basis of gel filtration and sedimentation studies, have a molecular weight of about 300,000.

Insulin receptors have also been solubilized from the surfaces of human leukocytes by using the nonionic detergent NP-40 (G3) or merely by incubating the cells in phosphate-buffered saline at 30°C (G4). Cuatrecasas (C15) has used affinity chromatography with insulin-agarose derivatives to purify detergent-solubilized insulin receptors from liver cell membranes and was able to achieve a purification factor of about 2×10^5. However, as the starting material contains such a minute proportion of receptor, isolation of sufficient amounts to permit detailed study presents a considerable problem.

4.8. GLUCAGON

The only established physiological action of glucagon is to enhance the output of glucose from the liver (B4), and Rodbell and co-workers (B3, P6, R5–R7) have studied the glucagon receptor in isolated liver membranes. The apparent affinity of the receptor for ^{125}I-labeled glucagon (about 3×10^8 M^{-1}) was found to be approximately equal to the apparent affinity for activation of membrane adenyl cyclase. The close link between receptor binding and membrane stimulation is emphasized by the observation that biologically inactive glucagon fragments do not bind to the receptor. Guanyl nucleotides appear to have a specific role in the activation of adenyl cyclase by glucagon. The nucleotides have been shown to bind to sites distinct from the glucagon receptor and regulate the response of adenyl cyclase to glucagon receptor binding.

Glucagon receptors have been extracted from homogenates of cat myocardium with the detergent Lubrol-PX (K8, L15, L16) and appear to have a molecular weight of 24,000–28,000 as judged by SDS polyacrylamide gel electrophoresis.

4.9. GROWTH HORMONE (GH)

Growth hormone affects a wide variety of tissues, and the hormone is involved in the control of glucose metabolism and protein synthesis.

Human growth hormone labeled with ^{125}I has been shown to bind to receptor sites on the surfaces of human peripheral blood leukocytes (L13) and membranes prepared from the livers of pregnant rabbits (S17, T4).

Radioreceptor assays based on the GH–GH receptor interaction have been used to study growth hormone levels in human serum (G9, H6, L14, T4).

The growth hormone receptor on human leukocytes consists of a single population of binding sites (4000 sites per cell) with an association constant of about $10^9 M^{-1}$ at 30°C (D2, D3). The human leukocyte receptor appears not to bind porcine, bovine, or ovine growth hormone (L13) whereas the rabbit liver receptor has been found to bind human, monkey, bovine, and ovine growth hormone. Human prolactin, placental lactogen, glucagon, insulin, gonadotropins, TSH, and ACTH show minimal receptor binding in both systems.

5. Antibodies to Hormone Receptors

5.1. THYROTROPIN RECEPTOR ANTIBODIES

5.1.1. Introduction

There is now considerable evidence that the hyperthyroidism associated with Graves' disease is due to antibodies to the thyrotropin receptor. The antibodies, sometimes described as thyroid-stimulating antibodies (TSAb) appear to mimic the effects of TSH by binding to the receptor and activating adenyl cyclase.

The presence of thyroid-stimulating antibodies in the serum of patients with Graves' disease was first described by Adams and Purves in 1956 (A1). The antibody activity is associated with a heterogeneous population of IgG (S11, S16), and the thyroid-stimulating site is formed by combination of heavy and light chains in the Fab part of the molecule (S12). The overall effect of TSAb on the thyroid is identical to that of TSH (D8), but the time course of action of TSAb appears to be prolonged relative to the TSH both *in vivo* and *in vitro* (K5, P5, S12).

The effects of both TSH and TSAb are mimicked by cAMP (K4) and both TSAb and TSH stimulate cAMP production in thyroid tissue slices (K5) and thyroid membranes (M13).

The first step in thyroid stimulation by TSAb, therefore, is probably contact with an adenyl cyclase-linked site on the thyroid cell surface. Leading from this, we can postulate that interaction of this site with the immune system is responsible for initiation of TSAb synthesis.

The binding of TSAb to thyroid tissue has been studied in considerable detail. The binding sites appear to be localized in the thyroid cell membrane (D8), and solubilization of the binding sites by freezing and thawing (D5, S10) indicates that they have a molecular weight of about 30,000 and isoelectric point of 4.5 (S11).

Subsequent to this work, it has been possible to study the binding of ^{125}I-labeled TSH to the thyrotropin receptor and relate the TSAb binding sites to the TSH binding sites. Lissitzky *et al.* (L18), Smith and Hall (S13), Manley *et al.* (M6), and Mehdi and Nussey (M10) have shown that TSAb competes with ^{125}I-labeled TSH for binding sites in human thyroid membranes. Further, in experiments with solubilized receptor preparations, Manley et al. (M6) and Hall et al. (H1) have shown that TSAb and TSH bind to the same receptor molecule. This work suggests that thyroid-stimulating antibodies are antibodies directed against the TSH receptor.

5.1.2. Hyperthyroidism and TSAb

The effect of TSAb on the binding of ^{125}I-labeled TSH to thyroid membranes has been used to develop a radioreceptor assay for TSAb (S13). Using this assay, Mukhtar et al. (M13) were able to detect TSAb in 57 out of 57 patients with untreated Graves' disease and hyperthyroidism and show a highly significant correlation between the serum TSH receptor-binding activity and early ^{131}I uptakes. These data provided good evidence for a causative role of TSAb in the hyperthyroidism of these patients.

Thyroid function in health is controlled by TSH. The serum level of TSH is principally regulated by the interaction of thyrotropin-releasing hormone (TRH), triiodothyronine (T_3), and probably thyroxine (T_4) at the pituitary level (H1). Thyroid hormones reduce serum TSH levels, and TRH increases serum TSH levels. The effect of exogenous TRH on serum TSH provides the basis of the TRH test of thyroid function. Administration of T_3 results in a fall in serum TSH with subsequent reduction in thyroidal radioiodine uptake, and this effect provides the basis of the T_3 suppression test.

Thyroid stimulators of nonpituitary origin, such as TSAb, clearly cannot be controlled by the TRH–thyroid hormone–TSH system, and we have recently studied the relationship between serum TSAb and the T_3 suppression and TRH tests in Graves' patients treated for hyperthyroidism (C11). In patients who were euthyroid or hyperthyroid after treatment, there was an excellent agreement between the levels of TSAb and the absence of TSH control of thyroid function as measured by the T_3 suppression and TRH tests. This again suggested that in the patients with detectable TSAb, the antibody was responsible for stimulating thyroid function.

5.1.3. The Effect of Treatment for Graves' Disease on Serum TSAb

In a recent study by Mukhtar et al. (M13) all patients with untreated Graves' disease and hyperthyroidism were found to have detectable levels of TSAb. Patients treated by partial thyroidectomy, antithyroid drugs, or radioiodine showed a frequency of detectable TSAb of 17%, 53%, and 50%, respectively. The change in frequency of detectable TSAb from 100% to about 50% in patients treated by drugs or radioiodine was probably due to spontaneous remission. In the case of subtotal thyroidectomy, however, the operation itself clearly had a dramatic effect on circulating TSAb levels. The mechanism of this effect is not clear at present, but the effect of thyroidectomy clearly indicates a major role for the thyroid in TSAb synthesis.

5.1.4. Thyroid-Stimulating Antibodies in Ophthalmic Graves' Disease, Carcinoma of the Thyroid, and Autoimmune Thyroiditis

5.1.4.1. *Ophthalmic Graves' Disease.*   Recent studies in our laboratory have shown that 23 out of 57 patients with ophthalmic Graves' disease (patients who have the eye signs of Graves' disease but are euthyroid or hypothyroid) had serum TSAb levels detectable in the receptor assay. The existence of serum TSAb in patients who are apparently euthyroid is difficult to explain. Further, in this group of patients, the presence or the absence of TSAb did not correlate well with results from T_3 suppression and TRH tests. This is in marked contrast to the excellent relationship between serum TSAb and T_3 suppression and TRH tests observed in patients treated for Graves' disease and hyperthyroidism (C11). At least two factors could contribute to the apparently anomalous presence of TSAb in patients with ophthalmic Graves' disease. First, the patients may have circulating antibodies that bind to the TSH receptor and give a positive result in the receptor assay, but because of some alteration in antibody specificity or binding affinity the binding reaction is unable to activate adenyl cyclase and stimulate the thyroid.

Second, the thyroids in some patients with ophthalmic Graves' disease may well suffer from considerable autoimmune destruction. Consequently TSAb, although capable of causing hyperthyroidism in patients with normal thyroid tissue, can only maintain normal or reduced levels of thyroid hormones.

A combination of these two factors could explain the apparent discrepancy between thyroid function and the presence of serum TSAb in patients with ophthalmic Graves' disease.

5.1.4.2. *Autoimmune Thyroiditis.*   About 14% of patients with autoimmune thyroiditis have levels of serum TSAb detectable by receptor assay (M13). The TSAb activity in these patients is quite distinct from antithyroglobulin and antimicrosomal antibodies (S13), but the presence of TSAb in patients with autoimmune thyroiditis emphasizes its close relationship to Graves' disease.

The reasons for the inability of TSAb to induce hyperthyroidism in these patients could be the same as those suggested for ophthalmic Graves' disease.

5.1.4.3. *Carcinoma of the Thyroid.*   Preliminary experiments in our laboratory indicated that the serum of one out of six patients with carcinoma of the thyroid contained TSAb activity detectable in the receptor assay (S13), and these results were in agreement with earlier studies of Le Marchand-Beraud *et al.* (L9), who used a bioassay to estimate TSAb. More recent and extensive studies with the receptor assay showed that the serum from 24 out of 84 patients with thyroid carcinoma contained detectable TSAb activity. There was no clear association between tumor type and the presence of TSAb.

It is possible that the production of TSAb in these patients is the result of tumor-induced changes in the thyroid or immune system. Alternatively, these patients may have Graves' disease quite independently of the carcinoma.

5.2. INSULIN-RECEPTOR ANTIBODIES

Flier *et al.* (F2) have reported the existence of antibodies to the insulin receptor in patients with a unique diabetic syndrome associated with the skin condition acanthosis nigricans. The plasma insulin levels in these patients are considerably elevated and their blood glucose levels show a markedly blunt response to injected insulin.

A study of the insulin binding characteristics of circulating monocytes from these patients indicated that their ability to bind the ^{125}I-labeled hormone was greatly reduced. This was found to be due to antibodies of the IgG class binding to the monocyte surface and blocking the binding of insulin. The antibodies presumably cause impaired insulin receptor binding *in vivo* resulting in a clinical syndrome of high insulin resistance.

The mechanism of action of the antibodies could be (a) direct binding to the insulin receptor; (b) binding to sites close to the receptor in such a way as to sterically hinder the hormone–receptor interaction; (c) interaction with sites distant from the receptor in such a way as to induce membrane changes that reduce the insulin binding activity of the receptor.

Studies with insulin receptors on human leukocytes, rat liver membranes, and avian erythrocytes indicated that the antibodies were more active in inhibiting insulin binding to human insulin receptors, but some antibodies were active in the rat and avian systems. This suggests that antbodies to the insulin receptor show some degree of phylogenetic specificity. A similar type of specificity has been observed with antibodies to the thyrotropin receptor (S13).

5.3. MYASTHENIA GRAVIS AND ANTIBODIES TO THE ACETYLCHOLINE RECEPTOR

Myasthenia gravis is a neuromuscular junction disease of man characterized by muscle weakness and fatigability. Simpson in 1960 (S8) first proposed that myasthenia was due to acetylcholine receptor antibodies that bound to the receptor and blocked the action of acetylcholine. Strong support for Simpson's hypothesis has recently come from studies with experimentally induced myasthenia.

Immunization of animals with acetylcholine receptor protein purified from the electric organs of *Electrophorus electricus* and *Torpedo californica* has led to the establishment of experimental models of myasthenia gravis (L12, P3, T1). The experimental disease resembles spontaneously occurring human myasthenia in every criterion so far examined. Clinically, muscle weakness, fatigability, and improvement by anticholinesterase drugs occurs. Electrophysiologically, the decreasing response of muscle to low-frequency motor nerve stimulation and the observation of post-activation facilitation followed by muscle exhaustion with rapid stimulation are characteristic of human myasthenia and are also found in the experimental disease. Furthermore, antibodies that bind to the acetylcholine receptor can be detected in both types of myasthenia (A2, A3, H5, L10, S19) and *in vitro* anti-acetylcholine receptor anitbodies have been shown to diminish acetylcholine sensitivity of muscle fibers, reduce the miniature end plate potential amplitudes and decrease the ability of the receptor to bind the specific acetylcholine inhibitor α-bungarotoxin (G13).

Recently, Lennon (L10) has reported the presence of anti-acetylcholine receptor antibody in the serum of 62 out of 71 patients with myasthenia gravis. Also the antibody was found in a newborn infant from a myasthenic woman. This is quite consistent with the well established transplacental passage of immunoglobulin G and is analogous to the transplacental passage of thyroid-stimulating antibodies in Graves' disease (D8). Passive transfer of experimental myasthenia gravis has been performed with lymph node cells from donor guinea pigs immunized with purified acetylcholine receptor (T2). The sensitized cells may have acted directly on the neuromuscular junction or indirectly by releasing antibodies or non-immunoglobulin mediators. The relative contributions of humoral and cellular immune systems remains to be determined, but the experiments provide excellent additional evidence for the autoimmune character of myasthenia gravis.

5.4. ANTIBODIES TO OTHER RECEPTORS

To date, there is good evidence for autoantibodies to the TSH receptor, the insulin receptor, and the acetylcholine receptor. The antibodies to the TSH receptor that are able to mimic the effects of thyrotropin and cause hyperthyroidism are probably unique. However, it is quite reasonable to suppose that autoantibodies to other receptors exist that merely block the effect of the hormone. For example, antibodies to gonadotropin receptors could be involved in certain types of ovarian and testicular failure. The radioreceptor assays for these and many other peptide hormones are now well established and provide a convenient method for detecting anti-receptor antibodies and investigating this possibility.

6. Radioreceptor Assays

Radioimmunoassays are now available for studying virtually all poly-peptide hormones. Radioreceptor assays have also been developed for many hormones, and in this section the two systems of measurement are compared.

Both radioreceptor and radioimmunoassays usually utilize ^{125}I-labeled hormones. The hormone's antigenic sites, which are used in the radio-immunoassay, are generally less susceptible to denaturation during label-ing than are the receptor-binding sites. Consequently labeling of hormones for use in a receptor system is generally more difficult.

Preparation of antisera for radioimmunoassay is usually a straight-forward procedure in the case of polypeptide hormones and can lead to antibodies with very high affinity and titer. For example, in my own laboratory guinea pig anti-TSH antisera can be used at a dilution of 1 in 10^6 and have average association constants in excess of $10^{11} M^{-1}$. Further-more, antisera are stable for several years at $4°C$, and certainly for several days at $37°C$. Hormone receptors are usually prepared by simple pro-cedures from tissue homogenates. However, the affinity and binding capacity of the hormone receptor are completely outside the investigator's control and are often inferior to a good antiserum. Also, hormone receptor preparations tend to be unstable, particularly at $37°C$.

The types of binding involved in hormone receptor and antigen–anti-body reactions are probably similar, as mentioned in Section 3.3. However, the relative instability of receptor preparations and receptor binding sites on labeled hormones can result in both receptor and hormone denaturation during the assay procedure.

Perhaps the most convenient method of separating free and antibody-bound hormone is the second antibody method, in which antibody-bound hormone is precipitated by addition of an antiantibody. In the case of radioreceptor assays, such a method cannot be used. Most receptor assays utilize particulate receptor preparations and use centrifugation to separate bound and free hormone. However, fairly high g values are often required to sediment the receptors, and conventional laboratory centrifuges are generally unsuitable.

The precision of radioreceptor and radioimmunoassay assays is similar, multiple determinations usually showing excellent agreement. In general, however, the radioimmunoassay has similar or superior sensitivity and is methodologically more convenient.

The principal disadvantage of the radioimmunoaasay is that it recognizes antigenic sites on the hormone, and these are not usually involved directly in the biological activity. Consequently, the radioimmunoassay may detect biologically inactive hormonelike materials and fail to detect hormonelike substances with modified antigenic determinants but intact receptor binding sites. The radioreceptor assay clearly does not have these disadvantages.

Perhaps the most important use of radioreceptor assays will be in the detection of antibodies to hormone receptors (see Section 5). The problems of producing a specific antiserum to an antireceptor antibody are formidable. Consequently, the radioreceptor assay in which the competition between antibody and labeled hormone for the receptor is used to estimate antireceptor activity is probably the only convenient method of studying these substances.

7. Concluding Statement

There is now preliminary information on the binding of many polypeptide hormones to target-tissue receptor sites. Hormone binding induces changes in the receptor itself, which are then transmitted through the membrane to an enzyme such as adenyl cyclase.

The nature of these secondary effects of receptor binding is completely unknown at present. However, when highly purified water-soluble hormone receptors become available, detailed kinetic, thermodynamic, and spectroscopic studies should permit an understanding of at least the first stages of hormone-induced changes in target cell membranes.

REFERENCES

A1. Adams, D. D., and Purves, H. D., Abnormal responses in the assay of thyrotropin. *Proc. Univ. Otago Med. Sch.* 34, 11–12 (1956).

A2. Aharonov, A., Abramsky, O., Tarrab-Hazdai, R., and Fuchs, S., Humoral antibodies to acetylcholine receptor in patients with myasthenia gravis. *Lancet* 2, 340–342 (1975).

A3. Almon, R. R., Andrew, C. G., and Appel, S. H., Serum globulin in myasthenia gravis: Inhibition of α-bungarotoxin binding to acetylcholine receptors. *Science* 186, 55–57 (1974).

B1. Bashford, C. L., Harrison, S. J., Radda, G. K., and Mehdi, Q., The relation between lipid mobility and the specific hormone binding of thyroid membranes. *Biochem. J.* 146, 473–479 (1975).

B2. Beall, R. J., and Sayers, G., Isolated adrenal cells: Steroidogenesis and cyclic AMP accumulation in response to ACTH. *Arch. Biochem. Biophys.* 148, 70–76 (1972).

B3. Birnbaumer, L., Pohl, S. L., and Rodbell, M., The glucagon sensitive adenyl cyclase system in plasma membranes of rat liver. II. Comparison between glucagon and fluoride stimulated activities. *J. Biol. Chem.* **246,** 1857–1860 (1971).

B4. Bloom, S. R., Glucagon. *Br. J. Hosp. Med.* **13,** 150–158 (1975).

B5. Butcher, R. W., Sneyd, J. G. T., Park, C. R., and Sutherland, E. W., Effect of insulin on adenosine 3′,5′-monophosphate in the rat epididymal fat pad. *J. Biol. Chem.* **241,** 1651–1653 (1966).

C1. Catt, K. J., and Dufau, M. L., Spare gonadotropin receptors in rat testis. *Nature (London), New Biol.* **244,** 219–221 (1973).

C2. Catt, K. J., Dufau, M. L., and Tsuruhara, T., Studies on a radioligand-receptor assay for luteinizing hormone and chorionic gonadotropin. *J. Clin. Endocrinol. Metab.* **32,** 860–863 (1971).

C3. Catt, K. J., Dufau, M. L., and Tsuruhara, T., Radioligand-receptor assay of luteinizing hormone and chorionic gonadotropin. *J. Clin. Endocrinol. Metab.* **34,** 123–132 (1972).

C4. Catt, K. J., Tsuruhara, T., and Dufau, M. L., Gonadotropin binding sites of the rat testis. *Biochim. Biophys. Acta* **279,** 194–201 (1972).

C5. Catt, K. J., Watanabe, K., and Dufau, M. L., Cyclic AMP released by rat testis during gonadotropin stimulation *in vitro. Nature (London)* **239,** 280–281 (1972).

C6. Channing, C. P., and Kammerman, S., Characteristics of gonadotropin receptors of porcine granulosa cells during follicle maturation. *Endocrinology* **92,** 531–540 (1973).

C7. Channing, C. P., and Kammerman, S., Effects of hCG, asialo-hCG and the subunits of hCG upon luteinization of monkey granulosa cell cultures. *Endocrinology* **93,** 1035–1043 (1973).

C8. Chase, L. R., Fedak, S. A., and Aurbach, G. D., Activation of skeletal adenyl cyclase by parathyroid hormone in vitro. *Endocrinology* **84,** 761–768 (1969).

C9. Cheng, K., Properties of follicle-stimulating-hormone receptor in cell membranes of bovine testis. *Biochem. J.* **149,** 123–132 (1975).

C10. Cheng, K., A radioreceptor for follicle-stimulating hormone. *J. Clin. Endocrinol. Metab.* **41,** 581–589 (1975).

C11. Clague, R., Mukhtar, E. D., Pyle, G. A., Nutt, J., Clark, F., Scott, M., Evered, D., Rees Smith, B., and Hall, R., Thyroid-stimulating immunoglobulins and the control of thyroid function. *J. Clin. Endocrinol. Metab.* **43,** 550–556 (1976).

C12. Cuatrecasas, P., Interaction of insulin with the cell membrane: The primary action of insulin. *Proc. Natl. Acad. Sci. U.S.A.* **63,** 450–457 (1969).

C13. Cuatrecasas, P., Insulin-receptor interaction in adipose tissue cells: Direct measurement and properties. *Proc. Natl. Acad. Sci. U.S.A.* **68,** 1264–1268 (1971).

C14. Cuatrecasas, P., Properties of the insulin receptor isolated from liver and fat cell membranes. *J. Biol. Chem.* **247,** 1980–1991 (1972).

C15. Cuatrecasas, P., Affinity chromatography and purification of the insulin receptor of liver cell membranes. *Proc. Natl. Acad. Sci. U.S.A.* **69,** 1277–1281 (1972).

C16. Cuatrecasas, P., Desbuquois, B., and Krug, F., Insulin-receptor interactions in liver cell membranes. *Biochem. Biophys. Res. Commun.* **44,** 333–339 (1971).

D1. Danzo, B. J., Characterization of a receptor for human chorionic gonadotrophin in luteinized rat ovaries. *Biochim. Biophys. Acta* **304,** 560–569 (1973).

D2. De Meyts, P., and Roth, J., Cooperativity in lingand binding: A new graphic analysis. *Biochem. Biophys. Res. Commun.* **66,** 1118–1126 (1976).

D3. De Meyts, P., Roth, J., Neville, D. M., Gavin, J. R., and Lesniak, M. A., Insulin interactions with its receptors: Experimental evidence for negative cooperativity. *Biochem. Biophys. Res. Commun.* **55,** 154–161 (1973).

D4. Di Bella, F. P., Douša, T. P., Miller, S. S., and Arnaud, C. D., Parathyroid hormone receptors of renal cortex: Specific binding of biologically active, ^{125}I-labelled hormone and relationship to adenylate cyclase activation. *Proc. Natl. Acad. Sci. U.S.A.* **71**, 723–726 (1974).

D5. Dirmikis, S., and Munro, D. S., Studies on the binding activity for the long-acting thyroid stimulator. *J. Endocrinol.* **58**, 577–590 (1973).

D6. Dorrington, J. H., and Fritz, I. B., Effects of gonadotropins on cyclic AMP production by isolated seminiferous tubule and interstitial cell preparations. *Endocrinology* **94**, 395–403 (1974).

D7. Dorrington, J. H., Vernon, R. G., and Fritz, I. B., The effect of gonadotrophins on the 3′,5′-AMP levels of seminiferous tubules. *Biochem. Biophys. Res. Commun.* **46**, 1523–1528 (1972).

D8. Dorrington, K. J., and Munro, D. S., The long-acting thyroid stimulator. *Clin. Pharmacol. Ther.* **7**, 788–806 (1966).

D9. Dufau, M. L., Charreau, E. H., and Catt, K. J., Characteristics of a soluble gonadotropin receptor from the rat testis. *J. Biol. Chem.* **248**, 6973–6982 (1973).

D10. Dufau, M. L., Ryan, D. W., Baukal, A. J., and Catt, K. J., Gonadotrophin receptors. Solubilization and purification by affinity chromatography. *J. Biol. Chem.* **250**, 4822–4824 (1975).

D11. Dufau, M. L., Watanabe, K., and Catt, K. J., Stimulation of cyclic AMP production by the rat testis during incubation with hCG in vitro. *Endocrinology* **92**, 6–11 (1973).

F1. Finn, F. M., Widnell, C. C., and Hofmann, K., Localization of an adrenocorticotropic hormone receptor on bovine adrenal cortical membranes. *J. Biol. Chem.* **247**, 5695–5702 (1972).

F2. Flier, J. S., Kahn, C. R., Roth, J., and Bar, R. S., Antibodies that impair insulin receptor binding in an unusual diabetic syndrome with severe insulin resistance. *Science* **190**, 63–65 (1975).

F3. Freychet, P., Roth, J., and Neville, D. M., Monoiodoinsulin: Demonstration of its biological activity and binding to fat cells and liver membranes. *Biochem. Biophys. Res. Commun.* **43**, 400–408 (1971).

G1. Gardiner, W. R., and Ottaway, J. H., Observations on programs to estimate the parameters of enzyme kinetics. *FEBS Lett.* **2**, Suppl., S34–S42 (1969).

G2. Gavin, J. R., Kahn, C. R., Gordon, P., Roth, J., and Neville, D. M. Radioreceptor assay of insulin: Comparison of plasma and pancreatic insulins and proinsulins. *J. Clin. Endocrinol. Metab.* **41**, 438–445 (1975).

G3. Gavin, J. R. III, Mann, D. L., Buell, D. N., and Roth, J., Preparation of solubilized insulin receptors from human lymphocytes. *Biochem. Biophys. Res. Commun.* **49**, 870–876 (1972).

G4. Gavin, J. R. III, Buell, D. N., and Roth, J., Water-soluble insulin receptors from human lymphocytes. *Science* **178**, 168–169 (1972).

G5. Gavin, J. R. III, Roth, J., Jen, P., and Freychet, P., Insulin receptors in human circulating cells and fibroblasts. *Proc. Natl. Acad. Sci. U.S.A.* **69**, 747–751 (1972).

G6. Gelato, M., Marshall, S., Boudreau, M., Bruni, J., Campbell, G. A., and Meites, J., Effects of thyroid and ovaries on prolactin binding activity in rat liver. *Endocrinology* **96**, 1292–1299 (1975).

G7. Gliemann, J., Gammeltoft, S., and Vinten, J., Time course of insulin receptor binding and insulin induced lipogenesis in isolated rat fat cells. *J. Biol. Chem.* **250**, 3368–3374 (1975).

G8. Goltzmann, D., Peytremann, A., Callahan, E., Tregear, G. W., and Potts, J. T., Analysis of the requirements for parathyroid hormone action in renal membranes with the use of inhibiting analogues. *J. Biol. Chem.* **250**, 3199–3203 (1975).

G9. Gordon, P., Lesniak, M. A., Hendricks, C. M., and Roth, J., Big growth hormone components from human plasma: Decreased reactivity demonstrated by radioreceptor assay. *Science* **182**, 829–831 (1973).

G10. Gospodarowicz, D., A comparative study of the lipolytic activity of thyroid-stimulating hormone and luteinizing hormone. *J. Biol. Chem.* **248**, 1314–1317 (1973).

G11. Gospodarowicz, D., Preparation and characterization of plasma membranes from bovine corpus luteum. *J. Biol. Chem.* **248**, 5050–5056 (1973).

G12. Grahame-Smith, D. G., Butcher, R. W., Ney, R. I., and Sutherland, E. W., Adenosine 3′,5′-monophosphate as the intracellular mediator of the action of adrenocorticotropic hormone on the adrenal cortex. *J. Biol. Chem.* **242**, 5535–5541 (1967).

G13. Green, D. P. L., Miledi, R., and Vincent, A., Neuromuscular transmission after immunization against acetylcholine receptors. *Proc. R. Soc. London, Ser. B* **189**, 57–68 (1975).

H1. Hall, R., Smith, B. R., and Mukhtar, E. D., Thyroid stimulators in health and disease. *Clin. Endocrinol.* **4**, 213–230 (1975).

H2. Haour, F., and Bertrand, J., Insulin receptors in the plasma membranes of human placenta. *J. Clin. Endocrinol. Metab.* **38**, 334–337 (1974).

H3. Haour, F., and Saxena, B. B., Characterization and solubilization of gonadotrophin receptor of bovine corpus luteum. *J. Biol. Chem.* **249**, 2195–2205 (1974).

H4. Hart, I. R., and McKenzie, J. M., Comparison of the effects of thyrotropin and long-acting thyroid stimulator on guinea pig adipose tissue. *Endocrinology* **88**, 26–30 (1971).

H5. Heilbronn, E., and Mattson, C., The nicotinic cholinergic receptor protein: Improved purification method, preliminary amino acid composition and observed autoimmune response. *J. Neurochem.* **22**, 315–317 (1974).

H6. Herrington, A. C., Jacobs, L. S., and Daughaday, W. H., Radioreceptor and radioimmunoassay quantitation of human growth hormone in acromegalic serum. Overestimation by immunoassay and systematic differences between antisera. *Clin. Endocrinol. Metab.* **39**, 257–262 (1974).

H7. Hill, A. V., The possible effect of the aggregation of the molecules of haemoglobin on its dissociation curves. *J. Physiol. (London)* **40**, iv–vii (1910).

H8. Hofmann, K., Wingender, W., and Finn, F. M., Correlation of adrenocorticotropic activity of ACTH analogs with degree of binding to an adrenal cortical particulate preparation. *Proc. Natl. Acad. Sci. U.S.A.* **67**, 829–836 (1970).

H9. House, P. D. R., and Weidemann, M. J., Characterizations of an [125I]-insulin binding plasma membrane fraction from rat liver. *Biochem. Biophys. Res. Commun.* **41**, 541–548 (1970).

H10. Hunter, W. M., and Greenwood, F. C., Preparation of iodine[181] labelled growth hormone of high specific activity. *Nature (London)* **194**, 495–496 (1962).

K1. Kammerman, S., Canfield, R. E., Kolena, J., and Channing, C. P., The binding of iodinated hCG to porcine granulosa cells. *Endocrinology* **91**, 65–74 (1972).

K2. Kammerman, S., and Ross, J., Increase in numbers of gonadotrophin receptors on granulosa cells during follicle maturation. *J. Clin. Endocrinol. Metab.* **41**, 546–550 (1975).

K3. Karush, F., Immunologic specificity and molecular structure. *Adv. Immunol.* **2**, 1–40 (1962).

K4. Kendall-Taylor, P., Adenyl cyclase activity in the mouse thyroid. *J. Endocrinol.* **52**, 533–540 (1972).

K5. Kendall-Taylor, P., Effects of long-acting thyroid stimulator (LATS) and LATS protector on human thyroid adenyl cyclase activity. *Br. Med. J.* **3**, 72–75 (1973).

K6. Kendall-Taylor, P., and Munro, D. S., Lipolytic activity of long-acting thyroid stimulator. *Biochim. Biophys. Acta* **231**, 314–319 (1971).

K7. Keutmann, H. T., Barling, P. M., Hendy, G. N., Segré, G. V., Niall, H. D., Aurbach, G. D., O'Riordan, J. L. H., and Potts, J. T., Isolation of human para-thyroid hormone. *Biochemistry* **13**, 1646–1652 (1974).

K8. Klein, I., Fletcher, M. A., and Levey, G. S., Evidence for a dissociable glucagon binding site in a solubilized preparation of myocardial adenylate cyclase. *J. Biol. Chem.* **248**, 5552–5554 (1973).

K9. Kono, T., and Barham, F. W., The relationship between the insulin-binding capacity of fat cells and the cellular response to insulin. *J. Biol. Chem.* **246**, 6210–6216 (1971).

K10. Kotani, M., Kariya, T., and Field, J. B., Studies of thyroid-stimulating hormone binding to bovine thyroid plasma membranes. *Metab., Clin. Exp.* **24**, 959–971 (1975).

L1. Labrosse, M. S., and Lakatua, D., A simple and sensitive radioreceptor assay for ACTH in human plasma. *Am. J. Clin. Pathol.* **63**, 285–286 (1975).

L2. Lee, C. Y., and Ryan, R. J., The uptake of human luteinizing hormone by slices of luteinized rat ovaries. *Endocrinology* **89**, 1515–1523 (1971).

L3. Lee, C. Y., and Ryan, R. J., Estrogen stimulation of human chorionic gona-dotropin binding by luteinized rat ovarian slices. *Endocrinology* **95**, 1691–1693 (1974).

L4. Lee, C. Y., Tateishi, K., Ryan, R. J., and Jiang, N. S., Binding of human chorionic gonadotropin by rat ovarian slices. Dependence on the functional state of the ovary. *Proc. Soc. Exp. Biol. Med.* **148**, 505–507 (1975).

L5. Lee Selinger, R. C., and Civen, M., ACTH diazotized to agarose: Effects on isolated adrenal cells. *Biochem. Biophys. Res. Commun.* **43**, 793–799 (1971).

L6. Lefkowitz, R. J., Roth, J., and Pastan, I., Radioreceptor assay of adrenocortico-tropic hormone: New approach to assay of polypeptide hormones in plasma. *Science* **170**, 633–635 (1970).

L7. Lefkowitz, R. J., Roth, J., Pricer, W., and Pastan, I., ACTH receptors in the adrenal: Specific binding of ACTH-^{125}I and its relation to adenyl cyclase. *Proc. Natl. Acad. Sci. U.S.A.* **65**, 745–752 (1970).

L8. Leidenberger, F. A., and Riechart, L. E., Species differences in luteinizing hormone as inferred from slope variations in a radioligand receptor assay. *Endocrinology* **92**, 646–649 (1973).

L9. Le Marchand-Beraud, T., Griessen, M., and Scazziga, B. R., Clinical signifi-cance of LATS and TSH in the blood. *Ann. Clin. Res.* **4**, 121–137 (1972).

L10. Lennon, V., Humoral factors in myasthenia gravis. *Nature (London)* **258**, 11–12 (1975).

L11. Lennon, V. A., and Carnegie, P. R., Immunopharmacological disease—a break in tolerance to receptor sites. *Lancet* **1**, 630–633 (1971).

L12. Lennon, V. A., Lindstrom, J. M., and Seybold, M. E., Experimental auto-immune myasthenia: A model of myasthenia gravis in rats and guinea pigs. *J. Exp. Med.* **141**, 1365–1375 (1975).

L13. Lesniak, M. A., Gordon, P., Roth, J., and Gavin, J. R., Binding of ^{125}I-human growth hormone to specific receptors in human cultured lymphocytes. *J. Biol. Chem.* **249**, 1661–1667 (1974).

L14. Lesniak, M. A., Roth, J., Gordon, P., and Gavin, J. R., Human growth hormone radioreceptor assay using cultured human lymphocytes. *Nature (London), New Biol.* **241**, 20–22 (1973).

L15. Levey, G. S., The glucagon receptor and adenylate cyclase. *Metab., Clin. Exp.* **24**, 301–310 (1975).

L16. Levey, G. S., Fletcher, M. A., Klein, I., Ruiz, E., and Schenk, A., Characterization of ^{125}I-glucagon binding in a solubilized preparation of cat myocardial adenylate cyclase. *J. Biol. Chem.* **249**, 2665–2673 (1974).

L17. Lineweaver, H., and Burk, D., The determination of enzyme dissociation constants. *J. Am. Chem. Soc.* **56**, 658–666 (1934).

L18. Lissitzky, S., Fayet, G., Verrier, B., Hennen, G., and Jaquet, P., Thyroid-stimulating hormone binding to cultured thyroid cells. *FEBS Lett.* **29**, 20–24 (1973).

L19. Loton, E. G., and Sneyd, J. G. T., An effect of insulin on adipose tissue adenosine 3′:5′-cyclic monophosphate phosphodiesterase. *Biochem. J.* **120**, 187–193 (1970).

M1. McIlhinney, R. A. J., and Schulster, D., Studies on the binding of ^{125}I-labelled corticotrophin to isolated rat adrenocortical cells. *J. Endocrinol.* **64**, 175–184 (1975).

M2. McIntosh, C. H. S., and Hesch, R. D., Labelled antibody membrane assay for parathyroid hormone. A new approach to the measurement of receptor bound hormone. *Biochem. Biophys. Res. Commun.* **64**, 376–383 (1975).

M3. Malbon, C. C., and Zull, J. E., Interactions of parathyroid hormone and plasma membranes from rat kidney. *Biochem. Biophys. Res. Commun.* **56**, 952–958 (1974).

M4. Manganiello, V., and Vaughan, M., An effect of insulin on cyclic adenosine 3′:5′-monophosphate phosphodiesterase activity in fat cells. *J. Biol. Chem.* **248**, 7164–7170 (1973).

M5. Manley, S. W., Bourke, J. R., and Hawker, R. W., The thyroptrophin receptor in guinea pig thyroid homogenate: General properties. *J. Endocrinol.* **61**, 419–436 (1974).

M6. Manley, S. W., Bourke, J. R., and Hawker, R. W., The thyrotrophin receptor in guinea pig thyroid homogenate: Interaction with the long-acting thyroid stimulator. *J. Endocrinol.* **61**, 437–445 (1974).

M7. Marchalonis, J. J., An enzymatic method for the trace iodination of immunoglobulins and other proteins. *Biochem. J.* **113**, 299–305 (1969).

M8. Marshall, R. N., Underwood, L. E., Voina, S. J., Foushee, D. B., and Van Wyk, J. J., Characterization of the insulin and somatomedin C receptors in human placental cell membranes. *J. Clin. Endocrinol. Metab.* **39**, 283–292 (1974).

M9. Marx, S. J., Fedak, S. A., and Aurbach, G. D., Preparation and characterization of a hormone-responsive renal plasma membrane fraction. *J. Biol. Chem.* **247**, 6913–6918 (1972).

M10. Mehdi, Q. S., and Nussey, S. S., A radio-ligand receptor assay for the long-acting thyroid stimulator. *Biochem. J.* **145**, 105–111 (1975).

M11. Mendelson, C. Dufau, M., and Catt, K., Gonadotropin binding and stimulation of cyclic adenosine 3′:5′-monophosphate and testosterone production in isolated Leydig cells. *J. Biol. Chem.* **250**, 8818–8823 (1975).

M12. Moore, W. V., and Wolff, J., Thyroid-stimulating hormone binding to beef thyroid membranes. Relation to adenylate cyclase activity. *J. Biol. Chem.* **249**, 6255–6263 (1974).

M13. Mukhtar, E. D., Smith, B. R., Pyle, G. A., Hall, R., and Vice, P., Relation of thyroid-stimulating immunoglobulin to thyroid function and effects of surgery, radioiodine and antithyroid drugs. *Lancet* **1**, 713–715 (1975).

N1. Nisonoff, A., and Pressman, D., Heterogeneity and average combining constants of antibodies from individual rabbits. *J. Immunol.* **80**, 417–428 (1958).

P1. Pahnke, V. G., Leidenberger, F. A., and Kunzig, H. J., Correlation between HCG (LH)-binding capacity, Leydig cell number and secretory activity of rat testis throughout pubescence. *Acta Endocrinol. (Copenhagen)* **79**, 610–618 (1975).

P2. Papainannou, S., and Gospodarowicz, D., Comparison of the binding of human chorionic gonadotropin to isolated bovine luteal cells and bovine luteal plasma membranes. *Endocrinology* **97**, 114–124 (1975).

P3. Patrick, J., and Lindstrom, J., Autoimmune response to acetylcholine receptor. *Science* **180**, 871–872 (1973).

P4. Pennock, B. E., A calculator for finding binding parameters from a Scatchard plot. *Anal. Biochem.* **56**, 306–309 (1973).

P5. Petersen, V. B., Rees Smith, B., and Hall, R., A study of thyroid stimulating activity in human serum with the highly sensitive cytochemical bioassay. *J. Clin. Endocrinol. Metab.* **41**, 199–202 (1975).

P6. Pohl, S. L., Birnbaumer, L., and Rodbell, M., The glucagon-sensitive adenyl cyclase system in plasma membranes of rat liver I. Properties. *J. Biol. Chem.* **246**, 1849–1856 (1971).

R1. Reichert, L. E., and Bhalla, V. K., Development of a radioligand tissue receptor assay for human follicle-stimulating hormone. *Endocrinology* **94**, 483–491 (1974).

R2. Reichert, L. E., Leidenberger, F., and Trowbridge, C. G., Studies on luteinizing hormone and its subunits: Development and application of a radioligand receptor assay and properties of the hormone-receptor interaction. *Recent Prog. Horm. Res.* **29**, 497–532 (1973).

R3. Reichert, L. E., Ramsey, R. B., and Carter, E. B., Application of a tissue receptor assay to measurement of serum follitropin (FSH). *J. Clin. Endocrinol. Metab.* **41**, 634–637 (1975).

R4. Richardson, M. C., and Schulster, D., Corticosteroidogenesis in isolated adrenal cells: Effect of adrenocorticotrophic hormone, adenosine 3′,5′-monophosphate and β^{1-24}-adrenocorticotrophic hormone diazotized to polyacrylamide. *J. Endocrinol.* **55**, 127–139 (1972).

R5. Rodbell, M., Birnbaumer, L., Pohl, S. L., and Krans, M. J., The glucagon sensitive adenyl cyclase system in plasma membranes of rat liver. V. An obligatory role of guanyl nucleotides in glucagon action. *J. Biol. Chem.* **246**, 1877–1882 (1971).

R6. Rodbell, M., Krans, M. J., Pohl, S. L., and Birnbaumer, L., The glucagon sensitive adenyl cyclase system in plasma membranes of rat liver. III. Binding of glucagon: Method of assay and specificity. *J. Biol. Chem.* **246**, 1861–1871 (1971).

R7. Rodbell, M., Krans, M. J., Pohl, S. L., and Birnbaumer, L., The glucagon sensitive adenyl cyclase system in plasma membranes of rat liver. IV. Effects of guanyl nucleotides on binding of ^{125}I-glucagon. *J. Biol. Chem.* **246**, 1872–1876 (1971).

R8. Rosenthal, H. E. A., A graphic method for the determination and presentation of binding parameters in a complex system. *Anal. Biochem.* **20**, 525–532 (1967).

S1. Scatchard, G., The attraction of proteins for small molecules and ions. *Ann. N.Y. Acad. Sci.* **51**, 660–672 (1949).

S2. Schwartz, R. H., Bianco, A. R., Handwerger, B. S., and Kahn, R. C., Demonstration that monocytes rather than lymphocytes are the insulin binding cells in preparations of human peripheral blood mononuclear leukocytes: Implications for studies of insulin resistant states in man. *Proc. Natl. Acad. Sci. U.S.A.* **72**, 474–478 (1975).

S3. Senft, G., Schultz, G., Munska, K., and Hoffman, M., Effects of glucocorticoids and insulin on 3′,5′-AMP phosphodiesterase activity in adrenalectomized rats. *Diabetologia* **4**, 330–335 (1968).

S4. Sharma, K., Ahmed, N. K., Sutliff, L. S., and Brush, J. S., Metabolic regulation of steroidogenesis in isolated adrenal cells of the rat. ACTH regulation of cGMP and cAMP levels and steroidogenesis. *FEBS Lett.* **45**, 107–110 (1974).

S5. Shiu, R. P. C., and Friesen, H. G., Properties of a prolactin receptor from the rabbit mammary gland. *Biochem. J.* **140**, 301–311 (1974).

S6. Shiu, R. P. C., and Friesen, H. G., Solubilization and purification of a prolactin receptor from the rabbit mammary gland. *J. Biol. Chem.* **249**, 7902–7911 (1974).

S7. Shiu, R. P. C., Kelly, P. A., and Friesen, H. G., Radioreceptor assay for prolactin and other lactogenic hormones. *Science* **180**, 968–971 (1973).

S8. Simpson, J. A., Myasthenia Gravis: A new hypothesis. *Scott. Med. J.* **5**, 419–436 (1960).

S9. Sips, R., On the structure of a catalyst surface. *J. Chem. Phys.* **16**, 490–495 (1948).

S10. Smith, B. R., The interaction of the long-acting thyroid stimulator with thyroid tissue in vitro. *J. Endocrinol.* **46**, 45–54 (1970).

S11. Smith, B. R., Characterization of long acting thyroid stimulator γ G binding protein. *Biochim. Biophys. Acta* **229**, 649–662 (1971).

S12. Smith, B. R., Dorrington, K. J., and Munro, D. S., The thyroid-stimulating properties of long-acting thyroid stimulator γ G-globulin subunits. *Biochim. Biophys. Acta* **192**, 277–285 (1969).

S13. Smith, B. R., and Hall, R., Thyroid-stimulating immunoglobulins in Graves' disease. *Lancet* **2**, 427–431 (1974).

S14. Smith, B. R., and Hall, R., Binding of thyroid-stimulators to thyroid membranes. *FEBS. Lett.* **42**, 301–304 (1974).

S15. Smith, B. R., and Munro, D. S., The nature of the interaction between thyroid stimulating γ G-globulin and thyroid tissue. *Biochim. Biophys. Acta* **208**, 285–293 (1970).

S16. Smith, B. R., Munro, D. S., and Dorrington, K. J., The distribution of the long-acting thyroid stimulator among γ G-immunoglobulins. *Biochim. Biophys. Acta* **188**, 89–100 (1969).

S17. Sneid, D. S., Jacobs, L. S., Weldon, V. V., Trivedi, B. L., and Daughaday, W. H., Radioreceptor inactive growth hormone associated with stimulated secretion in normal subjects. *J. Clin. Endocrinol. Metab.* **41**, 471–474 (1975).

S18. Solomon, S. S., Effect of insulin and lipolytic hormones on cyclic AMP phosphodiesterase activity in normal and diabetic rat adipose tissue. *Endocrinology* **96**, 1366–1373 (1975).

S19. Sugiyama, H., Benda, P., Meunier, J.-C., and Changeux, J.-P., Immunological characteristics of the cholinergic receptor protein from Electrophorus Electricus. *FEBS Lett.* **35**, 124–128 (1973).

S20. Sutcliffe, H. S., Martin, T. J., Eisman, J. A., and Pilczyk, R., Binding of parathyroid hormone to bovine kidney-cortex plasma membranes. *Biochem. J.* **134,** 913–921 (1973).

T1. Tarrab-Hazdi, R., Aharonov, A., Abramsky, O., Yaar, I., and Fuchs, S., Passive transfer of experimental autoimmune myasthenia by lymph node cells in inbred guinea pigs. *J. Exp. Med.* **142,** 785–789 (1975).

T2. Tarrab-Hazdai, R., Aharonov, A., Silman, I., Fuchs, S., and Abramsky, O., Experimental autoimmune myasthenia induced in monkeys by purified acetyl choline receptor. *Nature (London)* **256,** 128–130 (1975).

T3. Teng, C. S., Rees Smith, B., Anderson, J., and Hall, R., Comparison of thyrotrophin receptors in membranes prepared from fat and thyroid tissue. *Biochem. Biophys. Res. Commun.* **66,** 836–841 (1975).

T4. Tsushima, T., and Friesen, H. G., Radioreceptor assay for growth hormone. *J. Clin. Endocrinol. Metab.* **37,** 334–337 (1973).

T5. Turkington, R. W., Stimulation of RNA synthesis in isolated mammary cells by insulin and prolactin bound to Sepharose. *Biochem. Biophys. Res. Commun.* **41,** 1362–1367 (1970).

T6. Turkington, R. W., Measurement of prolactin activity in human plasma by new biological and radioreceptor assays. *J. Clin. Invest.* **50,** 94a (1971).

V1. Verrier, B., Fayet, G., and Lissitzky, S., Thyrotrophin binding properties of isolated thyroid cells and their purified plasma membranes. *Eur. J. Biochem.* **42,** 355–365 (1974).

W1. Wolfsen, A. R., McIntyre, H. B., and Odell, W. D., Adrenocorticotropin measurement by competitive binding receptor assay. *J. Clin. Endocrinol. Metab.* **34,** 684–689 (1972).

VITAMIN D ENDOCRINE SYSTEM

Hector F. DeLuca

Department of Biochemistry, College of Agricultural and Life Sciences,
University of Wisconsin-Madison, Madison, Wisconsin

1. Introduction

Almost since its discovery in 1919, vitamin D has been assumed to have the role of a typical vitamin, namely, that it is required in the diet and that it functions in a catalytic role similar to the water-soluble vitamins. This viewpoint undoubtedly contributed to the conceptual lag in vitamin D action that was ended only recently with the introduction of the concept of vitamin D as a prohormone.

If one examines the question of whether vitamin D represents a true vitamin or not, the answer is equivocal. We realize that if children raised in the temperate climates are deprived of dietary sources of vitamin D, many of them would suffer the debilitating disease of rickets. Furthermore, we also realize that adult man deprived of vitamin D would eventually develop the symptoms of osteomalacia. However, these diseases are unheard of in climates where there is sufficient exposure to sunlight and where there is adequate nutrition, not including a dietary source of vitamin D. We also know that a vitamin D-active substance is produced in the skin upon unltraviolet irradiation, and, therefore, we can conclude that if man or animals receive sufficient amounts of ultraviolet irradiation, vitamin D is not required and thus cannot be considered a vitamin. However, since man lives in areas where there is marginal sunlight, either because of climatic conditions or because of industrial pollution or both, and since man covers his body with clothing and spends much of his time inside structures he has erected, insufficient amounts of vitamin D are produced in the skin, making it a dietary essential. This situation is unlike that with any other vitamin, and hence vitamin D must be considered a special case of a vitamin that in reality is a prohormone. It is the purpose of this chapter to illustrate recent developments that demonstrate quite conclusively that vitamin D is the precursor of a hormone of central importance in the control of serum calcium and phosphorus, which are in turn necessary for mineralization of bone, muscle contraction, nerve function, etc.

Because vitamin D is the precursor of a hormone that functions in the mobilization of calcium and phosphorus and because other hormonal factors interact with vitamin D in these functions, it will become evident that a disturbance of vitamin D conversion to its active hormone may result in a variety of pathological situations, only two of which are the well recognized symptoms of rickets and osteomalacia. The hormone derived from vitamin D must, therefore, be viewed in a broad context, and the implications of its failure to be produced are much wider than the narrow concepts of vitamin D function held in the past several decades.

In at least one sense vitamin D should be considered as a substance analogous to cholesterol, which is converted to a hormone by a system that is analogous to the adrenal system in production of the adrenal steroids. So far, however, only one hormone derived from vitamin D is known, although it is possible that others will be found. By keeping this analogy in mind, the organization of concepts to follow may be facilitated.

2. Historical

The disease rickets, which is illustrated in Fig. 1, has reportedly been described even in ancient times. However, the first clear description of the disease appeared in 1645 by Whistler, an English physician (S10). The etiology of the disease remained unknown, and a variety of treatments had been used, some of which were successful. Cod liver oil and sunlight were among those used, but without proof of success. With the industrialization of the countries of Northern Europe came increased elimination of ultra-

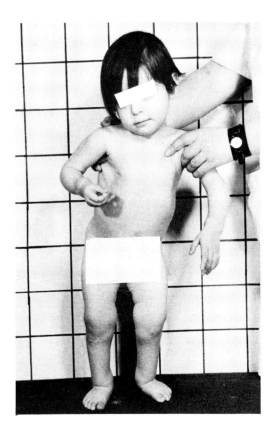

FIG. 1. Child suffering from vitamin D deficiency rickets. By courtesy of Dr. Sonia Balsan, Hôpital des Enfants Malades, Paris, France.

violet irradiation of the population. This was due primarily to the change from an agrarian to urban society and the emission of smoke and other industrial pollutants that prevented adequate ultraviolet penetration to the population. Undoubtedly these two factors and perhaps others led to the appearance of rickets in almost epidemic proportions in Europe by the beginning of the 20th century. An understanding of the development of the disease or of the treatment was lacking until this disease could be produced experimentally. The discovery of the vitamins by McCollum, especially the discovery of the fat-soluble vitamin A, opened up the possibility that dietary deficiencies could result in disease (M3). This undoubtedly inspired Sir Edward Mellanby to produce the disease rickets by dietary means. In 1919 he successfully produced the disease rickets in dogs by feeding them a diet primarily of plant material (plant material is extremely deficient in vitamin D compounds) and by keeping them away from ultraviolet light (M7).

Sir Edward Mellanby was able to prevent and cure the disease by the administration of cod liver oil and concluded that this was due to a vitamin, presumably vitamin A, which had been discovered by McCollum. McCollum and his co-workers recognized that the substance described by Sir Edward Mellanby had biological effects different from those reported for vitamin A. Knowing the stability of vitamin A, McCollum was able to destroy that substance by aeration and heating whereas the antirachitic substance remained stable to this treatment. He, therefore, clearly demonstrated the existence of a new vitamin, which he called vitamin D (M4). At about the same time Mellanby could cure the disease in experimental animals by cod liver oil, others, particularly physicians, were able to treat the human disease rickets by exposure of children to sunlight or artificially produced ultraviolet light (H28). A dichotomy of information, therefore, existed at that time in which cod liver oil in some way equaled sunlight in alleviation of the disease rickets. An important experiment by Goldblatt and Soames (G10) demonstrated that livers from rats irradiated with ultraviolet light contained an antirachitic substance that could cure rickets in other rachitic rats. It was Steenbock and his associates who were able to demonstrate clearly that ultraviolet light could induce in diets and other biological materials antirachitic activity (S14). He and Hess were then able to demonstrate that the activatable material was found in the nonsaponifiable or sterol fraction (H13, S15). The discovery of the irradiation process permitted the introduction of vitamin D into a wide variety of foods and led directly to the elimination of the disease rickets and undoubtedly osteomalacia among children and adults, respectively, of the Western civilizations. This discovery also paved the way for the isolation and identification of the vitamin D structures.

In 1931 Askew and his collaborators successfully isolated vitamin D_2 from ergosterol activated by ultraviolet irradiation (A2). Although Windaus and his collaborators had isolated what they believed to be vitamin D_1, this later proved to be a mixture of vitamin D_2 and one of the other irradiation products, tachysterol. However, Windaus and his collaborators realized their error and successfully isolated and identified vitamin D_2 independent of Askew and collaborators (W6).

Although it was assumed, therefore, that the vitamin D structure was known, strange results with birds were obtained by Steenbock and collaborators, who demonstrated that irradiated ergosterol was not equivalent to cod liver oil or irradiated cholesterol samples in curing rickets in chicks, whereas they were equivalent in curing rickets in rats (S17). This led

Waddell to suggest that another vitamin D compound, which is derived from the cholesterol compounds, must exist (W1). Windaus and his collaborators successfully synthesized 7-dehydrocholesterol (W5) chemically, and from this substance they isolated vitamin D_3 after ultraviolet irradiation (S4). Vitamin D_3 was, therefore, structurally elucidated, which essentially closed the book on the isolation and identification of the dietary vitamin D compounds. At that time, however, Windaus and his collaborators were not aware that they had discovered the truly natural form of the vitamin. Figure 2 illustrates the structure of the two vitamin D precursors and vitamin D_2 as well as vitamin D_3.

The fortification of foods by ultraviolet light was discontinued when an adequate supply of crystalline vitamin D_2 became available, simply because ultraviolet irradiation of foods produced off-flavors that were difficult to deal with. Fortification of foods now takes place with crystalline vitamin D_2 and crystalline vitamin D_3.

Although additional chemical work has been done, including the total synthesis of vitamin D_3, there has been little additional activity on the

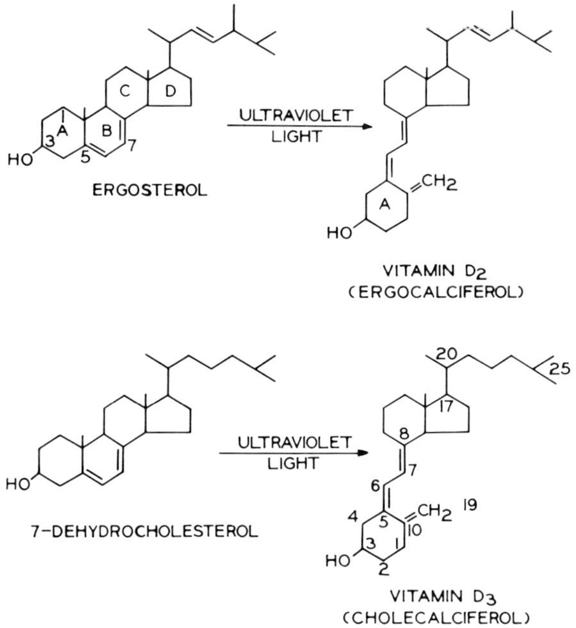

FIG. 2. The conversion of the provitamin D sterols to their respective vitamin D compounds by ultraviolet irradiation. The upper portion represents the conversion of ergosterol to the vitamin D_2, or ergocalciferol, and the lower portion represents the conversion of 7-dehydrocholesterol to vitamin D_3, or cholecalciferol.

chemistry and biochemistry of the vitamin itself. Instead, during the ensuing decades, considerable work was carried out to describe the physiological functions of the vitamin. In 1937 it was clearly established that vitamin D improved intestinal calcium absorption directly and that this in part played a role in the healing of the rachitic lesions (N2). In the 1950s there came the realization that vitamin D functions in the mobilization of calcium from previously formed bone (C1). Although it had been believed that this was primarily the result of excessive amounts of vitamin D, Carlsson and his collaborators were able to show that at physiologic doses the vitamin plays an important role in the mobilization of calcium from the skeleton. In the late 1950s, Schachter and his collaborators demonstrated that vitamin D activates the active calcium transport across the intestinal membrane (S2), whereas Harrison and Harrison illustrated that vitamin D improves intestinal absorption of phosphate independently of an improvement of intestinal calcium absorption (H8). It was not until the last decade that there came the realization that vitamin D did not act directly but must be converted to at least one hormone, which is believed to carry out the multiple functions of the vitamin in intestine, bone, and elsewhere to produce a large number of physiologic effects (D2). There has also been considerable advance in the realization that there is an intimate relationship between vitamin D and the parathyroid hormone, which will be described in this chapter. The possibilities of utilizing this new information on the metabolism and function of vitamin D in understanding and treating disease are immense. This is especially true since disturbances either in a source of vitamin D, or in its metabolism to the active form, or in the hormonal signals that bring about the synthesis of the active form of vitamin D could bring about a large number of pathological states, which may or may not have associated failure of bone mineralization (rickets and osteomalacia).

3. Physiologic Functions of the Vitamin

Although it is often believed that a deficiency of vitamin D results only in a failure of bone mineralization and hence the disease rickets in the young and osteomalacia in adult, it is now clear that we must expand our view of the functions of the vitamin. There is no doubt that a major function of the vitamin is to bring about normal mineralization of newly forming bone collagen. We can therefore say that, in the absence of vitamin D, mineralization of bone collagen does not occur and hence the disease rickets in the young and osteomalacia in the adult occurs. However, it is also clear that a deprivation of vitamin D brings about the acute disease state of hypocalcemic tetany. Although parathyroid hormone is involved in the etiology of hypocalcemic tetany, it is also clear that vitamin D plays a basic role in preventing this disturbance and that there is an interlocking function between the parathyroid hormone and vitamin D in this capacity. A chronic and suboptimal amount of vitamin D could also bring about chronic deterioration of bone without drastic failure of new mineralization and contribute to such diseases as osteoporosis. Finally, it is now believed that vitamin D plays an important role in muscle function (D4).

3.1. PREVENTION OF RICKETS AND OSTEOMALACIA

Bone is composed of three major components: collagen, mucopolysaccharide, and hydroxyapatite mineral. Although a discussion of the generation of new bone is beyond the scope of this chapter, it is known that osteoblasts and chondroblasts elaborate newly formed collagen into the extracellular space. Collagen by itself is a soft and pliable structure, and it is the deposit of hydroxyapatite mineral among the collagen fibrils at particular sites that cement the collagen fibrils in such a way as to impart the structural rigidity necessary for the structural role of the skeleton. In rickets and osteomalacia, osteoblasts and chondrocytes elaborate the collagen fibrils, but they fail to calcify. An intriguing idea is that vitamin D might play a role in the mineralization process, which in itself is not well understood and remains controversial. One view holds that the collagen fibrils, properly prepared, nucleate a supersaturated solution of calcium and phosphate that catalyzes crystallization of hydroxyapatite on collagen fibrils (G7). Another view is that the osteoblasts and chondrocytes accumulate calcium and phosphorus in vesicles and that vesicles carrying the mineral are elaborated into the extracellular space and are utilized for mineralization of collagen (A1). Whatever the mechanism, so far no role for vitamin D has been demonstrated in either of the two processes. However, the possibility must remain that vitamin D may play a role in the mineralization process either by stimulating the pumping of calcium and/or phosphorus into the extracellular bone fluid compartment or by functioning in some way in the packaging of calcium and phosphate in vesicles. However, this is mere speculation and there is no experimental evidence yet to support the idea. We, therefore, leave open the possibility that vitamin D plays a role in the mineralization process.

It is known that blood taken from vitamin D-deficient animals or children has insufficient supplies of calcium and phosphorus to support mineralization of bone. At least a major defect in vitamin D deficiency is an inadequate supply of calcium and phosphorus to the calcification sites. It can, therefore, be considered that an important function of vitamin D is to elevate plasma calcium and plasma phosphorus to levels required to support normal mineralization of bone. By carrying out these functions, the vitamin also provides calcium to prevent hypocalcemic tetany and provides phosphorus to support other functions, such as growth and cellular functions depending on phosphorus.

The elevation of calcium and phosphorus in the blood is the result of the activation of at least three, and possibly more, processes; the best known is that vitamin D stimulates intestinal calcium absorption. This is an active transport process requiring metabolic energy to facilitate the uphill transfer of calcium from the lumen of intestine to the extracellular fluid compartment (M2, S1). Phosphate is the normal accompanying anion for this transport process. In addition, vitamin D stimulates the transport of phosphate across intestinal membrane by a separate mechanism not involving calcium (C7, H8, K5, W3). In addition to the two mechanisms of absorption in the small intestine, vitamin D plays a role in the mobilization of calcium from previously formed bone (C1, R2). Although this mechanism is not well understood, it is believed that vitamin D, acting together with the parathyroid hormone, causes osteoblasts and osteoclasts to transfer calcium into the extracellular fluid compartment from the bone fluid compartment (O5). It must be borne in mind, however, that the possible participation of osteocytes in this process cannot be excluded.

Although the mobilization of calcium from previously formed bone might appear to be diametrically opposite to the calcification function of the vitamin, it must be borne in mind that old bone mineral represents a source of calcium and phosphorus that can be utilized to support adequate levels of calcium and phosphorus in the blood, which are in turn necessary for normal mineralization of bone. Unless there is a complete absence of calcium and phosphorus in the intestine, it is clear that the net effect of vitamin D is to cause mineralization of bone even though one of the sources of calcium and phosphorus might be previously formed bone.

It is possible that vitamin D stimulates renal reabsorption of calcium and of phosphorus. Although there is some evidence to support both ideas, additional work is needed. It seems clear that there is an improvement in renal reabsorption of calcium in response to vitamin D and/or its metabolites (G11, S13), although it must be borne in mind that 99% of the filtered calcium is reabsorbed in vitamin D-deficient animals. Therefore, the improvement in renal reabsorption of calcium is very small in response to the vitamin D compounds.

There is considerable controversy whether vitamin D improves renal reabsorption of phosphorus. Recently, there have been two reports that suggest an improvement in renal reabsorption of phosphate by vitamin D and its metabolites (G4, P6). However, there does not appear to be universal agreement on this point at the present time.

The function of vitamin D in muscle remains unknown although there has been a recent report that the 25-hydroxyvitamin D_3 (25-OH-D_3)[1] improves DNA synthesis and increases ATP levels in muscle (B9). The results of this study, however, are not convincing, and additional work is necessary before there is any insight regarding the role of vitamin D in muscle. The best evidence is clinical, in which it is known that vitamin D given to rachitic children produces a rapid and immediate response in increase in muscle strength and tone.

It is now certain that for all the functions, with the possible exception of muscle, vitamin D must be metabolized to its active hormone, as will be discussed in the ensuing section.

4. Sources of Vitamin D and Biogenesis

From a dietary point of view, vitamin D is not widely distributed (S5). In fact, vitamin D is rarely found in plant materials utilized for food. Thus a completely vegetarian diet, except under unusual circumstances, could not provide adequate amounts of vitamin D if the biosynthetic processes were not operative. Although it is common belief that milk represents an excellent source of vitamin D, this would hardly be true if milk were not fortified with crystalline vitamin D, as has been the case in many countries since 1924. Milk in fact possesses only about 40 units of vitamin D per quart even from cows receiving substantial amounts of vitamin D. Skeletal muscle or meats possess small amounts of vitamin D whereas glandular meats contain substantially greater quantities. However, the best sources are the fish liver oils and shark liver oils, which are rarely consumed except in a therapeutic or prophylactic sense for the prevention or cure of rickets.

With the discovery of the vitamin D irradiation process, described below, has come fortification of foods. In the United States the primary fortification is found in milk and dairy products in which there is an addition of 400 units of vitamin D_2 or vitamin D_3 per quart. In other countries, the fortification of milk is substantially below that figure, and it is not entirely clear what the true requirement of vitamin D is to prevent rachitic or osteomalacic lesions. It does appear, however, that the 400 IU per day level will prevent rickets whereas at levels of 200 units rickets will be prevented in most cases, although an occasional case will then appear. Fortifi-

---

[1] Abbreviations used: 25-OH-D_3, 25-hydroxyvitamin D_3; 1,25-(OH)$_2D_3$, 1,25-dihydroxyvitamin D_3; 24,25-(OH)$_2D_3$, 24,25-dihydroxyvitamin D_3; 1,24,25-(OH)$_3D_3$, 1,24,25-trihydroxyvitamin D_3; 25-OH-D_2, 25-hydroxyvitamin D_2; 1,25-(OH)$_2D_2$, 1,25-dihydroxyvitamin D_2; 24,25-(OH)$_2D_2$, 24,25-dihydroxyvitamin D_2; 1α-OH-D_3, 1α-hydroxyvitamin D_3; 1α-OH-D_2, 1α-hydroxyvitamin D_2; 24-OH-D_3, 24-hydroxyvitamin D_3.

cation of bread has been known, as has fortification of butter, but this has largely disappeared in recent years.

Of considerable interest is the biosynthetic source of vitamin D_3 (D5). Although often thought of as providing insignificant amounts of vitamin D, it is indeed possible that even in the temperate zones sunlight or ultraviolet irradiation of skin may still be responsible for the largest source of vitamin D. An exact figure of the efficiency of production of antirachitic activity in skin upon ultraviolet irradiation is lacking at the present time. In fact, it is not clear at the present time whether vitamin D_3 is the substance produced in the skin or not, although this can be surmised from information at hand.

It is beyond the scope of this chapter to describe the biosynthesis of cholesterol and its product, 7-dehydrocholesterol (D5). It is known, however, that 7-dehydrocholesterol, which is shown in Fig. 2, is produced in substantial quantities in the epidermis of skin. This sterol is found in the epidermis at a level to which 300 nm ultraviolet light will readily penetrate (D1). It is known that the ultraviolet irradiation of skin taken from rachitic animals will acquire the ability to cure rickets. Because of the existence of 7-dehydrocholesterol in skin, it is surmised that the product produced is vitamin D_3 because it is known that the irradiation of 7-dehydrocholesterol in organic solvents will produce not only vitamin D_3, but a number of other photoisomers. However, it must be made clear that the product vitamin D_3 has never been isolated in pure form from skin, nor has its production been unequivocally demonstrated in that tissue, although it seems highly probable that this is what occurs.

It is not known whether the production of vitamin D_3 in the skin is regulated or not. It would appear that tanning of skin or the existence of a high degree of pigmentation filters out some of the ultraviolet light, preventing or decreasing production of vitamin D_3. This concept has led Loomis (L8) to suggest that black races have evolved primarily because of their skin protection against production of vitamin D_3, which can be toxic in large amounts. By the same token, he has postulated that white-skinned individuals have evolved because of their efficient production of vitamin D_3. Whether or not this is the case remains to be determined, however. It is believed that the vitamin D_3 produced in the skin then appears in the circulation and is channeled into the metabolic pathways to be described.

Of considerable practical importance is the production of vitamin D_2 by commercial processes (S5). It is unlikely that vitamin D_2 represents a form of the vitamin that is produced in any substantial amounts in nature. However, because ergosterol was the first activatable sterol to be isolated, and because this sterol can be obtained cheaply and in large quantities from molds and microorganisms, it assumed the central position for vitamin D production early in vitamin D history. As a result, the major form of vitamin D that has appeared in supplemented diets in the past has been vitamin D_2. Its production from ergosterol by ultraviolet irradiation is also shown in Fig. 2. As will be shown, vitamin D_2, although being the unnatural form of vitamin D, as far as can be seen at the present time is equally as active as vitamin D_3 in man and other mammals, but is much less active than vitamin D_3 in birds (C3) and New-World monkeys (H29).

5. The Absorption and Transport of Vitamin D

Vitamin D is quite efficiently absorbed. It has been estimated that as much as 75% of orally administered vitamin D is absorbed in the rat (K3, N3). It has long been known that the absorption of vitamin D requires the presence of bile salts (G14). This has recently been reaffirmed but was clearly demonstrated by early works of Greaves and Schmidt. There has been little substantive work carried out on the site and mechanism of vitamin D absorption. In work on the disappearance of radioactive vitamin D from the intestines of rats, it appears that the distal small intestine is likely involved in absorption of vitamin D when it is dissolved in oils or fats (K3, N3). Apparently when vitamin D is presented to the intestine in bile salt solutions, it is more rapidly absorbed in the upper segments of the small intestine (S3). Presumably vitamin D enters together with the lipids through the lymphatic system and the blood system as chylomicrons, which are removed from the circulation by the liver. Vitamin D injected into the bloodstream becomes associated initially with both an α-globulin and a β-lipoprotein (R7). Upon more prolonged exposure, the vitamin D is found bound to the α-globulin; although there has been one report describing a specific vitamin D transport protein in birds, this has not proved to be the case in man or in rats. It seems likely that the major blood transport protein for vitamin D is an α-globulin of approximately 52,000 MW which has been isolated from rats (B11) and from man (P2). Little more is known about the transport protein, and little is known concerning the regulation of its biosynthesis.

6. Metabolism of Vitamin D

In this section the path of vitamin D metabolism will be described as it is currently known without reference to the functional forms of vitamin D and without reference to their participation in the functions of the vitamin; these will be described in a later section.

Initially vitamin D is rapidly removed from the plasma by the liver. As much as 60–80% of injected vitamin D is rapidly removed from the plasma by the liver within 60 minutes after administration (O4, P3). This is unlike other forms of vitamin D, which do not rapidly accumulate in the liver. Therefore, an important first mechanism is the uptake of vitamin D by the liver in substantial amounts. In the liver, vitamin D undergoes its first modification. In cells yet to be described it is known that vitamin D is hydroxylated on carbon-25 to produce 25-OH-D₃, as shown in Fig. 3 (H26, P4). This reaction occurs predominantly in the microsomal fraction of liver homogenates in both chicks and rats (B7, H25). Molecular oxygen is used as the source of oxygen and the reaction requires NADPH as well as magnesium ions. The reaction is not inhibited by carbon monoxide or other cytochrome P-450 inhibitors, nor is it inhibited by such lipid peroxidation inhibitors as diphenylparaphenylenediamine. The chemical mechanism of this hydroxylation, therefore, remains largely unknown and the subject of future investigation. In agreement with the inhibitor data, current evidence suggests that the feeding of phenobarbital, which increases microsomal P-450 dependent enzyme content in the liver, does not substantially affect the vitamin D-25-hydroxylase. In addition to the vitamin

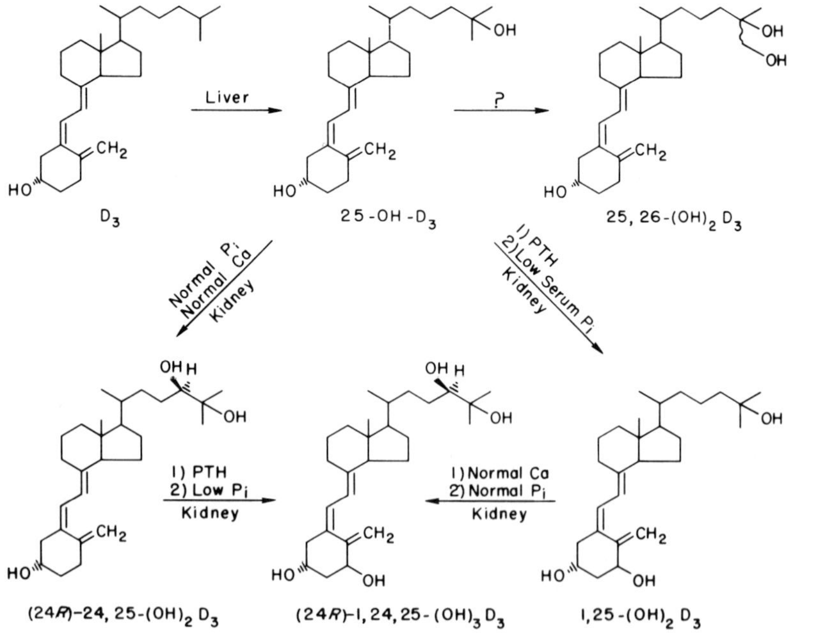

FIG. 3.   The known metabolic pathways of vitamin D conversion and the factors that regulate the conversion. PTH, parathyroid hormone.

D-25-hydroxylase, another rather nonspecific 25-hydroxylase appears to exist in liver tissues primarily in mitochondria (B7). This reaction appears to hydroxylate cholesterol on the 25 position and may act on vitamin D when it is present in large concentrations. The importance of this 25-hydroxylase to vitamin D metabolism remains unknown at the present time. The 25-OH-D_3 is secreted into the bloodstream from the liver and is bound to an α^2-globulin (B4, B11, P2). The level of 25-OH-D_3 in the bloodstream is remarkably constant, being in the neighborhood of 15–30 ng/ml, depending upon the method of assay used and the nutritional status of the population being sampled. The level of 25-OH-D_3 in the blood does not rise in proportion to the dosage of vitamin D given. In fact, there appears to be a feedback regulation on 25-hydroxylation by the hepatic level of 25-OH-D_3 itself (B5, B8). The mechanism of this regulation is not known, but it is believed that the microsomal reaction is inhibited either by product inhibition or by some allosteric means by 25-OH-D_3 of the liver and, as this is removed into the bloodstream, the hydroxylase is released to produce additional supplies of 25-OH-D_3. In the presence of large amounts of vitamin D, however, this regulation can be overcome either by competition or by the nonspecific mitochondrial 25-hydroxylase, which begins to function at higher substrate concentrations. Thus the circulating level of 25-OH-D_3 can be increased from the 20-ng range to several hundred nanograms per milliliter by giving large amounts of vitamin D (B10, H2).

The 25-OH-D_3 is specifically bound by the α-globulin described above for vitamin D_3. This globulin of 52,000 MW binds 25-OH-D_3 with a K_d of 1.8×10^{-9} M. It appears to bind one molecule of 25-OH-D per molecule of protein (B11, P2). The 25-OH-D_3 can be regarded as the major circulating form of vitamin D, being often in excess of vitamin D itself. The 25-OH-D_3 is picked up by the kidney, where it is converted to one of two products. As will be shown in the regulation section, if there is a need for calcium or for phosphorus, the kidneys have exclusively an enzyme called 25-OH-D_3-1-hydroxylase. This enzyme is found exclusively in the mitochondria and hydroxylates 25-OH-D_3 in the 1 position to produce $1\alpha,25$-dihydroxyvitamin D_3 ($1\alpha,25$-$(OH)_2D_3$) (F3, G12, G13). No evidence for 1-hydroxylation has been found in any other tissue and nephrectomized animals do not show an ability to carry out the 1-hydroxylation reaction. This enzyme has received considerable attention, and it is now known that it is highly specific for 25-OH-D_3, showing no activity whatsoever on vitamin D_3 itself or any analog that does not have a 25-hydroxyl function (G13). It does not hydroxylate 25-hydroxydihydrotachysterol or analogs of 25-OH-D_3, which apparently have a group that sterically hinders 1-hydroxylation. This mitochondrial enzyme has been solubilized, and its components were separated and reconstituted (G6). There is no question that the active hydroxylating enzyme is a cytochrome P-450 which has been proved both by spectral means and by isolation. The cytochrome P-450 incorporates one molecule of molecular oxygen into the 1-hydroxyl position, showing it to be a mixed-function oxidase (G5). In order for this cytochrome P-450 to operate, it must have an iron-sulfur protein, and recently it has been possible to isolate in relatively pure form the iron-sulfur protein, which is called a renal ferredoxin (P1). This substance is reduced by a renal ferredoxin reductase which is a flavoprotein and analogous to the adrenal adrenodoxin reductase. This is in turn reduced by NADPH. The NADPH is generated inside the mitochondria by energy-dependent transhydrogenation reaction. Thus in intact mitochondria, Krebs cycle substrates, electron transport, and oxidative phosphorylation generate sufficient amounts of NADPH to produce the hydroxylation of 25-OH-D_3 to 1,25-$(OH)_2D_3$, which is considered to be the hormonal form of the vitamin. A diagrammatic sketch of the mechanism of the 1-hydroxylase enzyme is shown in Fig. 4.

If the animal shows no need for calcium or for phosphorus, the kidney possesses predominantly another hydroxylase instead of the 1-hydroxylase, namely, the 25-OH-D_3-24-hydroxylase (H23, T6). Apparently this enzyme is not exclusively located in the kidney (G3), although within the kidney it apparently is exclusively located in the mitochondrial fraction. It is not clear whether this reaction is a mixed-function oxidase, nor is it clear whether it is dependent upon a cytochrome P-450 enzyme since it is not inhibited by carbon monoxide-oxygen mixtures, whereas the 1-hydroxylase is. This enzyme has a similar substrate specificity to the 1-hydroxylase; namely, it requires 25-hydroxyl function on a vitamin D backbone (T6). It is unknown whether the reaction will hydroxylate dihydrotachysterol, but it certainly does not hydroxylate vitamin D_3 itself. The product of the reaction is 24,25-dihydroxyvitamin D_3 (24,25-$(OH)_2D_3$) (H23), and it is immediately apparent that there are two stereo-

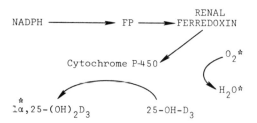

Fig. 4. Mechanism of 25-OH-D_3-1-hydroxylation by the chick kidney mitochondrial 1-hydroxylase system.

isomers possible with the hydroxyl function sticking either in or out of the plane. With the hydroxyl function sticking out of the plane, the configuration is designated as 24R,25-$(OH)_2D_3$, and it has been clearly demonstrated that the natural product has the 24R configuration (T6). The 24-hydroxylase will act not only on 25-OH-D_3, but on 1,25-$(OH)_2D_3$ to produce 1,24,25-trihydroxyvitamin D_3 (1,24,25-$(OH)_3D_3$) (K2, T7a). In vitamin D-deficient animals, the 24-hydroxylase is absent or is present in extremely low concentrations such that the predominant enzymic activity is the 25-OH-D_3-1-hydroxylase (T3, T5). After the administration of 1,25-$(OH)_2D_3$, there is a rapid appearance of the 24-hydroxylase, and it now appears that 1,25-$(OH)_2D_3$ may induce the appearance of the 25-OH-D_3-24-hydroxylase. The fate of the 24-hydroxylated vitamins remains unknown, although they appear to be rapidly metabolized and excreted, especially in the chicken and probably in mammals, at least when normal amounts of vitamin D are present (H21). Although the conversion of 24,25-$(OH)_2D_3$ to 1,24,25-$(OH)_3D_3$ can be shown by injection of the 24,25-$(OH)_2D_3$ into vitamin D-deficient animals or by incubation of the compound with kidney preparations from rachitic chickens, it is not clear whether this pathway has any significance *in vivo* inasmuch as conditions under which 24,25-$(OH)_2D_3$ is formed there is little or no 1-hydroxylase present. On the other hand, when 1,25-$(OH)_2D_3$ is produced, this substance immediately induces the appearance of the 24-hydroxylase, and it is indeed possible that 1,24,25-$(OH)_3D_3$ may represent an important route of 1,25-$(OH)_2D_3$ metabolism.

Recently it has been demonstrated clearly that 1,25-$(OH)_2D_3$ undergoes a reaction in which the side chain is oxidized (H6, K8). By labeling 1,25-$(OH)_2D_3$ on carbons 26 and 27 with carbon 14, it has been possible to show the appearance of carbon dioxide in the expired air of animals. This conversion is independent of serum calcium and phosphorus and dietary calcium and phosphorus levels. The exact nature of this pathway is not known and is currently under investigation. The site of this reaction is not known but is believed to be the intestine, and it may well have functional importance.

The major route of excretion of vitamin D and its metabolites is the bile (B2, N3), with less than 4% appearing in the urine (A3). Although the biliary metabolites have been studied and there has been the suggestion that there exist sulfates as well as glucuronides, so far no product has been clearly identified.

Sulfates of vitamin D have been isolated and identified from rabbits given large amounts of vitamin D (H14), and the vitamin D sulfates have been described in milk (L7). It is not clear what their importance is physiologically or whether they represent a major excretory pathway.

The metabolism of vitamin D_2, in contrast to vitamin D_3, has been studied very little. However, both 25-hydroxyvitamin D_2 (25-OH-D_2) and 1,25-dihydroxyvitamin D_2 (1,25-$(OH)_2D_2$) have been isolated in pure form and their structures identified (J1, S20). Similarly, 24,25-dihydroxyvitamin D_2 (24,25-$(OH)_2D_2$) has also been isolated and identified (G. Jones, H. K. Schnoes, and H. F. DeLuca, unpublished results). The path of vitamin D_2 apparently is identical in both the rat and the bird (J2). It certainly appears at this time that 1,25-$(OH)_2D_2$ represents the hormonal form of vitamin D_2 and as far as can be determined for man, vitamin D_2 undergoes identical reactions and appears to be equivalent biologically to the vitamin D_3 series. In the bird, however, it has long been known that vitamin D_2 or ergocalciferol is much less biologically active than is vitamin D_3. This interesting divergence of biological activity in these species has been pursued. It has been shown that radioactive vitamin D_2 disappears very rapidly from the circulation of birds and appears in the biliary and fecal excretion products (I1). An examination of the enzymes which carry out the 25-hydroxylation and the 1- and 24-hydroxylation reactions demonstrate that the chick enzymes act identically on the vitamin D_2 compounds as they do on the vitamin D_3 compounds (J2). However, when the metabolites are given to vitamin D-deficient chicks, it is apparent that the vitamin D_2 metabolites are approximately one-tenth as active as their vitamin D_3 counterparts (J3). Furthermore, they are also rapidly metabolized and excreted, which suggests that the mechanism of discrimination is likely a reaction which rapidly conjugates or inactivates the vitamin D_2 compounds and prepares them for biliary excretion. This, however, has not been firmly established.

7. Vitamin D as a Prohormone

In all the functions described under Section 3, vitamin D does not act immediately to produce those responses, but instead there is a substantial time lag between administration and response. This led initially to an investigation in the author's laboratory in search of the reason for the delay. It soon became apparent that vitamin D is rapidly metabolized prior to these responses, and the metabolites that could be separated from vitamin D by column chromatography were shown to be more active and could act much more rapidly than the parent vitamin (L10, M8). This led to a substantial effort in the isolation and identification of the biologically active metabolites of vitamin D, yielding the compounds listed in the preceding section (B10, H22, J1, S20). Thus, as shown in Fig. 5, 25-OH-D_3 acts much more rapidly than vitamin D_3 in producing an intestinal response, whereas 1,25-$(OH)_2D_3$ is the most rapidly acting form

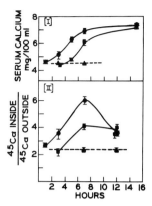

Fig. 5. The time course of response of intestinal calcium transport (lower panel) and bone calcium mobilization system (upper panel) to the metabolites (650 pmoles intravenously) of vitamin D. In the case of each of the two responses, vitamin D_3 itself at the same dosage level would not produce a response until 10–12 hours after intravenous administration. Intestinal calcium transport was measured by the everted-sac technique in the upper segment of the duodenum whereas bone calcium mobilization was measured by the elevation of serum calcium concentration of rats maintained on a vitamin D-deficient low-calcium diet (M1, T1). ●——●, 1,25-dihydroxyvitamin D_3; ■——■, 25-hydroxyvitamin D_3; ▲---▲, control.

of vitamin D known, producing a clear and measurable response by 3 hours, which reaches a maximum at 6 hours after dosage. When the metabolites are examined for their biological activity, it is apparent when they are administered each day parenterally that $1,25\text{-}(OH)_2D_3$ is ten times and $25\text{-}OH\text{-}D_3$ is three times more active than the parent vitamin in curing rickets, in initiating intestinal calcium absorption, and in mobilizing calcium from bone (T4). Furthermore, the $1,25\text{-}(OH)_2D_3$ is active when added directly to tissue cultures, whereas $25\text{-}OH\text{-}D_3$ is active at very large concentrations and vitamin D_3 itself is inactive or much less active (R1, R4, S19, T12).

Although these results suggested very clearly that $1,25\text{-}(OH)_2D_3$ is probably the biologically active form, proof was lacking. The fact that the kidney is the sole site of 1-hydroxylation of $25\text{-}OH\text{-}D_3$ made possible certain experiments that show conclusively that at physiologic doses or concentrations, $1,25\text{-}(OH)_2D_3$, or a further metabolite, must be the active form. Thus nephrectomized, vitamin D-deficient animals do not show an intestinal calcium transport response (B13), a bone calcium mobilization response (H16), or an intestinal phosphate transport response (C7) to $25\text{-}OH\text{-}D_3$ at physiologic concentrations. These animals, on the other hand, respond to $1,25\text{-}(OH)_2D_3$ equally well whether kidneys are present or not. It is, therefore, clear that $1,25\text{-}(OH)_2D_3$ or a further metabolite is the metabolically active form, at least in these systems. Since 1,25-$(OH)_2D_3$ is produced in the kidney and has its target of action in intestine and bone, it can be regarded as a hormone. As a hormone, its biogenesis should be regulated in a feedback manner by the physiologic products it seeks to affect. Vitamin D-deficient animals, however, have substantial amounts of 25-OH-D_3-1-hydroxylase and no measurable vitamin D_3-24-hydroxylase (B12, T3, T5). This is true regardless of the dietary calcium and phosphorus levels and regardless of the serum calcium and phosphorus levels of the animal. Thus the 1-hydroxylase enzyme is not subject to regulation in the vitamin D-deficient animal. However, as pointed out in the previous section on metabolism, 1,25-$(OH)_2D_3$ when given to vitamin D-deficient animals will cause the appearance of the 25-OH-D_3-24-hydroxylase, and as this hydroxylase appears in kidney tissue, the 25-OH-D_3-1-hydroxylase begins to diminish (T5). Thus it seems that the 1,25-$(OH)_2D_3$ induces the appearance of the 24-hydroxylase. It is after such an induction has taken place that the renal vitamin D hydroxylases become subject to regulation by the need for calcium and the need for phosphorus. The nature of the induction process, if it is such, by 1,25-$(OH)_2D_3$ is not known although 1,25-$(OH)_2D_3$ does stimulate RNA synthesis in the kidney, which may suggest such an induction (C4).

7.1. REGULATION OF THE RENAL VITAMIN D HYDROXYLASES BY THE NEED FOR CALCIUM

Normal calcemic animals produce both 1,25-$(OH)_2D_3$ and 24,25-$(OH)_2D_3$. If there is a reduction in serum calcium concentration by calcium deprivation or other means, there is a stimulation of 1,25-$(OH)_2D_3$ synthesis and a suppression of 24,25-$(OH)_2D_3$ synthesis (Fig. 6). On the other side of the coin, when plasma calcium rises above normal, the production of 1,25-$(OH)_2D_3$ is shut down and the production of 24,25-$(OH)_2D_3$ is stimulated. Since 1,25-$(OH)_2D_3$ is a calcium-mobilizing hormone, it is reasonable therefore that the need for calcium regulates the biosynthesis of this calcium-mobilizing hormone. Inasmuch as the rise in serum calcium levels above normal stimulates production of 24,25-$(OH)_2D_3$, one can logically ask what the function of this metabolite might be. An examination of the biological activity of the 24-hydroxylated forms of vitamin D as compared to their non-24-hydroxylated counterparts in both rats and chicks has revealed that the 24-hydroxylated compounds have markedly lower biological activity than their non-24-hydroxylated counterparts (H21, T6, T7). Furthermore, they are rapidly metabolized and excreted, suggesting that 24-hydroxylation may be an inactivation mechanism (H21). Recently there has been the suggestion that this compound may participate in suppression of parathyroid hormone secretion,

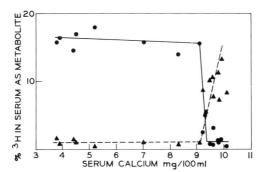

FIG. 6. The relationship of serum calcium concentration to the accumulation of 1,25-(●——●) and 24,25-(▲---▲) dihydroxyvitamin D₃ in the serum of young grow-ing rats. Serum calcium concentration was adjusted by means of dietary manipulations, and, after appropriate adjustment, conversion of radioactive 25-OH-D₃ to the two metabolites indicated during the 12-hour period was measured (B12).

although the evidence for this idea is far from convincing. At the present time the best approximation is that 24-hydroxylation is important for help-ing regulate the 1-hydroxylase and probably represents the mechanism utilized in the inactivation of the vitamin D molecule.

The regulation of 1,25-(OH)₂D₃ synthesis by the serum calcium level is mediated by the parathyroid glands (F4, G2). In response to hypocal-cemia the parathyroid glands secrete parathyroid hormone, which in some unknown way stimulates production of 1,25-(OH)₂D₃; this in turn stimu-lates the mobilization of calcium from bone and intestine. The parathyroid hormone, therefore, appears to act in a manner analogous to adrenal corticotropin for steroidogenesis; i.e., the need for calcium stimulates the production of parathyroid hormone, which in turn stimulates production of the major calcium-mobilizing hormone of the body—1,25-(OH)₂D₃.

7.2. 1,25-(OH)₂D₃ IN CALCIUM HOMEOSTASIS

Because of the finding that parathyroid hormone stimulates production of 1,25-(OH)₂D₃, a calcium-mobilizing hormone, it has been possible to reevaluate the relationship between the peptide hormone and vitamin D in regard to their relative roles in calcium homeostasis. It is now suffi-ciently clear that the parathyroid hormone stimulates intestinal calcium absorption by stimulating production of 1,25-(OH)₂D₃ in the kidney (G2, R5, R6). Once 1,25-(OH)₂D₃ is produced, the parathyroid hormone does not function on the intestine directly. The response of intestine from vita-min D-deficient, parathyroidectomized rats to 1,25-(OH)₂D₃ is identical whether parathyroid hormone is present or not. In fact, radioactive para-thyroid hormone does not bind to the intestine *in vivo* (Z1). On the other hand, the parathyroid hormone does bind to bone, and it can be demonstrated that the bone calcium mobilization system does not respond to $1,25\text{-}(OH)_2D_3$ unless the parathyroid hormone is also present. It is, therefore, clear that to mobilize calcium from bone both parathyroid hormone and $1,25\text{-}(OH)_2D_3$ are necessary whereas in the intestine only $1,25\text{-}(OH)_2D_3$ appears to be essential. Besides these functions of the parathyroid hormone, it is also known that the parathyroid hormone causes a phosphate diuresis in the kidney and is also known to improve renal reabsorption of calcium. Putting together these relationships, the calcium homeostatic mechanism can be substantially revised as shown in Fig. 7. In this system, when serum calcium falls below 10 mg/100 ml, which is considered the normal level of serum calcium in man, the parathyroid glands are stimulated to secrete parathyroid hormone. The parathyroid hormone progresses to bone and to kidney, where they can both be shown to have specific receptor sites. In the kidney the parathyroid hormone causes a phosphate diuresis not shown in that figure. It also stimulates production of $1,25\text{-}(OH)_2D_3$ and improves renal reabsorption of calcium. The $1,25\text{-}(OH)_2D_3$ proceeds to the intestine where it, without parathyroid hormone, stimulates intestinal calcium absorption. It also progresses to the bone where, together with parathyroid hormone, calcium is mobilized. Calcium from bone, intestine, and kidney, therefore, causes an elevation of extracellular fluid calcium resulting in a suppression of parathyroid hormone secretion, which in turn shuts down $1,25\text{-}(OH)_2D_3$ production, completing the calcium homeostatic mechanism.

When serum calcium rises above normal, the "C" cells, or parafollicular cells of the thyroid, are stimulated to secrete the peptide hormone, calcitonin, which proceeds to the bone and possibly intestine, where it suppresses calcium mobilization, bringing about a fall in plasma calcium concentration.

From this revised calcium homeostatic mechanism, it is evident that patients completely devoid of parathyroid hormone cannot mobilize calcium from bone even though they may have exogenous supplies of $1,25\text{-}(OH)_2D_3$. Hypoparathyroidism, therefore, represents a disease whereby the active form of vitamin D is not produced in sufficient quantities in response to the need for calcium. It is, therefore, clear that besides osteomalacia and rickets, a disturbance of vitamin D metabolism can also be observed in hypoparathyroidism, giving as a result hypocalcemic tetany.

7.3. $1,25\text{-}(OH)_2D_3$ AS A PHOSPHATE-MOBILIZING HORMONE

As pointed out in the preceding section, vitamin D plays an important role in the elevation of plasma phosphorus concentration by stimulating intestinal phosphate absorption and by stimulating mobilization of phos-

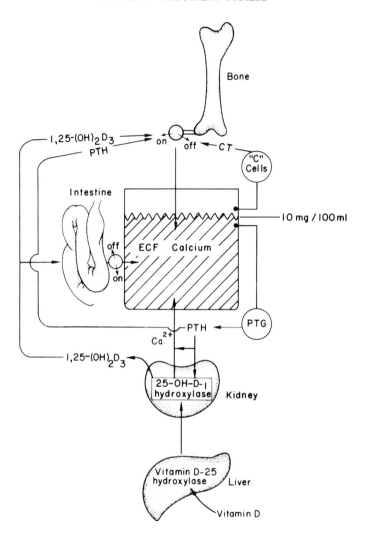

FIG. 7. Diagrammatic representation of the calcium homeostatic mechanism as it is presently understood, including the vitamin D endocrine system. PTG, parathyroid gland; PTH, parathyroid hormone; ECF, extracellular fluid; CT, calcitonin; 1,25-(OH)₂ D₃, 1,25-dihydroxyvitamin D₃.

phate from bone (C2). It may also stimulate renal tubular reabsorption of phosphate. Therefore, an important function of vitamin D is to stimulate phosphate transport reactions. Of considerable importance is the fact that rickets cannot be produced in rats unless they are deprived both of phosphate and vitamin D. Furthermore, Fraser and Scriver have described the sequence of rachitogenesis in man, which reveals that the bony lesions of rickets appear only after hypophosphatemia begins to appear (F1). In addition, one can substantially reverse the bony lesions of rickets both in children and in rats by the provision of adequate amounts of inorganic phosphorus. It may be, therefore, that the elevation of serum phosphorus concentration is primarily responsible for the mineralization of bone in the curing of rickets and osteomalacia.

As might be expected, since 1,25-(OH)$_2$D$_3$ has a substantial role in the elevation of plasma phosphate, the plasma inorganic phosphorus concentration plays an important role in the regulation of 1,25-(OH)$_2$D$_3$ biosynthesis (T2). By removing the thyroparathyroid glands, it is possible to study the relationship of serum phosphorus concentration to the production of 1,25-(OH)$_2$D$_3$ as shown in Fig. 8 (T2). Thyroparathyroidectomized rats having normal serum phosphorus concentrations produce 24,25-(OH)$_2$D$_3$ and little 1,25-(OH)$_2$D$_3$. If, however, they are made hypophosphatemic by phosphate deprivation, one can stimulate the production of 1,25-(OH)$_2$D$_3$ and suppress 24,25-(OH)$_2$D$_3$ synthesis. Thus the need for phosphorus can stimulate 1,25-(OH)$_2$D$_3$ production by a mechanism not involving parathyroid hormone secretion. The relationship of plasma phosphorus concentration to the level of kidney 25-OH-D$_3$-1-hydroxylase can be clearly demonstrated in the chick (B1). Since 1,25-(OH)$_2$D$_3$ production is controlled by serum phosphorus concentration in part, and

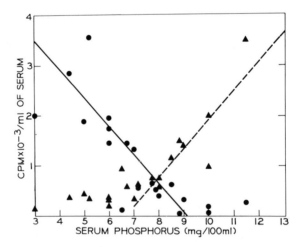

FIG. 8. The relationship of serum inorganic phosphorus concentration to the accumulation of 1,25-dihydroxyvitamin D$_3$ (●) or 24,25-dihydroxyvitamin D$_3$ (▲) in plasma of thyroparathyroidectomized rats. Serum inorganic phosphorus concentration was adjusted by dietary deprivation or by administration of glucose. After adjustment, the conversion of radioactive 25-hydroxyvitamin D$_3$ to the appropriate metabolite was studied *in vivo* as described by Tanaka and DeLuca (T2).

since it has a function in stimulating intestinal phosphate transport, we can regard 1,25-$(OH)_2D_3$ as a phosphate-mobilizing, as well as a calcium-mobilizing, hormone.

Because 1,25-$(OH)_2D_3$ can be considered to have two functions—calcium mobilization and phosphate mobilization—and its production is regulated by two signals, it is difficult to understand how a single hormone can correct the appropriate and specific signal. It is indeed possible to demonstrate that 1,25-$(OH)_2D_3$, by interacting with the parathyroid hormone, can satisfy both requirements (D2). If one examines the sequence of events following a hypocalcemic stimulus, it becomes clear that hypocalcemia results in parathyroid hormone secretion. The parathyroid hormone stimulates 1,25-$(OH)_2D_3$ production and the 1,25-$(OH)_2D_3$ in turn stimulates the intestine to absorb calcium and stimulates the bone to mobilize calcium, which is possible because of the presence of the parathyroid hormone. However, 1,25-$(OH)_2D_3$ also stimulates phosphate absorption and mobilization from bone, but because of the parathyroid hormone causes a phosphate diuresis, the loss of phosphate in the urine essentially cancels the phosphate-elevating effect of the 1,25-$(OH)_2D_3$ in the serum. Thus under hypocalcemic stimulus, the 1,25-$(OH)_2D_3$ system, together with parathyroid hormone, results in a rise in serum calcium with little or no change in serum phosphorus.

On the other hand, a hypophosphatemic stimulus does not involve parathyroid hormone secretion, and in fact parathyroid hormone secretion is probably suppressed. Low serum phosphorus stimulates 1,25-$(OH)_2D_3$ production; and 1,25-$(OH)_2D_3$ cannot mobilize calcium from bone because parathyroid hormone is absent. It does stimulate intestinal calcium absorption, but, because parathyroid hormone is lacking, some of the calcium absorbed will not be reabsorbed in the kidney. 1,25-$(OH)_2D_3$ will stimulate mobilization of phosphorus both from intestine and bone, and since there is no parathyroid hormone present, there will be no loss of phosphorus in the urine; thus the hypophosphatemic stimulus brings about an elevation in serum phosphorus with only a slight increase in serum calcium concentration. Thus 1,25-$(OH)_2D_3$ can act as a calcium-mobilizing hormone and as a phosphate-mobilizing hormone.

There has been considerable attention focused recently on the idea that 1,25-$(OH)_2D_3$ or other vitamin D metabolites might feedback suppress the secretion of parathyroid hormone. In fact, work has been done that would demonstrate that there is an accumulation of 1,25-$(OH)_2D_3$ in the parathyroid gland (H12), and more recently evidence for the existence of a receptor for 1,25-$(OH)_2D_3$ in parathyroid glands has been presented (B17). However, physiologic experiments that might support the idea that parathyroid hormone secretion is suppressed directly by

vitamin D metabolites is at least controversial. There is need for considerable and substantial physiologic experiments to examine the question in
some detail before this idea can be accepted; although it may be intellectu-
ally appealing.

7.4. Mechanism of Regulation of the Vitamin D Hydroxylases

As has been pointed out earlier, it is not known how $1,25\text{-}(OH)_2D_3$
brings about the appearance of the $25\text{-}OH\text{-}D_3\text{-}24$-hydroxylase, nor is there
any evidence as to how this may result in a suppression of the $25\text{-}OH\text{-}D_3$-
1-hydroxylase. However, because low blood phosphorus as well as parathyroid hormone secretion stimulates $1,25\text{-}(OH)_2D_3$ production, a hypothesis
has appeared that may have physiologic merit (D3). It has been suggested
that the renal cell level of inorganic phosphorus may be the determinant
as to whether the 1-hydroxylase functions or whether the 24-hydroxylase
functions. If the renal cell level of inorganic phosphorus falls below a
given figure of approximately 400 $\mu g/g$, the 1-hydroxylase is favored,
whereas if it rises above that figure, the 24-hydroxylase is favored. Renal
cell level of inorganic phosphorus can be lowered by either phosphate
deprivation, which provides less phosphorus to be absorbed in the renal
tubules, resulting in lowered renal cell level of inorganic phosphorus, or
it could be lowered by parathyroid hormone, which blocks renal tubule
reabsorption of phosphorus. This hypothesis is supported by direct measurements of renal cortical levels of inorganic phosphorus (T2), but it
must be regarded as a hypothesis without further substantiation. Other
than this, the actual mechanism whereby the 1-hydroxylase or the 24-hy-
droxylase is stimulated or suppressed remains largely unknown. The
changeover in the hydroxylases from a physiologic point of view requires
many hours. Evidence has been presented against the idea that the
changeover is the result of a direct ionic inhibition or activation of the
enzymes, but rather because the lifetime of the enzymes is on the order
of 2–3 hours, the mechanism may involve the regulation of enzyme synthesis or degradation.

8. Analogs of $1,25\text{-}(OH)_2D_3$

With the discovery that vitamin D is converted to $1,25\text{-}(OH)_2D_3$ before
it can function has come renewed interest in the possibility that analogs
(Fig. 9) of vitamin D can be prepared which would either have enhanced
biological activity, specific biological activity or antivitamin activity. So
far none of these ends have been achieved, although there are analogs of
particular interest that are worthy of discussion.

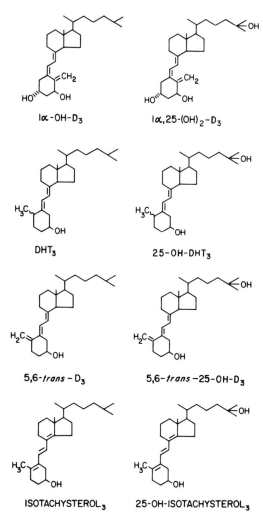

FIG. 9. Analogs of 1,25-dihydroxyvitamin D_3 (1,25-$(OH)_2D_3$). DHT$_3$, dihydrotachysterol$_3$.

Long before it was realized that vitamin D must be metabolically altered, an analog of 1,25-$(OH)_2D_3$ was prepared. Dihydrotachysterol, from either the vitamin D_2 or the vitamin D_3 series, was prepared by reduction of irradiation mixtures, primarily to stabilize the preparations. The active product from this treatment proved to be dihydrotachysterol, the structure of which is shown in Fig. 9. This compound, which is still widely used in the treatment of hypocalcemic diseases and in some cases in the treatment of vitamin D-resistant rickets, proved to have interesting properties long before there appeared a biochemical rationale for its effectiveness. At low concentrations or doses, the dihydrotachysterols are much less active than vitamin D_3, having antirachitic activity somewhere between 1/250 and 1/500 (S21). However, at high doses commonly used in therapy of vitamin D-resistant disease, the dihydrotachysterols appear to be much more effective than vitamin D itself. This empirical observation and the fact that its activity had a much shorter half-life than large doses of vitamin D led to its wide acceptance and use in disease.

In 1971, when it was realized that the metabolically active form of vitamin D is $1,25-(OH)_2D_3$, it was recognized that the dihydrotachysterol structure is analogous to the $1,25-(OH)_2D_3$ inasmuch as the A ring of this compound is rotated 180° relative to vitamin D (H3, H4). This placed the 3-hydroxyl function in a spatial position similar to that occupied by the 1-hydroxyl of $1,25-(OH)_2D_3$. Thus it became obvious that dihydrotachysterols could be functioning as analogs of $1,25-(OH)_2D_3$ rather than of the vitamin itself. Radioactive dihydrotachysterol$_3$ was chemically synthesized and shown to be rapidly converted to 25-hydroxydihydrotachysterol, primarily by liver preparations (H3). The conversion of the dihydrotachysterol to the 25-hydroxydihydrotachysterol, however, is not feedback inhibited by either $25-OH-D_3$ or 25-hydroxydihydrotachysterol itself (B6). Likely the dihydrotachysterol is hydroxylated on carbon 25 by the mitochondrial enzyme, as described in the previous section. Thus the dihydrotachysterol is rapidly converted to 25-hydroxydihydrotachysterol and then functions directly on intestine and bone. Nephrectomized, vitamin D-deficient animals respond just as well to 25-hydroxydihydrotachysterol or dihydrotachysterol as do intact animals (H3, H7), illustrating that the kidney is not involved in its function, and furthermore studies with radioactive dihydrotachysterol, both *in vivo* and *in vitro*, have failed to show any 1-hydroxylation by the kidney enzyme which hydroxylates $25-OH-D_3$ in the 1 position (G13, H3, H4). The dihydrotachysterol is rapidly metabolized and excreted, thereby accounting for its short-lived biological activity. Because it is available and has been cleared through the various Food and Drug Administration authorities, the dihydrotachysterol is currently the best available compound as a substitute for $1,25-(OH)_2D_3$.

With the discovery that dihydrotachysterol and 25-hydroxydihydrotachysterol are analogs of $1,25-(OH)_2D_3$ came the search for other possible analogs that are easy to prepare. It is possible to isomerize vitamin D_3 to its 5,6-*trans* isomer, and furthermore it can be further isomerized to the isotachysterol form. In addition, the $25-OH-D_3$ can be isomerized to form the 5,6-*trans*-25-OH-D_3 (H15, H17). All these compounds function analogously to the dihydrotachysterols; namely, they are just as active in the absence of kidneys as in their presence, which illustrates that the compounds are not 1-hydroxylated before function. However, from a biological point of view they are approximately 1/1000 to 1/10,000 times less active than their analog, 1,25-$(OH)_2D_3$. Nevertheless they can be given in large amounts and can be considered as analogs of 1,25-$(OH)_2D_3$ by virtue of their rapid conversion to the 25-hydroxy derivative in the liver. Although the 5,6-*trans*-vitamin D_3 has been used in the treatment of hypocalcemia and impaired intestinal calcium absorption in renal failure (R8), it is not likely that these compounds will be useful from a therapeutic point of view; but they do represent important and curious analogs that may have significance in vitamin D toxicity.

Perhaps the most important of the analogs of 1,25-$(OH)_2D_3$ prepared to date are the 1α-hydroxyvitamin D_3 (1α-OH-D_3) and 1α-hydroxyvitamin D_2 (1α-OH-D_2). The 1α-OH-D_3 was prepared as a chemical synthetic exercise in the author's laboratory when a procedure for the chemical synthesis of 1,25-$(OH)_2D_3$ was first devised (H20). This compound proved to be extremely interesting, having biological activity approximately one-half that of 1,25-$(OH)_2D_3$ in the rat (H19) and almost equal activity to 1,25-$(OH)_2D_3$ in the chicken (H10). Several chemical syntheses have been devised for the compound, illustrating its ease of preparation, and hence it represents a viable alternative to 1,25-$(OH)_2D_3$ as a therapeutic agent. 1α-OH-D_2 has also been prepared and appears to be identical with 1α-OH-D_3 in biological activity in mammals (L1); however, the 1α-OH-D_2 is much less active than the 1α-OH-D_3 in birds (J3), representing once again the side-chain discrimination for the vitamin D_2 structure by these species. Because of the rapidity with which 1α-OH-D_3 functions and because it has biological activity equal to 1,25-$(OH)_2D_3$ in the bird, it has been suggested that 1α-OH-D_3 is not hydroxylated before it can function, and that the 25-hydroxyl function might be necessary only to direct the 1-hydroxylase enzyme and then is no longer necessary for function in the target tissue. However, recently 1α-OH-D_3 labeled in the 6 position with tritium has been chemically synthesized, and with this material it has been possible to demonstrate that this compound is converted rapidly to 1,25-$(OH)_2D_3$ in the liver before the target tissues respond (H24). In the case of the bird, the 1α-OH-D_3 is converted to some degree also in the intestine to 1,25-$(OH)_2D_3$, which perhaps accounts for its more effective activity in birds versus mammals (H25). In any case, it appears that the 25-hydroxyl function is necessary not only to direct 1-hydroxylation, but also for final function of the compound in intestine and bone.

Another interesting exercise in preparation of analogs of 1,25-$(OH)_2D_3$ has been the chemical synthesis of the 3-deoxy-1-hydroxylated vitamin

D's. The rationale behind these preparations is to examine the question of whether the 3-hydroxyl function is necessary for biological activity, especially since dihydrotachysterol has activity, and, if one can assume that the 3-hydroxyl in that compound is in the spatial position occupied by the 1-hydroxyl of 1,25-$(OH)_2D_3$, it might appear that the 3-hydroxyl might not be important in final biological activity. 3-Deoxy-1α-OH-D_3 has been prepared because it would appear that the absence of the hydroxyl on the 3 position would fix very strongly the 1-hydroxyl in the axial position on carbon 1. Chemical synthesis of the 3-deoxy-1α-OH-D_3 (L2, O3) and 3-deoxy-1α,25-$(OH)_2D_3$ (O2) has been achieved. The 3-deoxy compounds do possess biological activity both in the stimulation of intestinal calcium absorption and in the stimulation of calcium mobilization from bone. However, both compounds are approximately 1/10 to 1/100 as active as their analogs possessing the 3-hydroxyl function, suggesting that the 3-hydroxyl group, although not essential to biological activity, must provide some structural contribution for its binding to the receptor molecules.

Another important foray into biological activity has been a study of the 24-hydroxylated vitamins, as has been discussed under metabolism. The 24-hydroxylated vitamins have two stereoisomers possible. They are designated as the S or R 24-hydroxy compounds, indicating hydroxyl functions projecting into or out of the plane. It is clear both in rats and in chicks that the 24S-hydroxyvitamin D_3 (24-OH-D_3) and the 24S,25-$(OH)_2D_3$ are much less biologically active than their corresponding 24R-hydroxylated counterparts (T6, T7). The primary reason for the discrimination is that the 1-hydroxylase enzyme of the kidney discriminates against the 24S configuration compounds (Y. Tanaka and H. F. DeLuca, unpublished results). The 1,24,25-$(OH)_3D_3$ S and R compounds are approximately equal in biological activity *in vivo*, although in bone organ cultures it seems that the S configuration is also slightly less active than the R configuration (S18).

Although in no case does 24-hydroxylation enhance biological activity, at least as far as is known to this author, the degree to which 24-hydroxylation diminishes biological activity differs between chicks and rats. In the chick, 24-hydroxylation markedly reduces biological activity to approximately one-tenth or less of its non-24-hydroxylated counterparts (H21). In the rat, however, biological activity of the 24-hydroxylated compound often approaches that of the non-24-hydroxylated compound. However, biological testing of these compounds is done in vitamin D-deficient animals where 24-hydroxylated compounds rarely exist. In both species the 24-hydroxylated compounds are rapidly excreted, at least in normal animals, suggesting that the 24-hydroxylation represents a signal for elimination of the biologically active vitamin D compounds.

There have been other 1-hydroxylated compounds prepared. The $2\alpha,25$-$(OH)_2D_3$ has been prepared, as has been the 3-epi-1,25-$(OH)_2D_3$. The 2α compound is totally without biological activity (K1) whereas the configuration markedly diminishes biological activity of the 1,25-$(OH)_2D_3$ (S6). It is likely that the 3α-hydroxyl interferes with binding of the 1,25-$(OH)_2D_3$ to the target tissue receptor sites, although this represents a speculation.

Studies have been carried out that examine the question of whether the length of side chain is critical to biological activity of the hydroxylated vitamin D compounds. So far, however, only shortened side chains have been prepared for 25-OH-D_3 and their 5,6-*trans* isomers (H18). Using this model, it is clear that even shortening the side chain by one carbon markedly diminishes biological activity. Preliminary results in our own laboratory have revealed that the 24-nor-1,25-$(OH)_2D_3$ has markedly diminished biological activity, illustrating the essentiality of a side chain of proper length. Other side chain derivatives include the 26-nor and 26,27-bisnor-25-OH-D_3 and their 5,6-*trans* isomers (H18). These compounds also have diminished biological activity, again suggesting the essentiality of the vitamin D side chain surrounding the 25-hydroxyl function. It is of interest, however, that vitamin D_2, which possesses a methyl group on carbon 24, is fully biologically active in mammals although not so in birds. The *epi*-25-OH-D_2 has been prepared and shown to be much less biologically active than the 25-OH-D_2 itself in mammals (J. A. Campbell and H. F. DeLuca, unpublished results). However, the 1-hydroxylated *epi*-25-OH-D_3 has not been prepared, so that one cannot examine the question of whether the methyl group on carbon 24 in the incorrect configuration interferes with 1-hydroxylation or with binding to the target tissue receptors.

The analogs described above have been examined not only in intact animals, but also in organ-culture experiments in which the mobilization of calcium from bone has been examined and in the binding of the compound to what is believed to be a cytosol receptor of chick small intestine. In these two isolated target-organ systems, 1,25-$(OH)_2D_3$ is clearly the most biologically active, approached very closely by 1,25-$(OH)_2D_2$ and within one order of magnitude by 1,24R,25-$(OH)_3D_3$, by two orders of magnitude by the 1α-OH-D_3 compounds, then the 25-OH-D_3 and finally the 24,25-$(OH)_2D_3$ compounds (S19).

Although it is premature to draw firm conclusions on the structural requirements for biological activity of the 1,25-$(OH)_2D_3$, it appears that all three hydroxyl functions are either essential or contribute greatly to the binding of the compound to its receptors and to its biological activity. The cis-triene structure apparently is extremely important, although biological activity can be obtained with analogs in which one of the double bonds is reduced or in which the configuration of the triene system is changed to the trans state. Finally, a fully extended side chain appears to be required for biological activity in which the environment surrounding the 25-hydroxyl function has very strict requirements. It is of interest that X-ray crystallography of the 25-OH-D has been completed, illustrating that in the crystalline form the 25-hydroxy compound possesses a fully extended side chain (L. Dahl, T. Toan, and H. F. DeLuca, unpublished results), and it is of interest that the A ring has been isolated in crystalline form in two conformations, which have been structurally elucidated by X-ray crystallography and by nuclear magnetic resonance NMR studies (T. Toan, L. Dahl, and H. F. DeLuca, unpublished results; L3, O1).

There has been much recent interest in the possibility that the plant kingdom possesses compounds that are either identical with or analogs of the $1,25$-$(OH)_2D_3$. A disease has appeared in grazing cattle in South America that produces wasting, calcification, and death. This disease has been related to the grazing of cattle on the leaves of a plant *Solanum malacoxylon* (W2). The active principle from the plant leaves has been extracted and tested biologically. In many respects this water-soluble extract acts identically to $1,25$-$(OH)_2D_3$, in that it stimulates intestinal calcium absorption in nephrectomized animals or in strontium-poisoned animals. Furthermore, this substance will directly stimulate the production of calcium-binding protein in cultures of small intestine. In addition, it will substitute for vitamin D in the stimulation of serum calcium and serum phosphorus elevation of vitamin D-deficient animals (U1). These biological activities have been used to suggest that the *Solanum malacoxylon* extract possesses $1,25$-$(OH)_2D_3$ in a soluble form. Recent work in the laboratory of Wasserman has provided evidence that this is in fact true, although identification of the compound as $1,25$-$(OH)_2D_3$ is not convincing. Work in our own laboratory has positively identified at least one component, $1,25$-$(OH)_2D_3$. In addition, there also may be other analogs that contribute to biological activity. However, the complete structural elucidation of the active principle has not yet been made and will undoubtedly be completed before this chapter is in print.

9. Diseases of Calcium and Phosphorus Metabolism Related to Defects in Vitamin D Metabolism

As has been pointed out in the preceding section, rickets and osteomalacia represent diseases that result from a deficiency of vitamin D building blocks for the vitamin D endocrine system. These two diseases are characterized by the elaboration of collagen matrix by the osteoblasts and chondrocytes of bone, but they fail to calcify in a normal fashion. As a result, large patches of osteoid tissue, which represents osteoblast elaborated organic matrix that has not calcified, can be found. There has been much discussion regarding how these diseases evolve. Although a major contributor may be a function of vitamin D directly on the mineralization process at the bone site, so far this has not been proved. Instead the primary mechanism for etiology of these diseases is a failure of supply of calcium and phosphorus to bone (H27, O5). There has been much discussion whether rachitogenesis is the result of a lack of calcium or a lack of phosphorus, or both. Inasmuch as parathyroidectomy diminishes the ability of the animal to produce $1,25\text{-}(OH)_2D_3$, one might expect that rachitic lesions would be observed in the parathyroidectomized state. Clearly such is not the case; obviously, therefore, something more is necessary for rachitogenesis other than a hypocalcemia and lack of $1,25\text{-}(OH)_2D_3$. Both in man and in rats deprived of phosphorus, rickets can be observed even in the presence of vitamin D and presumably of adequate amounts of $1,25\text{-}(OH)_2D_3$. Furthermore, Fraser $et\ al.$ (F1) have described the sequence of events resulting in rachitogenesis in man, in which it is believed that, initially, partial vitamin D depletion results in depressed intestinal calcium absorption and a hypocalcemia but no bone disease. Hypocalcemia stimulates parathyroid hormone secretion and hypertrophy, giving rise to excessive phosphate diuresis. Therefore, in the second stage of bone disease parathyroid hormone present in large amounts and together with remaining amounts of vitamin D in bone will mobilize calcium from bone, restoring the blood to normal calcemia. However, the secondary hyperparathyroidism results in excessive loss of phosphate in the urine, giving rise to a hypophosphatemia. At this stage rachitic lesions begin to develop in the bone (F1). This is followed by a third stage of rachitogenesis in which the bone becomes depleted in vitamin D compounds, giving rise to a resistance of the bone to parathyroid hormone stimulation and a hypocalcemia. The large amounts of circulating parathyroid hormone still stimulate phosphate diuresis giving a severe hypophosphatemia. Under these conditions, severe bone disease results. In rats (M5, S16) and in children (F1), phosphate administration, even in the absence of vitamin D, will produce mineralization of bone, although imperfect and incomplete. These results suggest that the primary defect in rachitogenesis and probably in osteomalaciogenesis is phosphate deficiency, perhaps coupled with a defect in the mineralization process due to the absence of the active form of vitamin D.

Another major group of patients which have defective vitamin D metabolism are those suffering from either acute or chronic renal disease. Although acute renal failure and the attendant hypocalcemia has not been adequately studied, it is virtually certain that chronic renal azotemic disease is associated with a deterioration of bone (S12). Although there is considerable discussion on the etiology of this disease, it seems certain that a rise in serum phosphorus due to failure of excretion is a contributing factor (S9). This rise in serum phosphorus may well give rise to high renal cortical levels of inorganic phosphorus, which suppress $1,25\text{-}(OH)_2D_3$ synthesis. Furthermore, the reduction in renal mass must also contribute to the failure of $1,25\text{-}(OH)_2D_3$ synthesis. This results in diminished intestinal calcium absorption and diminished bone calcium mobilization, giving rise to hypocalcemia. Furthermore, the absence of the active form of vitamin D at the mineralization sites may also retard mineralization. The hypocalcemia stimulates the parathyroid glands into excessive secretion and hypertrophy giving rise to severe secondary hyperparathyroidism. With the presence of even small amounts of active vitamin D, the excessive amounts of parathyroid hormone bring about excessive bone erosion giving rise to osteitis fibrosa cystica on one hand and the absence of the active form of vitamin D giving rise to osteomalacia on the other. Severe bone disease is, therefore, well recognized in varying degrees at various dialysis clinics serving azotemic renal patients.

There have been numerous studies in which the treatment of the renal osteodystrophy has been attempted with $1,25\text{-}(OH)_2D_3$ or its analog $1\alpha\text{-}OH\text{-}D_3$. The results of these studies are uniformly excellent, as might be expected, in which there is an improvement of intestinal calcium absorption, correction of the hypocalcemia, suppression of parathyroid hormone secretion and mineralization of bone. Treatment of patients even with severe bone disease with $1,25\text{-}(OH)_2D_3$ for about a year gives remarkable improvement and often results in the return of the skeleton to approximately normal (B14, S8).

Patients suffering from the absence of the parathyroid glands can no longer sense hypocalcemia, and as a result they are unable to receive the signal or stimulus to produce $1,25\text{-}(OH)_2D_3$ when there are obvious calcium needs in the patient. As a result, these patients develop hypocalcemia, diminished intestinal calcium absorption, and hypocalcemic tetany. Obviously treatment with human parathyroid hormone is not practical since it is not available, and even if it were, since it is a peptide hormone, routine injections would be necessary. However, inasmuch as the parathyroids stimulate $1,25\text{-}(OH)_2D_3$ synthesis and $1,25\text{-}(OH)_2D_3$ can act on intestine without the presence of the parathyroid hormone, these patients can be adequately managed by the administration of small amounts of $1,25\text{-}(OH)_2D_3$ and sufficient amounts of oral calcium (K4, N1). It is evident that hypocalcemic hypoparathyroid patients cannot be managed with the idea of utilizing bone calcium to maintain serum calcium levels because of the absence of the parathyroid hormone. In any case, hypocalcemic hypoparathyroid patients treated with small amounts of either 1,25-$(OH)_2D_3$ or 1α-OII-D_3 have been successfully managed with the possible exception of one or two cases. Direct analysis of the plasma levels of 1,25-$(OH)_2D_3$ in such patients has revealed them to be low (N1, J. Eisman and H. F. DeLuca, unpublished results).

Another class of patients are the pseudo-hypoparathyroid group, which secrete excessive amounts of parathyroid hormone in response to hypocalcemic stimuli. However, the parathyroid hormone lacks in its ability to function in the target organs in such patients. They suffer hypocalcemia, retarded intestinal calcium absorption, as well as defective bone growth in such bones as the fourth metacarpal. These patients can also be treated with 1,25-$(OH)_2D_3$ plus oral calcium to correct their hypocalcemia. An examination of the serum levels of 1,25-$(OH)_2D_3$ in hypoparathyroid patients, pseudohypoparathyroid patients, and hyperparathyroids, has revealed that the pseudo- and hypoparathyroid patients have low circulating levels of 1,25-$(OH)_2D_3$ whereas the primary hyperparathyroid patients have very high circulating levels of the vitamin D hormone (N1, J. Eisman and H. F. DeLuca, unpublished results).

A disease of major significance in terms of numbers, is osteoporosis. Osteoporosis has many possible causes; there is an idiopathic osteoporosis, which affects very young patients, and the mechanism remains unknown at the present time. There are steroid-induced osteoporotic symptoms, which also are of unknown etiology, although there is some evidence that the steroid hormones can interfere with vitamin D metabolism. Preliminary results revealed that the bone disease in the latter case can be at least partially corrected by the administration of 50–100 μg of 25-OH-D_3 daily plus oral calcium (T. Hahn, personal communication). By far the largest number of patients of concern are those who suffer either senile osteoporosis or postmenopausal osteoporosis. Again, there is no universal agreement as to how the disease develops although it is almost certain that this is a multicomponent disease in which many factors contribute to its development. Certainly in the case of postmenopausal osteoporosis, the lack of sex hormones must aggravate this already developing bone disease, although there is considerable disagreement as to the mechanism of this development. There appears to be general agreement that a chronic lack of calcium predisposes man to the development of osteoporosis since such a person becomes very markedly dependent upon bone calcium for maintenance of his serum calcium level. This must bring about continual insult to the bone by small amounts of parathyroid hormone seeking to raise serum calcium levels. Another contributing factor might be high-phosphate diets, which interfere to some degree with intestinal calcium absorption and tend to repress ionized calcium levels in the blood. This could also bring about secretion of parathyroid hormone and continual attack of the hormone on bone on a chronic basis. Although it would be difficult to see the small changes in short experimental or study periods, osteoporosis is a disease that develops continually and chronically over a period of 30 years. The disease is characterized by a lack of total bone mass, which is likely the result of slightly excessive bone destruction and inadequate replacement with newly forming bone. Another possibility is that the kidneys lose their sensitivity to the parathyroid hormone in the biogenesis of $1,25\text{-}(OH)_2D_3$. This has clearly been demonstrated in the case of old rats, which lack the ability to produce $1,25\text{-}(OH)_2D_3$ in response to hypocalcemic stimuli (R. Horst, N. Jorgensen, and H. F. DeLuca, unpublished results). However, their intestine and bones are responsive to exogenous $1,25\text{-}(OH)_2D_3$. Recently preliminary results have revealed that patients suffering from diagnosed osteoporosis have significantly lower serum $1,25\text{-}(OH)_2D_3$ levels than their normal age-matched counterparts. Possibly inadequate production of $1,25\text{-}(OH)_2D_3$ in response to the need for calcium is a contributing factor. On a chronic basis this reduced amount of $1,25\text{-}(OH)_2D_3$ would retard intestinal calcium absorption and again predispose the organism to maintaining serum calcium at the expense of bone. Furthermore, the chronically low level of $1,25\text{-}(OH)_2D_3$ would not be able to stimulate new bone formation. A distinct possibility, therefore, is that this disease may have a component of defective vitamin D metabolism and its treatment may involve at least in part $1,25\text{-}(OH)_2D_3$ or one of its analogs (G1, L9).

Of special interest is the group of patients suffering from vitamin D-resistant rickets. Dent has reported that there are approximately thirty distinct types of vitamin D-resistant rickets (D6). It would be impossible to decide at this stage which of these diseases might represent a defect in vitamin D metabolism although there have been two major groups of patients that have been studied. The well known X-linked dominant familial hypophosphatemic vitamin D-resistant rickets has received much attention. So far, however, this disease has not been shown to be a defect in vitamin D metabolism, and current evidence suggests that it is in fact a defect in phosphate transport reactions, both in intestine (S7) and kidney (G8). Treatment of this disease with $1,25\text{-}(OH)_2D_3$ has not been successful, at least at physiologic doses (G9). The most successful treatment has been the administration of frequent doses of oral phosphate, as much as the patient can tolerate, and the addition of $1\alpha\text{-}OH\text{-}D_3$ or $1,25\text{-}(OH)_2D_3$ to prevent the secondary hyperparathyroidism that would result from phosphate administration.

Vitamin D-dependency rickets, which is also known as Prader's disease or pseudo-vitamin D-deficiency rickets, is a disease in which children present at an early age with rickets despite adequate amounts of vitamin D. These children also are completely healed by the administration of large amounts of vitamin D at a level of anywhere from 50,000 to 150,000 units per day. This disease can be treated with small and physiologic amounts of 1,25-(OH)$_2$D$_3$ (F2) or small amounts of its analog 1α-OH-D$_3$ (R3), which has led to the suggestion that this disease represents a defect in the conversion of 25-OH-D$_3$ to the 1,25-(OH)$_2$D$_3$. Treatment with 25-OH-D$_3$ is also successful, although superphysiologic amounts of this compound are required. Additional work must be carried out before this can be considered a true genetic block in 1,25-(OH)$_2$D$_3$ biosynthesis, but it appears at the present time that these patients have a defective 1-hydroxylase enzyme possessing a large Michaelis constant for 25-OH-D$_3$ (F2).

There are other types of diseases that appear to be a defect in vitamin D metabolism, one of which is the phenobarbital–dilantin-induced osteo-malacia (K7). There is disagreement as to the extent of the osteomalacia that occurs in patients being treated with these antiepileptic drugs, although there is no doubt that some centers see clear evidence of the disease in approximately 30% of the cases. Successful treatment has been reported with larger amounts of vitamin D$_2$ and of vitamin D$_3$ (S11). Additional work must be carried out in this important area before clear conclusions can be drawn regarding the mode of treatment of the disease and the etiology of the development of the bone disease.

Throughout these discussions of bone disease it is apparent that a defect in vitamin D metabolism does not always result in rickets and osteo-malacia as has been previously surmised from the deficiency diseases caused by insufficient amounts of vitamin D. Instead it is obvious that a disruption of vitamin D metabolism could contribute to a large variety of diseases and that the vitamin D metabolites or analogs could be of great use in judicious management of the diseases.

10. Mechanism of Action of 1,25-(OH)$_2$D$_3$

Throughout the past decade, the metabolism of vitamin D has been investigated primarily because of the interest in understanding how the vitamin might function. We must now transfer our attentions to the question of how 1,25-(OH)$_2$D$_3$ must function if it in fact functions directly without further metabolism—a question that has not been totally answered to date. Assuming, however, that the 1,25-(OH)$_2$D$_3$ functions directly, there has been only one system which has been studied in great detail regarding function of the vitamin, that is, the mechanism whereby 1,25-(OH)$_2$D$_3$ increases intestinal calcium absorption. It is safe to say at the present time that there is no universal agreement regarding the mechanism whereby 1,25-$(OH)_2D_3$ initiates intestinal calcium absorption or the actual mechanism whereby calcium is transported across the intestine. To begin our discussion here, we will consider first the path and site of 1,25-$(OH)_2D_3$ function and finally the ideas concerning the mechanism whereby calcium is transported across intestine.

There seems to be little doubt that 1,25-$(OH)_2D_3$ is found predominantly in the intestinal nuclear fraction as separated by differential centrifugation methods (C5, C6, L5). As much as 80% of the tissue radioactivity will be found in this fraction. However, it is not altogether certain whether all of this radioactivity is located in the nuclei or in a fraction that sediments with the nuclei. Thus far an adequate preparation of pure nuclei from intestine has not been made. In fact, the best methods yield anywhere between 20 and 30% of the total cellular DNA in the nuclear fraction (C6, L6). Using this approach, only 20–30% of the total tissue radioactivity can be accounted for in the nuclear fraction; however, one is not certain whether the method of isolation of the nuclei specifically excludes the nuclei of interest. Chromatin has been isolated from the intestine and, depending upon the mode of preparation, anywhere from 30% (C5) to all of the nuclear radioactivity can be located in this fraction (H9). When chromatin is prepared by the method of Marushige and Bonner, no more than 20 or 30% of the cellular radioactivity can be found in that fraction (C6). On the other hand, if the procedure is modified as described by Haussler and Norman, virtually all the radioactivity can be found in that fraction (H9). However, under these circumstances the fraction called chromatin is far from being only chromatin—it contains virtually every other type of cell component describable (C6, L4). Thus it is not clear whether the 1,25-$(OH)_2D_3$ that enters the intestinal cell is found in total in the nuclear fraction. Certainly some of the radioactivity appears in the nuclear fraction, which makes feasible the idea that the 1,25-$(OH)_2D_3$ functions by some induction mechanism.

The most popular concept is that 1,25-$(OH)_2D_3$ becomes associated with a 3.0–3.5 S protein, which then is transferred into the nuclear fraction and initiates transcription of specific genes that code for calcium transport protein (B15). Evidence for the existence of such a protein has been put forth for chicken intestine (B15, B16, K6), but the same protein cannot be found in the rat intestine (K6). In the rat intestine, instead a 6 S protein can be found that binds both 25-OH-D_3 and 1,25-$(OH)_2D_3$. This protein, in fact, prefers 25-OH-D_3 to the 1,25-$(OH)_2D_3$, which makes it unlikely that it is a receptor protein. Brumbaugh and Haussler have shown that the 3.0–3.5 S protein can bind to nuclei (B15), an observation that has been confirmed in Norman's laboratory (P5). The existence of a 3.7 S protein in the cytosol of chick intestine has been confirmed in our laboratory and the 3.0–3.5 S proteins of Brumbaugh and Haussler are probably degraded forms of the 3.7 S protein. The 3.7 S protein has been successfully stabilized and is now used in a radioreceptor assay for 1,25-$(OH)_2D_3$ (E1). Haussler and his collaborators have also utilized the chromatin-binding procedure as a radioreceptor assay (B18).

Emtage and Lawson have studied the polysomes derived from vitamin D-deficient chicks and from chicks given vitamin D for their ability to produce proteins *in vitro*. Using this approach they have demonstrated that the polysomes from vitamin D-repleted animals produce a radioactive protein, which is precipitated by an antibody to the calcium binding protein of intestine (E2). Emtage and Lawson believe that the nuclei make a message in response to the 1,25-$(OH)_2D_3$, which then directs polysomes to produce a calcium-binding protein. Although these experiments are interesting and important, they do not conclusively demonstrate that the mode of action of 1,25-$(OH)_2D_3$ is to unmask or direct transcription of a gene which codes for the Wasserman calcium-binding protein. Certainly intestines from vitamin D-treated animals at the steady-state level would be producing calcium-binding protein, and these experiments are a more elegant way of demonstrating that principle.

The only protein that has so far been discovered and isolated that can possibly play a role in vitamin D-induced intestinal calcium transport is a calcium-binding protein discovered by Taylor and Wasserman (T9). This protein, which has a molecular weight of 24,000 when isolated from chick and approximately 8000–12,000 when isolated from mammals (W4), binds four molecules of calcium per mole of protein and appears only after the administration of vitamin D or one of its metabolites. The kinetics of its appearance may not correlate exactly with intestinal calcium transport, and furthermore calcium transport does not always correlate with whether calcium-binding protein is present in intestine or not (H5). However, factors that appear to affect calcium transport also appear to affect calcium-binding protein levels in an appropriate manner. The exact way in which the calcium binding protein is assembled in a calcium transport system has not been determined. Taylor and Wasserman demonstrated originally that the location of calcium binding protein is primarily goblet cells and on the surface of the brush border of the intestinal epithelial cells (T10). There is some disagreement as to this subcellular location and hence new developments can be expected.

There is uniform agreement that the site of vitamin D function on calcium transport is at the brush border surface of the intestinal epithelial cells. There has been evidence that the 1,25-$(OH)_2D_3$ increases a calcium-dependent adenosine triphosphatase (M6) which has been equated to intestinal alkaline phosphatase. However, the correlation between calcium transport and this system does not appear to be convincing either. Recently the existence of a calcium-binding complex of 230,000 molecular weight in the brush border following vitamin D administration has been observed (M9). This derives probably from a 200,000 molecular weight protein in the brush border which does not bind calcium. The appearance of this calcium-binding complex correlates well with intestinal calcium transport; whether this is in fact the calcium carrier remains unknown. The calcium undoubtedly crosses the epithelial or microvillous membrane and is either packaged in vesicles in the terminal web region or is picked up by mitochondria which scavenge calcium at any concentration above 10^{-7} M. The vesicles could be extruded at the basal–lateral membrane by a sodium-dependent process (M1), or alternatively there is a sodium dependency of calcium extrusion at the basal–lateral membrane, perhaps by an exchange mechanism. Because the sodium is high in extracellular fluid, as a result of the sodium–potassium ATPase pump system, the down-hill sodium gradient could provide energy to deplete calcium from the basal–lateral membrane region of the cell and to extrude it in the serosal fluid (O5). It is, therefore, possible then that mitochondria would release calcium in such an environment, completing the calcium shuttle system (Fig. 10). The sodium dependence of calcium extrusion across intestinal epithelium has been adequately demonstrated (M1), but beyond that the intestinal calcium-transport mechanism is a highly experimental subject in which few facts are available. One can expect major developments in this area in the next decade, perhaps leading ultimately to a solution of how the hormone derived from vitamin D functions in this system.

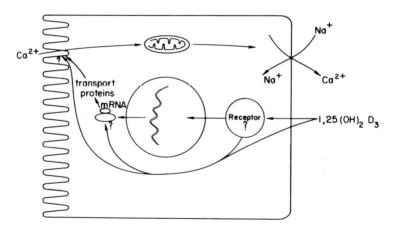

FIG. 10. Diagrammatic representation of the postulated mechanisms whereby 1,25-dihydroxyvitamin D_3 (1,25-(OH)$_2$D$_3$) initiates intestinal calcium transport.

In the mobilization of calcium from bone, little is known beyond the fact that 1,25-$(OH)_2D_3$ initiates bone calcium mobilization both *in vivo* and *in vitro* by an actinomycin D-sensitive process (R1, R4, S19, T1). Thus, in this system 1,25-$(OH)_2D_3$ functions in the classical steroid mechanism in which nuclear activity is involved. A receptor has not yet been reported for bone tissue, nor is there any clear evidence as to the mechanism of the calcium mobilization system. It seems clear that the system requires parathyroid hormone *in vivo*, although *in vitro* 1,25-$(OH)_2D_3$ brings about bone resorption without addition of parathyroid hormone. The dichotomy of these experiments must be resolved eventually, although animals in a hypophosphatemic state will also mobilize their bone in response to 1,25-$(OH)_2D_3$ in the absence of parathyroid hormone. Thus, inasmuch as bone cultures are studied in hypophosphatemic medium, it is possible that this is the reason for the lack of requirement for parathyroid hormone in that system versus *in vivo* systems.

The role of vitamin D in the transport of intestinal phosphate has not received very much attention. It is clear that in the intestinal phosphate transport mechanism calcium is not involved and sodium is required (C7, T8). According to Taylor, sodium is required for the uptake of calcium by its brush border surface rather than extrusion into the scrosal surface as is the case with the calcium transport system. Little is known about the phosphate transport mechanism except that it appears to respond specifically to 1,25-$(OH)_2D_3$ rather than 25-OH-D_3 or vitamin D_3 itself (C7).

The mechanism of action of 1,25-$(OH)_2D_3$ in the kidney is even less well understood except that there appears to be a vitamin D-dependent calcium binding protein which appears in the kidney as well (T11). Exactly how this functions and where it functions remains unknown at the present time.

11. Assessment of Vitamin D Hormonal Status

It is obvious from the above chapter that a measurement of vitamin D and its metabolites in disease states will be of extreme importance in diagnosis and perhaps in intelligent management of the disease. So far the clinical chemistry of vitamin D measurements is in a primitive stage. The measurement of vitamin D_3 itself is limited by the fact that it can be adequately carried out only by biological assay. The 25-OH-D_3 can be measured by radioligand assay methods involving either a plasma binding protein for 25-OH-D_3 (B3) or a cytosol-binding protein derived from rachitic rat kidneys (H1). Both methods appear to be convenient and easily applied. Some question exists as to the specificity of the methods, especially when high doses of vitamin D are studied. Recently methods have been developed that involve the measurement of 25-OH-D_3 in serum by means of high-pressure liquid chromatography utilizing the cis-triene chromophore for measurement (J. Eisman and H. F. DeLuca, unpublished results). In this method radioactive 25-OH-D_3 is added to a plasma sample to permit monitoring of recovery of the 25-OH-D_3. It is then extracted, chromatographed on two different column systems and ultimately injected into a high-pressure liquid column and the optical density at 254 nm recorded. An aliquot of the injected material is counted to reveal the recovery of radioactivity, and the optical density in the 25-OH-D_3 peak on high-pressure liquid chromatography is used to assess the 25-OH-D_3 levels. With this method, plasma levels in the neighborhood of 20 ng/ml have been found in normal man.

The measurement of 1,25-$(OH)_2D_3$ is a much more difficult one since it involves measurement of picogram amounts of metabolite per milliliter of plasma. Brumbaugh and Haussler have developed a radioreceptor assay involving the chick intestinal cytosol and the chick intestinal chromatin to specifically bind the radioactive 1,25-$(OH)_2D_3$ after extensive purification (B18). Their methods have been successful, although normal values reported from that group have been decreasing steadily as the technology of the system has been improved. Currently the recent reports reveal plasma levels on the order of 40 pg/ml in normal man. The 3.7 S chicken intestinal cytosol protein has been utilized for a direct radioreceptor ligand assay after extraction and purification by two column procedures (E1). This more rapid procedure has been developed such that it is sensitive to 10 pg of metabolite. It is now possible to determine 1,25-$(OH)_2D_3$ levels on 2–5 ml of serum. Normal values by this method are in the range of 29 pg/ml with zero levels for chronic renal failure patients or nephrectomized patients. Another assay involves extraction, purification by two column methods including high-pressure liquid chromatography and measurement by biological assay by bone resorption techniques (P. Stern, A. Hamstra and H. F. DeLuca, unpublished results). This method has revealed similar levels of 1,25-$(OH)_2D_3$ in the plasma of normal patients. The technology of all these methods is difficult, but it is likely that within the next few years at least the simpler radioreceptor assays will be set up in a variety of clinical laboratories that will lead to an assessment of vitamin D status in a wide variety of bone diseases and will probably lead to the monitoring of 1,25-$(OH)_2D_3$ levels during treatment of the diseases.

12. Conclusion

Vitamin D can no longer be regarded simply as a vitamin, but rather as a building block for one hormone, which has its endocrine system located in the kidney and the targets of hormone action in intestine, bone, and kidney. The realization of the existence of this system has had a great impact on our understanding of calcium and phosphorus metabolism and on our understanding of the etiology of a variety of bone diseases. Furthermore, it has provided the tools for the treatment of bone diseases in which there is a defect in vitamin D metabolism. Finally, from the clinical point of view, methods for assessment of vitamin D metabolism and hormonal status are under development that will usher into the clinical chemistry area a new era of bone disease in treatment, diagnosis, and evaluation of treatment.

ACKNOWLEDGMENT

Some of the original investigations reported in this review were supported by a program-project grant from the National Institutes of Health, No. AM-14881 and the Harry Steenbock Research Fund.

REFERENCES

A1. Anderson, H. C., Vesicles associated with calcification in the matrix of epiphyseal cartilage. *J. Cell. Biol.* **41**, 59–72 (1969).

A2. Askew, F. A., Bourdillon, R. B., Bruce, H. M., Jenkins, R. G. C., and Webster, T. A., The distillation of vitamin D. *Proc. R. Soc. London, Ser. B* **107**, 76–90 (1931).

A3. Avioli, L. V., Lee, S. W., McDonald, J. E., Lund, J., and DeLuca, H. F., Metabolism of vitamin D_3-^{3}H in human subjects: Distribution in blood, bile, feces, and urine. *J. Clin. Invest.* **46**, 983–992 (1967).

B1. Baxter, L. A., and DeLuca, H. F., Stimulation of 25-hydroxyvitamin D_3-1α-hydroxylase by phosphate depletion. *J. Biol. Chem.* **251**, 3158–3161 (1976).

B2. Bell, P. A., and Kodicek, E., Investigations on metabolites of vitamin D in rat bile. Separation and partial identification of a major metabolite. *Biochem. J.* **115**, 663–669 (1969).

B3. Belsey, R. E., DeLuca, H. F., and Potts, J. T., Jr., A rapid assay for 25-OH-vitamin D_3 without preparative chromatography. *J. Clin. Endocrinol. Metab.* **38**, 1046–1051 (1974).

B4. Belsey, R. E., Clark, M. B., Bernat, M., Glowacki, J., Holick, M. F., DeLuca, H. F., and Potts, J. T., Jr., The physiologic significance of plasma transport of vitamin D and metabolites. *Am. J. Med.* **57**, 50–56 (1974).

B5. Bhattacharyya, M. H., and DeLuca, H. F., The regulation of rat liver calciferol-25-hydroxylase. *J. Biol. Chem.* **248**, 2969–2973 (1973).

B6. Bhattacharyya, M. H., and DeLuca, H. F., Comparative studies on the 25-hydroxylation of vitamin D_3 and dihydrotachysterol$_3$. *J. Biol. Chem.* **248**, 2974–2977 (1973).

B7. Bhattacharyya, M. H., and DeLuca, H. F., Subcellular location of rat liver calciferol-25-hydroxylase. *Arch. Biochem. Biophys.* **160**, 58–62 (1974).

B8. Bhattacharyya, M. H., and DeLuca, H. F., The regulation of calciferol-25-hydroxylase in the chick. *Biochem. Biophys. Res. Commun.* **59**, 734–741 (1974).

B9. Birge, S. J., and Haddad, J. G., 25-Hydroxycholecalciferol stimulation of muscle metabolism. *J. Clin. Invest.* **56**, 1100–1107 (1975).

B10. Blunt, J. W., DeLuca, H. F., and Schnoes, H. K., 25-Hydroxycholecalciferol. A biologically active metabolite of vitamin D_3. *Biochemistry* **7**, 3317–3322 (1968).

B11. Botham, K. M., Ghazarian, J. G., Kream, B. E., and DeLuca, H. F., Isolation of a potent inhibitor of 25-hydroxyvitamin D_3-1-hydroxylase from rat serum. *Biochemistry* **15**, 2130–2135 (1976).

B12. Boyle, I. T., Gray, R. W., and DeLuca, H. F., Regulation by calcium of *in vivo* synthesis of 1,25-dihydroxycholecalciferol and 21,25-dihydroxycholecalciferol. *Proc. Natl. Acad. Sci. U.S.A.* **68**, 2131–2134 (1971).

B13. Boyle, I. T., Miravet, L., Gray, R. W., Holick, M. F., and DeLuca, H. F., The response of intestinal calcium transport to 25-hydroxy and 1,25-dihydroxy vitamin D in nephrectomized rats. *Endocrinology* **90**, 605–608 (1972).

B14. Brickman, A. S., Sherrard, D. J., Jowsey, J., Singer, F. R., Baylink, D. J., Maloney, N., Massry, S. G., Norman, A. W., and Coburn, J. W., 1,25-Dihydroxycholecalciferol. Effect on skeletal lesions and plasma parathyroid hormone levels in uremic osteodystrophy. *Arch. Intern. Med.* **134**, 883–888 (1974).

B15. Brumbaugh, P. F., and Haussler, M. R., 1α,25-Dihydroxycholecalciferol receptors in intestine. II. Temperature-dependent transfer of the hormone to chromatin via a specific cytosol receptor. *J. Biol. Chem.* **249**, 1258–1262 (1974).

B16. Brumbaugh, P. F., and Haussler, M. R., Nuclear and cytoplasmic binding components for vitamin D metabolites. *Life Sci.* **16**, 353–362 (1975).

B17. Brumbaugh, P. F., Hughes, M. R., and Haussler, M. R., Cytoplasmic and nuclear binding components for 1α,25-dihydroxyvitamin D_3 in chick parathyroid glands. *Proc. Natl. Acad. Sci. U.S.A.* **72**, 4871–4875 (1975).

B18. Brumbaugh, P. F., Haussler, D. H., Bressler, R., and Haussler, M. R., Radio-receptor assay for 1α,25-dihydroxyvitamin D_3. *Science* **183**, 1089–1091 (1974).

C1. Carlsson, A., Tracer experiments on the effect of vitamin D on the skeletal metabolism of calcium and phosphorus. *Acta Physiol. Scand.* **26**, 212–220 (1952).

C2. Castillo, L., Tanaka, Y., and DeLuca, H. F., The mobilization of bone mineral by 1,25-dihydroxyvitamin D_3 in hypophosphatemic rats. *Endocrinology* **97**, 995–999 (1975).

C3. Chen, P. S., Jr., and Bosmann, H. B., Effect of vitamin D_2 and D_3 in serum calcium and phosphorus in rachitic chicks. *J. Nutr.* **83**, 133–139 (1964).

C4. Chen, T. C., and DeLuca, H. F., Stimulation of [³H]uridine incorporation into nuclear RNA of rat kidney by vitamin D metabolites. *Arch. Biochem. Biophys.* **156**, 321–327 (1973).

C5. Chen, T. C., and DeLuca, H. F., Receptors of 1,25-dihydroxycholecalciferol in rat intestine. *J. Biol. Chem.* **248**, 4890–4895 (1973).

C6. Chen, T. C., Weber, J. C., and DeLuca, H. F., On the subcellular location of vitamin D metabolites in intestine. *J. Biol. Chem.* **245**, 3776–3780 (1970).

C7. Chen, T. C., Castillo, L., Korycka-Dahl, M., and DeLuca, H. F., Role of vitamin D metabolites in phosphate transport of rat intestine. *J. Nutr.* **104**, 1056–1060 (1974).

D1. Daniels, F., Jr., Man and radiant energy: Solar radiation. *Hand. Physiol., Sec. 4: Adapt. Environ.* pp. 969–987 (1964).

D2. DeLuca, H. F., Vitamin D: The vitamin and the hormone. *Fed. Proc., Fed. Am. Soc. Exp. Biol.* **33**, 2211–2219 (1974).

D3. DeLuca, H. F., The role of the kidney in the metabolism of vitamin D. *Proc. Int. Congr. Nephrol., 5th, 1972* pp. 127–136 (1974).

D4. DeLuca, H. F., Recent advances in our understanding of the vitamin D endocrine system. *J. Lab. Clin. Med.* **87**, 7–26 (1976).

D5. DeLuca, H. F., Blunt, J. W., and Rikkers, H., Biogenesis. *In* "The Vitamins" (W. H. Sebrell, Jr. and R. S. Harris, eds.), Vol. 3, pp. 213–230. Academic Press, New York, 1971.

D6. Dent, C. E., Metabolic forms of rickets (and osteomalacia). *Treat. Inborn Errors Metab., Proc. Symp. Soc. Study Inborn Errors Metab. 12th, 1976*, pp. 124–129 (1976).

E1. Eisman, J. A., Hamstra, A. J., Kream, B. E., and DeLuca, H. F., A sensitive, precise and convenient method for determination of 1,25-dihydroxyvitamin D in human plasma. *Arch. Biochem. Biophys.* (in press).

E2. Emtage, J. S., Lawson, D. E. M., and Kodicek, E., Vitamin D-induced synthesis of mRNA for calcium-binding protein. *Nature (London)* **246**, 100–101 (1973).

F1. Fraser, D., Kooh, S. W., and Scriver, C. R., Hyperparathyroidism as the cause of hyperaminoaciduria and phosphaturia in human vitamin D deficiency. *Pediatr. Res.* **1**, 425–435 (1967).

F2. Fraser, D., Kooh, S. W., Kind, H. P., Holick, M. F., Tanaka, Y., and DeLuca, H. F., Pathogenesis of hereditary vitamin D dependent rickets: An inborn error of vitamin D metabolism involving defective conversion of 25-hydroxyvitamin D to 1α,25-dihydroxyvitamin D. *N. Engl. J. Med.* **289**, 817–822 (1973).

F3. Fraser, D. R., and Kodicek, E., Unique biosynthesis by kidney of a biologically active vitamin D metabolite. *Nature (London)* **228**, 764–766 (1970).

F4. Fraser, D. R., and Kodicek, E., Regulation of 25-hydroxycholecalciferol-1-hydroxylase activity in kidney by parathyroid hormone. *Nature (London), New Biol.* **241**, 163–166 (1973).

G1. Gallagher, C., Riggs, L., Eisman, J., Arnaud, S., and DeLuca, H. F., Impaired intestinal calcium absorption in postmenopausal osteoporosis: Possible role of vitamin D metabolites and PTH. *Clin. Res.* **24**, 360A (1976).

G2. Garabedian, M., Holick, M. F., DeLuca, H. F., and Boyle, I. T., Control of 25-hydroxycholecalciferol metabolism by the parathyroid glands. *Proc. Natl. Acad. Sci. U.S.A.* **69**, 1673–1676 (1972).

G3. Garabedian, M., Pavlovitch, H., Fellot, C., and Balsan, S., Metabolism of 25-hydroxyvitamin D₃ in anephric rats: A new active metabolite. *Proc. Natl. Acad. Sci. U.S.A.* **71**, 554–557 (1974).

G4. Gekle, D., Ströder, J., and Rostock, D., The effect of vitamin D on renal inorganic phosphate reabsorption of normal rats, parathyroidectomized rats, and rats with rickets. *Pediatr. Res.* **5**, 40–52 (1971).

G5. Ghazarian, J. G., Schnoes, H. K., and DeLuca, H. F., Mechanism of 25-hydroxycholecalciferol 1α-hydroxylation. Incorporation of oxygen-18 into the 1α position of 25-hydroxycholecalciferol. *Biochemistry* **12**, 2555–2558 (1973).

G6. Ghazarian, J. G., Jefcoate, C. R., Knutson, J. C., Orme-Johnson, W. H., and DeLuca, H. F., Mitochondrial cytochrome P₄₅₀: A component of chick kidney 25-hydroxycholecalciferol-1α-hydroxylase. *J. Biol. Chem.* **249**, 3026–3033 (1974).

G7. Glimcher, M. J., Macromolecular aggregation stage and reactivity of collagen in calcification. *Soc. Gen. Physiol.* **6**, 53–84 (1959).

G8. Glorieux, F., and Scriver, C. R., Loss of a parathyroid-sensitive component of phosphate transport in X-linked hypophosphatemia. *Science* **175**, 997–1000 (1972).

G9. Glorieux, F., Scriver, C. R., Holick, M. F., and DeLuca, H. F., X-Linked hypophosphatemic rickets: Inadequate therapeutic response to 1,25-dihydroxycholecalciferol. *Lancet* **2**, 287–289 (1973).

G10. Goldblatt, H., and Soames, K. M., Studies on the fat soluble growth-promoting factor (I) storage (II) synthesis. *Biochem. J.* **17**, 446–453 (1923).

G11. Gran, F. C., The retention of parenterally injected calcium in rachitic dogs. *Acta Physiol. Scand.* **50**, 132–139 (1960).

G12. Gray, R., Boyle, I., and DeLuca, H. F., Vitamin D metabolism: The role of kidney tissue. *Science* **172**, 1232–1234 (1971).

G13. Gray, R. W., Omdahl, J. L., Ghazarian, J. G., and DeLuca, H. F., 25-Hydroxy-cholecalciferol-1-hydroxylase: Subcellular location and properties. *J. Biol. Chem.* **247**, 7528–7532 (1972).

G14. Greaves, J. D., and Schmidt, C. L. A., The role played by bile in the absorption of vitamin D in the rat. *J. Biol. Chem.* **102**, 101–112 (1933).

H1. Haddad, J. G., and Chyu, K. J., Competitive protein-binding radioassay for 25-hydroxycholecalciferol. *J. Clin. Endocrinol. Metab.* **33**, 992–995 (1971).

H2. Haddad, J. G., and Stamp, T. C. B., Circulating 25-hydroxyvitamin D in man. *Am. J. Med.* **57**, 57–62 (1974).

H3. Hallick, R. B., and DeLuca, H. F., 25-Hydroxydihydrotachysterol$_3$-biosynthesis *in vivo* and *in vitro*. *J. Biol. Chem.* **246**, 5733–5738 (1971).

H4. Hallick, R. B., and DeLuca, H. F., Metabolites of dihydrotachysterol$_3$ in target tissues. *J. Biol. Chem.* **247**, 91–97 (1972).

H5. Harmeyer, J., and DeLuca, H. F., Calcium-binding protein and calcium absorption after vitamin D administration. *Arch. Biochem. Biophys.* **133**, 247–254 (1969).

H6. Harnden, D., Kumar, R., Holick, M. F., and DeLuca, H. F., Side chain metabolism of 25-hydroxy-[26,27-^{14}C]vitamin D$_3$ and 1,25-dihydroxy-[26,27-^{14}C]vitamin D$_3$ *in vivo*. *Science* **193**, 493–494 (1976).

H7. Harrison, H. C., and Harrison, H. E., Comparison of activity of 25-hydroxy-cholecalciferol and dihydrotachysterol$_2$ in the thyroparathyroid-ectomized rat. *Proc. Soc. Exp. Biol. Med.* **136**, 411–414 (1971).

H8. Harrison, H. E., and Harrison, H. C., Intestinal transport of phosphate: Action of vitamin D, calcium, and potassium. *Am. J. Physiol.* **201**, 1007–1012 (1961).

H9. Haussler, M. R., Myrtle, J. F., and Norman, A. W., The association of a metabolite of vitamin D$_3$ with intestinal mucosa chromatin *in vivo*. *J. Biol. Chem.* **243**, 4055–4064 (1968).

H10. Haussler, M. R., Zerwekh, J. E., Hesse, R. H., Rizzardo, E., and Pechet, M. M., Biological activity of 1α-hydroxycholecalciferol, a synthetic analog of the hormonal form of vitamin D$_3$. *Proc. Natl. Acad. Sci. U.S.A.* **70**, 2248–2252 (1973).

H11. Haussler, M. R., Baylink, D. J., Hughes, M. R., Brumbaugh, P. F., Wergedal, J. E., Shen, F. H., Nielsen, R. L., Counts, S. J., Bursac, K. M., and McCain, T. A., The assay of 1α,25-dihydroxyvitamin D$_3$: Physiologic and pathologic modulation of circulating hormone levels. *Clin. Endocrinol. (Oxford)* **5**, 151s–165s (1976).

H12. Henry, H. L., and Norman, A. W., Studies on the mechanism of action of calciferol. VII. Localization of 1,25-dihydroxy-vitamin D$_3$ in chick parathyroid glands. *Biochem. Biophys. Res. Commun.* **62**, 781–788 (1975).

H13. Hess, A. F., Weinstock, M., and Helman, F. D., The antirachitic value of irradiated phytosterol and cholesterol. I. *J. Biol. Chem.* **63**, 305–308 (1925).

H14. Higaki, M., Takahashi, M., Suzuki, T., and Sahashi, Y., Metabolic activities of vitamin D in animals. III. Biogenesis of vitamin D sulfate in animal tissue. *J. Vitaminol.* **11**, 261–265 (1965).

H15. Holick, M. F., Garabedian, M., and DeLuca, H. F., 5,6-Trans isomers of cholecalciferol and 25-hydroxycholecalciferol. Substitutes for 1,25-dihydroxychole-calficerol in anephric animals. *Biochemistry* 11, 2715–2719 (1972).

H16. Holick, M. F., Garabedian, M., and DeLuca, H. F., 1,25-Dihydroxycholecalciferol: Metabolite of vitamin D_3 active on bone in anephric rats. *Science* 176, 1146–1147 (1972).

H17. Holick, M. F., DeLuca, H. F., Kasten, P. M., and Korycka, M. B., Isotachysterol₃ and 25-hydroxyisotachysterol₃: Analogs of 1,25-dihydroxyvitamin D_3. *Science* 180, 964–966 (1973).

H18. Holick, M. F., Garabedian, M., Schnoes, H. K., and DeLuca, H. F., Relationship of 25-hydroxyvitamin D_3 side chain structure to biological activity. *J. Biol. Chem.* 250, 226–230 (1975).

H19. Holick, M. F., Kasten-Schraufrogel, P., Tavela, T., and DeLuca, H. F., Biological activity of 1α-hydroxyvitamin D_3 in the rat. *Arch. Biochem. Biophys.* 166, 63–66 (1975).

H20. Holick, M. F., Semmler, E. J., Schnoes, H. K., and DeLuca, H. F., 1α-Hydroxy derivative of vitamin D_3: A highly potent analog of 1α,25-dihydroxyvitamin D_3. *Science* 180, 190–191 (1973).

H21. Holick, M. F., Baxter, L. A., Schraufrogel, P. K., Tavela, T. E., and DeLuca, H. F., Metabolism and biological activity of 24,25-dihydroxyvitamin D_3 in the chick. *J. Biol. Chem.* 251, 397–402 (1976).

H22. Holick, M. F., Schnoes, H. K., DeLuca, H. F., Suda, T., and Cousins, R. J., Isolation and identification of 1,25-dihydroxycholecalciferol. A metabolite of vitamin D active in intestine. *Biochemistry* 10, 2799–2804 (1971).

H23. Holick, M. F., Schnoes, H. K., DeLuca, H. F., Gray, R. W., Boyle, I. T., and Suda, T., Isolation and identification of 24,25-dihydroxycholecalciferol: A metabolite of vitamin D_3 made in the kidney. *Biochemistry* 11, 4251–4255 (1972).

H24. Holick, M. F., Tavela, T. E., Holick, S. A., Schnoes, H. K., DeLuca, H. F., and Gallagher, B. M., Synthesis of 1α-hydroxy[6-³H]vitamin D_3 and its metabolism of 1α,25-dihydroxy[6-³H]vitamin D_3 in the rat. *J. Biol. Chem.* 251, 1020–1024 (1976).

H25. Holick, S. A., Holick, M. F., Tavela, T. E., Schnoes, H. K., and DeLuca, H. F., Metabolism of 1α-hydroxyvitamin D_3 in the chick. *J. Biol. Chem.* 251, 1025–1028 (1976).

H26. Horsting, M., and DeLuca, H. F., *In vitro* production of 25-hydroxycholecalciferol. *Biochem. Biophys. Res. Commun.* 36, 251–256 (1969).

H27. Howland, J., and Kramer, B., Calcium and phosphorus in the serum in relation to rickets. *Am. J. Dis. Child.* 22, 105–119 (1921).

H28. Huldshinsky, M., Heilung von Rachitis durch künstliche Höhensonne. *Dsch. Med. Wochenschr.* 45, 712–713 (1919).

H29. Hunt, R. D., Garcia, F. G., and Hegsted, D. M., A comparison of vitamin D_2 and D_3 in new world primates. I. Production and regression of osteodystrophia fibrosa. *Lab. Anim. Care* 17, 222–234 (1967).

I1. Imrie, M. H., Neville, P. F., Snellgrove, A. W., and DeLuca, H. F., Metabolism of vitamin D_2 and vitamin D_3 in the rachitic chick. *Arch. Biochem. Biophys.* 120, 525–532 (1967).

J1. Jones, G., Schnoes, H. K., and DeLuca, H. F., Isolation and identification of 1,25-dihydroxyvitamin D_2. *Biochemistry* 14, 1250–1256 (1975).

J2. Jones, G., Schnoes, H. K., and DeLuca, H. F., An *in vitro* study of vitamin D_2 hydroxylases in the chick. *J. Biol. Chem.* 251, 24–28 (1976).

J3. Jones, G., Baxter, L. A., DeLuca, H. F., and Schnoes, H. K., Biological activity of 1,25-dihydroxyvitamin D_2 in the chick. *Biochemistry* 15, 713–716 (1976).

K1. Kaneko, C., Yamada, S., Sugimoto, A., Ishikawa, M., Suda, T., Suzuki, M., and Sasaki, S., Synthesis and biological activity of 2α-hydroxyvitamin D_3. *J. Chem. Soc., Perkin Trans.* 1 pp. 1104–1107 (1975).

K2. Kleiner-Bossaller, A., and DeLuca, H. F., Formation of 1,24,25-trihydroxyvitamin D_3 from 1,25-dihydroxyvitamin D_3. *Biochim. Biophys. Acta* 338, 489–495 (1974).

K3. Kodicek, E., Metabolic studies on vitamin D. Symposium on *Bone Struct. Metab., Ciba Found. Symp., 1955* pp. 161–174 (1956).

K4. Kooh, S. W., Fraser, D., DeLuca, H. F., Holick, M. F., Belsey, R. E., Clark, M. B., and Murray, T. M., Treatment of hypoparathyroidism and pseudohypoparathyroidism with metabolites of vitamin D: Evidence for impaired conversion of 25-hydroxyvitamin D to 1α,25-dihydroxyvitamin D. *N. Engl. J. Med.* 293, 840–844 (1975).

K5. Kowarski, S., and Schachter, D., Effects of vitamin D on phosphate transport and incorporation into mucosal constituents of rat intestinal mucosa. *J. Biol. Chem.* 244, 211–217 (1969).

K6. Kream, B. E., Reynolds, R. D., Knutson, J. C., Eisman, J. A., and DeLuca, H. F., Intestinal cytosol binders of 1,25-dihydroxyvitamin D_3 and 25-hydroxyvitamin D_3. *Arch. Biochem. Biophys.* (in press).

K7. Kruse, R., Osteopathien bei antiepileptischer Langzeittherapie. *Monatsschr. Kinderheilkd.* 116, 378–381 (1968).

K8. Kumar, R., and DeLuca, H. F., Side chain oxidation of 25-hydroxy-[26,27-^{14}C] vitamin D_3 and 1,25-dihydroxy-[26,27-^{14}C]vitamin D_3 *in vivo* by chickens. *Biochem. Biophys. Res. Commun.* 69, 197–200 (1976).

L1. Lam, H.-Y., Schnoes, H. K., and DeLuca, H. F., 1α-Hydroxyvitamin D_2: A potent synthetic analog of vitamin D_2. *Science* 186, 1038–1040 (1974).

L2. Lam, H.-Y., Onisko, B. L., Schnoes, H. K., and DeLuca, H. F., Synthesis and biological activity of 3-deoxy-1α-hydroxyvitamin D_3. *Biochem. Biophys. Res. Commun.* 59, 845–849 (1974).

L3. LaMar, G. N., and Budd, D. L., Elucidation of the solution conformation of the A ring in vitamin D using proton coupling constants and a shift reagent. *J. Am. Chem. Soc.* 96, 7317–7324 (1974).

L4. Lawson, D. E. M., and Wilson, P. W., Intranuclear localization and receptor proteins for 1,25-dihydroxyvitamin D_3 in chick intestine. *Biochem. J.* 144, 573–583 (1974).

L5. Lawson, D. E. M., Wilson, P. W., and Kodicek, E., Metabolism of vitamin D. A new cholecalciferol metabolite, involving loss of hydrogen at C-1, in chick intestinal nuclei. *Biochem. J.* 115, 269–277 (1969).

L6. Lawson, D. E. M., Wilson, P. W., Barker, D. C., and Kodicek, E., Isolation of chick intestinal nuclei. Effect of vitamin D_3 on nuclear metabolism. *Biochem. J.* 115, 263–268 (1969).

L7. le Boulch, N., Gulat-Marnay, C., and Raoul, Y., Vitamin D_3 derivatives of human and cow's milk: Cholecalciferol sulfate ester and hydroxy-25-cholecalciferol. *Int. J. Vitam. Nutr. Res.* 44, 167–179 (1974).

L8. Loomis, W. F., Skin-pigment regulation of vitamin D biosynthesis in man. *Science* 157, 501–506 (1967).

L9. Lund, B., Hjorth, L., Kjaer, I., Reimann, I., Friis, T., Anderson, R. B., and Sørensen, O. H., Treatment of osteoporosis of ageing with 1α-hydroxycholecalciferol. *Lancet* 2, 1168–1171 (1975).

L10. Lund, J., and DeLuca, H. F., Biologically active metabolite of vitamin D₃ from bone, liver, and blood serum. *J. Lipid Res.* **7**, 739–744 (1966).

M1. Martin, D. L., and DeLuca, H. F., Influence of sodium on calcium transport by the rat small intestine. *Am. J. Physiol.* **216**, 1351–1359 (1969).

M2. Martin, D. L., and DeLuca, H. F., Calcium transport and the role of vitamin D. *Arch. Biochem. Biophys.* **134**, 139–148 (1969).

M3. McCollum, E. V., and Davis, M., The necessity of certain lipins in the diet during growth. *J. Biol. Chem.* **15**, 167–175 (1913).

M4. McCollum, E. V., Simmonds, N., Becker, J. E., and Shipley, P. G., Studies on experimental rickets. XXI. An experimental demonstration of the existence of a vitamin which promotes calcium deposition. *J. Biol. Chem.* **53**, 293–312 (1922).

M5. McCollum, E. V., Simmonds, N., Shipley, P. G., and Park, E. A., Studies on experimental rickets. XV. The effect of starvation on the healing of rickets. *Bull. Johns Hopkins Hosp.* **33**, 31 (1922).

M6. Melancon, M. J., Jr., and DeLuca, H. F., Vitamin D stimulation of calcium-dependent adenosine triphosphatase in chick intestinal brush borders. *Biochemistry* **9**, 1658–1664 (1970).

M7. Mellanby, E., A further determination of the part played by accessory food factors in the aetiology of rickets. *J. Physiol. (London)* **52**, liii (1919).

M8. Morii, H., Lund, J., Neville, P. F., and DeLuca, H. F., Biological activity of a vitamin D metabolite. *Arch. Biochem. Biophys.* **120**, 508–512 (1967).

M9. Moriuchi, S., and DeLuca, H. F., The effect of vitamin D₃ metabolites on membrane proteins of chick duodenal brush borders. *Arch. Biochem. Biophys.* **174**, 367–372 (1976).

N1. Neer, R. M., Holick, M. F., DeLuca, H. F., and Potts, J. T., Jr., Effects of 1α-hydroxyvitamin D₃ and 1,25-hydroxyvitamin D₃ on calcium and phosphorus metabolism in hypoparathyroidism. *Metab. Clin. Exp.* **24**, 1403–1413 (1975).

N2. Nicolaysen, R., Studies upon the mode of action of vitamin D. III. The influence of vitamin D on the absorption of calcium and phosphorus in the rat. *Biochem. J.* **31**, 122–129 (1937).

N3. Norman, A. W., and DeLuca, H. F., The preparation of H³-vitamins D₂ and D₃ and their localization in the rat. *Biochemistry* **2**, 1160–1168 (1963).

O1. Okamura, W. H., Norman, A. W., and Wing, R. M., Vitamin D: Concerning the relationship between molecular topology and biological function. *Proc. Natl. Acad. U.S.A.* **71**, 4194–4197 (1974).

O2. Okamura, W. H., Mitra, M. N., Procsal, D. A., and Norman, A. W., Studies on vitamin D and its analogs. VIII. 3-Deoxy-1α,25-dihydroxyvitamin D₃, a potent new analog of 1α,25-(OH)₂D₃. *Biochem. Biophys. Res. Commun.* **65**, 24–30 (1975).

O3. Okamura, W. H., Mitra, M. N., Wing, R. M., and Norman, A. W., Chemical synthesis and biological activity of 3-deoxy-1α-hydroxyvitamin D₃ an analog of 1α,25-dihydroxyvitamin D₃, the active form of vitamin D₃. *Biochem. Biophys. Res. Commun.* **60**, 179–185 (1974).

O4. Olson, E. B., Jr., Knutson, J. C., Bhattacharyya, M. H., and DeLuca, H. F., The effect of hepatectomy on the synthesis of 25-hydroxyvitamin D₃. *J. Clin. Invest.* **57**, 1213–1220 (1976).

O5. Omdahl, J. L., and DeLuca, H. F., Regulation of vitamin D metabolism and function. *Physiol. Rev.* **53**, 327–372 (1973).

P1. Pedersen, J. I., Ghazarian, J. G., Orme-Johnson, N. R., and DeLuca, H. F., Isolation of chick renal mitochondrial ferredoxin active in the 25-hydroxyvitamin D₃-1α-hydroxylase system. *J. Biol. Chem.* **251**, 3933–3941 (1976).

P2. Peterson, P. A., Isolation and partial characterization of a human vitamin D-binding plasma protein. *J. Biol. Chem.* **246**, 7748–7754 (1971).

P3. Ponchon, G., and DeLuca, H. F., The role of the liver in the metabolism of vitamin D. *J. Clin. Invest.* **48**, 1273–1279 (1969).

P4. Ponchon, G., Kennan, A. L., and DeLuca, H. F., "Activation" of vitamin D by the liver. *J. Clin. Invest.* **48**, 2032–2037 (1969).

P5. Procsal, D. A., Okamura, W. H., and Norman, A. W., Structural requirements for the interaction of $1\alpha,25$-$(OH)_2$-vitamin D_3 with its chick intestinal receptor system. *J. Biol. Chem.* **250**, 8382–8388 (1975).

P6. Puschett, J. B., Beck, W. S., Jr., and Jelonek, A., Parathyroid hormone and 25-hydroxyvitamin D_3: Synergistic and antagonistic effects on renal phosphate transport. *Science* **190**, 473–475 (1975).

R1. Raisz, L. G., Trummel, C. L., Holick, M. F., and DeLuca, H. F., 1,25-Dihydroxycholecalciferol: A potent stimulator of bone resorption in tissue culture. *Science* **175**, 768–769 (1972).

R2. Rasmussen, H. DeLuca, H., Arnaud, C., Hawker, C., and von Stedingk, M., The relationship between vitamin D and parathyroid hormone. *J. Clin. Invest.* **42**, 1940–1946 (1963).

R3. Reade, T. M., Scriver, C. R., Glorieux, F. H., Nogrady, B., Delvin, E., Poirier, R., Holick, M. F., and DeLuca, H. F., Response to crystalline 1α-hydroxyvitamin D_3 in vitamin D dependency. *Pediatr. Res.* **9**, 593–599 (1975).

R4. Reynolds, J. J., Holick, M. F., and DeLuca, H. F., The effects of vitamin D analogues on bone resorption. *Calcif. Tissue Res.* **15**, 333–339 (1974).

R5. Ribovich, M. L., and DeLuca, H. F., The influence of dietary calcium and phosphorus on intestinal calcium transport in rats given vitamin D metabolites. *Arch. Biochem. Biophys.* **170**, 529–535 (1975).

R6. Ribovich, M. L., and DeLuca, H. F., Intestinal calcium transport: Parathyroid hormone and adaptation to dietary calcium. *Arch. Biochem. Biophys.* **175**, 256–261 (1976).

R7. Rikkers, H., and DeLuca, H. F., An *in vivo* study of the carrier proteins of ^{3}H-vitamins D_3 and D_4 in rat serum. *Am. J. Physiol.* **213**, 380–386 (1967).

R8. Rutherford, W. E., Hruska, K., Blondin, J., Holick, M., DeLuca, H., Klahr, S., and Slatopolsky, E., The effect of 5,6-*trans*-vitamin D_3 on calcium absorption in chronic renal disease. *J. Clin. Endocrinol. Metab.* **40**, 13–18 (1975).

S1. Schachter, D., Vitamin D and the active transport of calcium by the small intestine. *In* "The Transfer of Calcium and Strontium Across Biological Membranes" (R. H. Wasserman, ed.), pp. 197–210. Academic Press, New York, 1963.

S2. Schachter, D., and Rosen, S. M., Active transport of Ca^{45} by the small intestine and its dependence on vitamin D. *Am. J. Physiol.* **196**, 357–362 (1959).

S3. Schachter, D., Finkelstein, J. D., and Kowarski, S., Metabolism of vitamin D. I. Preparation of radioactive vitamin D and its intestinal absorption in the rat. *J. Clin. Invest.* **43**, 787–796 (1964).

S4. Schenck, F., Über das Kristallisierte Vitamin D_3. *Naturwissenschaften* **25**, 159 (1937).

S5. Sebrell, W. H., Jr., and Harris, R. S., eds., "The Vitamins," 1st ed., Vol. 2. Academic Press, New York, 1954.

S6. Semmler, E. J., Holick, M. F., Schnoes, H. K., and DeLuca, H. F., The synthesis of $1\alpha,25$-dihydroxycholecalciferol—a metabolically active form of vitamin D_3. *Tetrahedron Lett.* **40**, 4147–4150 (1972).

S7. Short, E. M., Binder, H. J., and Rosenberg, L. E., Familial hypophosphatemic rickets: Defective transport of inorganic phosphate by intestinal mucosa. *Science* 179, 700–702 (1973).

S8. Silverberg, D. S., Bettcher, K. B., Dossetor, J. B., Overton, T. R., Holick, M. F., and DeLuca, H. F., Effect of 1,25-dihydroxycholecalciferol in renal osteodystrophy. *Can. Med. Assoc. J.* 112, 190–195 (1975).

S9. Slatopolsky, E., Rutherford, W. E., Hoffsten, P. E., Elkan, I. O., Butcher, H. R., and Bricker, N. S., Non-suppressible secondary hyperparathyroidism in chronic progressive renal disease. *Kidney Int.* 1, 38–46 (1972).

S10. Smerdon, G. T., Daniel Whistler and the English disease. A translation and biographical note. *J. Hist. Med. Allied Sci.* 5, 397–415 (1950).

S11. Stamp, T. C. B., Round, J. M., Rowe, D. J. F., and Haddad, J. G., Plasma levels and therapeutic effect of 25-hydroxycholecalciferol in epileptic patients taking anticonvulsant drugs. *Br. Med. J.* 4, 9–12 (1972).

S12. Stanbury, S. W., Bone disease in uremia. *Am. J. Med.* 44, 714–724 (1968).

S13. Steele, T. H., Engle, J. E., Tanaka, Y., Lorenc, R. S., Dudgeon, K. L., and DeLuca, H. F., Phosphatemic action of 1,25-dihydroxyvitamin D₃. *Am. J. Physiol.* 229, 489–495 (1975).

S14. Steenbock, H., and Black, A., Fat-soluble vitamins. XVII. The induction of growth-promoting and calcifying properties in a ration by exposure to ultraviolet light. *J. Biol. Chem.* 61, 405–422 (1924).

S15. Steenbock, H., and Black, A., Fat-soluble vitamins. XXIII. The induction of growth-promoting and calcifying properties in fats and their unsaponifiable constituents by exposure to light. *J. Biol. Chem.* 64, 263–298 (1925).

S16. Steenbock, H., and Herting, D. C., Vitamin D and growth. *J. Nutr.* 57, 449–468 (1955).

S17. Steenbock, H., Kletzien, S. W. F., and Halpin, J. G., The reaction of the chicken to irradiated ergosterol and irradiated yeast as contrasted with the natural vitamin D in fish liver oil. *J. Biol. Chem.* 97, 249–264 (1932).

S18. Stern, P. H., DeLuca, H. F., and Ikekawa, N., Bone resorbing activities of 24-hydroxy stereoisomers of 24-hydroxyvitamin D₃ and 24,25-dihydroxyvitamin D₃. *Biochem. Biophys. Res. Commun.* 67, 965–971 (1975).

S19. Stern, P. H., Trummel, C. L., Schnoes, H. K., and DeLuca, H. F., Bone resorbing activity of vitamin D metabolites and cogeners *in vitro*: Influence of hydroxyl substituents in the A ring. *Endocrinology* 97, 1552–1558 (1975).

S20. Suda, T., DeLuca, H. F., Schnoes, H. K., and Blunt, J. W., The isolation and identification of 25-hydroxyergocalciferol. *Biochemistry* 8, 3515–3520 (1969).

S21. Suda, T., Hallick, R. B., DeLuca, H. F., and Schnoes, H. K., 25-Hydroxydihydrotachysterol₃. Synthesis and biological activity. *Biochemistry* 9, 1651–1657 (1970).

T1. Tanaka, Y., and DeLuca, H. F., Bone mineral mobilization activity of 1,25-dihydroxycholecalciferol, a metabolite of vitamin D. *Arch. Biochem. Biophys.* 146, 574–578 (1971).

T2. Tanaka, Y., and DeLuca, H. F., The control of 25-hydroxyvitamin D metabolism by inorganic phosphorus. *Arch. Biochem. Biophys.* 154, 566–574 (1973).

T3. Tanaka, Y., and DeLuca, H. F., Stimulation of 24,25-dihydroxyvitamin D₃ production by 1,25-dihydroxyvitamin D₃. *Science* 183, 1198–1200 (1974).

T4. Tanaka, Y., and DeLuca, H. F., Biological activity of 1,25-dihydroxyvitamin D₃ in the rat. *Endocrinology* 92, 417–422 (1973).

T5. Tanaka, Y., Lorenc, R. S., and DeLuca, H. F., The role of 1,25-dihydroxyvitamin D_3 and parathyroid hormone in the regulation of chick renal 25-hydroxy-vitamin D_3-24-hydroxylase. *Arch. Biochem. Biophys.* **171**, 521–526 (1975).

T6. Tanaka, Y., DeLuca, H. F., Ikekawa, N., Morisaki, M., and Koizumi, N., Determination of stereochemical configuration of the 24-hydroxyl group of 24,25-dihydroxyvitamin D_3 and its biological importance. *Arch. Biochem. Biophys.* **170**, 620–626 (1975).

T7. Tanaka, Y., Frank, H., DeLuca, H. F., Koizumni, N., and Ikekawa, N., Importance of the stereochemical position of the 24-hydroxyl to biological activity of 24-hydroxyvitamin D_3. *Biochemistry* **14**, 3293–3296 (1975).

T7a. Tanaka, Y., and DeLuca, H. F., in preparation.

T8. Taylor, A. N., *In vitro* phosphate transport in chick ileum: Effect of cholecalciferol, calcium, sodium and metabolic inhibitors. *J. Nutr.* **104**, 489–494 (1974).

T9. Taylor, A. N., and Wasserman, R. H., Correlations between the vitamin D-induced calcium binding protein and intestinal absorption of calcium. *Fed. Proc., Fed. Am. Soc. Exp. Biol.* **28**, 1834–1838 (1969).

T10. Taylor, A. N., and Wasserman, R. H., Immunofluorescent localization of vitamin D-dependent calcium-binding protein. *J. Histochem. Cytochem.* **18**, 107–115 (1970).

T11. Taylor, A. N., and Wasserman, R. H., Vitamin D-induced calcium-binding protein: Comparative aspects in kidney and intestine. *Am. J. Physiol.* **223**, 110–114 (1972).

T12. Trummel, C. L., Raisz, L. G., Blunt, J. W., and DeLuca, H. F., 25-Hydroxycholecalciferol: Stimulation of bone resorption in tissue culture. *Science* **163**, 1450–1451 (1969).

U1. Uribe, A., Holick, M. F., Jorgensen, N. A., and DeLuca, H. F., Action of *Solanum malacoxylon* on calcium metabolism in the rat. *Biochem. Biophys. Res. Commun.* **58**, 257–262 (1974).

W1. Waddell, J., The provitamin D of cholesterol. I. The antirachitic efficacy of irradiated cholesterol. *J. Biol. Chem.* **105**, 711–739 (1934).

W2. Wasserman, R. H., Active vitamin D-like substances in *Solanum malacoxylon* and other calcinogenic plants. *Nutr. Rev.* **33**, 1–5 (1975).

W3. Wasserman, R. H., and Taylor, A. N., Intestinal absorption of phosphate in the chick: Effect of vitamin D_3 and other parameters. *J. Nutr.* **103**, 586–599 (1973).

W4. Wasserman, R. H., Taylor, A. N., and Fulmer, C. S., Vitamin D induced calcium binding protein and the intestinal absorption of calcium. *Biochem. Soc. Spec. Publ.* **3**, 55–74 (1974).

W5. Windaus, A., Lettre, H., and Schenck, F., 7-Dehydrocholesterol. *Justus Liebigs Ann. Chem.* **520**, 98–106 (1935).

W6. Windaus, A., Linsert, O., Lüttringhaus, A., and Weidlich, G., Crystalline vitamin D_2. *Justus Liebigs Ann. Chem.* **492**, 226–241 (1932).

Z1. Zull, J. E., and Repke, D. W., The tissue localization of tritiated parathyroid hormone in thyroparathyroidectomized rats. *J. iBol. Chem.* **247**, 2195–2199 (1972).

ADVANCES IN QUALITY CONTROL

T. P. Whitehead

Department of Clinical Chemistry, University of Birmingham,
Queen Elizabeth Medical Center, Edgbaston, Birmingham, England

1. Introduction

Using the language of those concerned with the mass media, the subject of quality control in clinical chemistry is suffering from "overexposure." Even those most devoted to the subject are becoming bored by the exponential growth in published papers and the innumerable symposia concerned with the subject. Despite this, and also because of it, the author

175

has written a chapter that attempts to sum up the present situation and also to highlight unsolved problems. The result is a personal and somewhat philosophical contribution to the subject. It attempts to answer several important questions: What evidence is there that all the endeavors of the profession have resulted in improved patient care? Is the present situation satisfactory? If it is not, for what reasons is it not?

A useful source of objective evidence concerning the quality of analytical performance of clinical chemistry laboratories is to be found in the results of interlaboratory surveys. Improvements in performance have been demonstrated over the last two decades in several countries. Such improvement is based upon the level of agreement between laboratories analyzing the same material and has been demonstrated both in the United States (G1) and the United Kingdom (W4). It is of considerable interest to compare the performance of United States laboratories in 1947, when probably the first interlaboratory survey was carried out by Belk and Sunderman (B2), with the present day results of such surveys. Using serum calcium determination as an example, in 1947 only 40% of laboratories obtained a result within ±10% of the mean result. Today surveys by the American College of Pathologists show that 95% of laboratories obtain results within ±10% of the mean value. Again using serum calcium as an example, in the United Kingdom a survey by Wootton and King published in 1953 (W9) showed that only 51% of laboratories obtained results within ±10% of the mean, whereas in recent surveys 95% of laboratories obtain results within that range. In both countries similar improvement can be shown for other substances.

There is no doubt that much of the improvement in performance has been brought about by the improvement in analytical techniques and equipment, particularly by the introduction of automation (W4). However, it is possible that the use of quality control techniques has also played an integral part. Is the present situation satisfactory? Are the majority of laboratories performing sufficiently well to meet clinical needs? This is a complex problem, and there is no simple answer. Not until a substance can be determined with reasonable precision can its use as an aid in the diagnostic process of classification of patients be truly assessed. With increasing precision and accuracy, the usefulness of a determination may be considerably increased. There are several important examples.

In the late 1950s and early 1960s the use of serum calcium determinations in the diagnosis of hyperparathyroidism was limited by the poor precision and accuracy of the techniques in common use. The majority of laboratories used techniques based upon precipitation of the calcium as oxalate and titration of the washed precipitate with permanganate solution. In the United Kingdom at the present time only three of the 428 laboratories practicing clinical chemistry use such a technique; it has been replaced by automated colorimetric or atomic absorption techniques. The direct result of the adoption of these newer techniques has been a considerable improvement in the uesfulness of serum calcium determinations in the diagnosis of hyperparathyroidism, and many of the additional and expensive methods of investigation used in earlier years, such as response to a low-calcium diet, have been dropped.

A second important example is the use of serum albumin determination. When the method of determination of albumin was predominantly based upon the difference in the determination of total protein and salt precipitation of the total globulins, the resultant precision and accuracy were responsible for the poor discriminating power of serum albumin. The usefulness of serum albumin determinations in such clinical conditions as liver dysfunction, malabsorption, and cancer of various sites is being demonstrated at the present time in the author's laboratory.

There have been a number of attempts in the past few years to assess the precision of the more common determinations necessary for present-day routine clinical purposes. Table 1 shows such values published by Tonks (T1), Barnett (B1), and Cotlove et al. (C1). Many laboratories can match the stringent requirements of Cotlove and his colleagues for all the listed determinations other than sodium. The precision of the author's laboratory assessed by control sera analyses during 1974 is also shown in the table and illustrates this point. Such levels of precision can be maintained only by continuous vigilance, using quality control techniques.

What about the situation in laboratories in general? Early in 1975, portions of the same blood serum were distributed to 312 hospital clinical chemistry laboratories in the United Kingdom taking part in the UK National Quality Control Scheme (W6). Again using serum calcium as an example, the results obtained by the participating laboratories are shown in the histogram in Fig. 1. Fourteen laboratories returned values below a commonly accepted reference interval ("normal range"), and twenty laboratories obtained values above it. The remaining 277 laboratories returned results spread through the reference range. Similar findings could be shown for many other substances, and surveys in other countries show a similar situation.

The situation with regard to enzymes is even more disturbing. Table 2 again shows the results returned by participants in the UK National Quality Control Scheme when asked to analyze the same material for aspartate aminotransferase (SGOT). The large number of different methods in use added to the problem, but the spread of results obtained by laboratories using the same method is unacceptably high.

TABLE 1
"ACCEPTABLE" COEFFICIENTS OF VARIATION COMPARED WITH THOSE ACHIEVED
AT THE DEPARTMENT OF CLINICAL CHEMISTRY, QUEEN ELIZABETH
MEDICAL CENTRE (QEMC), BIRMINGHAM, U.K.

| Determination | Coefficients of variation regarded as acceptable | | | CV achieved at QEMC (1974) |
	Tonks (T1)	Barnett (B1)	Cotlove et al. (C1)	
Sodium (140 mmoles/liter)	1.8	1.5	0.4	0.7
Potassium (4.2 mmoles/liter)	10.0	6.2	3.4	1.1
Chloride (100 mmoles/liter)	2.0	2.2	0.9	—
Calcium (2.5 mmoles/liter)	6.0	2.3	1.6	1.2
Phosphate (4.5 mg/100 ml; 140 mmoles/liter)	10.0	5.6	6.6	—
Bilirubin (1.8 mg/100 ml; 30 μmoles/liter)	10.0	20.0	—	3.3
Total protein (7 g/100 ml)	7.0	4.3	3.2	2.6
Albumin (4.0 g/100 ml)	10.0	7.1	3.5	3.1
Glucose (100 mg/100 ml; 5.5 mmoles/liter)	10.0	5.0	4.7	2.1
Uric acid (6.0 mg/100 ml; 0.36 mmoles/liter)	10.0	8.3	12.3	2.2
Urea (40 mg/100 ml; 6.7 mmoles/liter)	10.0	7.4	7.5	2.3
Cholesterol (200 mg/100 ml; 5.1 mmoles/liter)	10.0	—	8.2	4.0

Radioimmunoassay is not practiced in every clinical chemistry laboratory and tends to be the province of the larger and specialized laboratories. There have been several interlaboratory surveys of radioimmunoassay techniques which indicate that some laboratories would be more usefully employed collecting random numbers. Although the situation has improved, there are still considerable problems that will have a direct bearing on patient care. In addition, there is every reason to believe that quality control is not correctly practiced in many laboratories. Such an impression has been confirmed by the author's visits to laboratories which had been shown to be performing poorly in the UK National Quality Control Scheme (W6) and in visits to laboratories in a number of countries on behalf of the World Health Organization.

Thus, despite the wide use of quality control techniques, the present situation is disturbing. Many laboratories appear to practice quality control techniques in a manner that falsely reassures them rather than re-

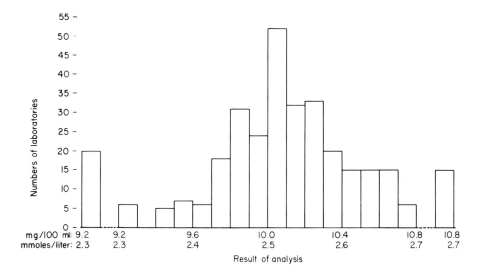

FIG. 1. Results of analyses of portions of the same serum by 312 laboratories in the United Kingdom. The distribution was made early in 1975. Twenty (6.4%) laboratories returned a result *below* the usually accepted reference (normal) range of 9.2 mg/100 ml (2.30 mmoles/liter); 15 (4.6%) laboratories returned a result *above* the usually accepted reference (normal) range.

flecting the true situation. This article is concerned with the possible reasons for such a situation.

2. The Terminology of Quality Control

The subject of quality control, and particularly its teaching, are bedeviled by problems of terminology. Terms are used that have different meanings to different authors. New terms are introduced without adequate definition or explanation of their use. Despite such proliferation of terms, it is the author's experience in writing about and teaching the subject that there are insufficient terms available.

The Expert Panel of the International Federation of Clinical Chemistry have produced Provisional Recommendations on Quality Control in Clinical Chemistry (B3). In Part 1, which is concerned with terminology, there are no fewer than 53 terms defined by the Panel. In writing a book on the subject (W4) the author has completely avoided 34 of the terms, but has used the following 19 terms in the manner advocated by the Panel:

TABLE 2

RESULTS FROM SURVEY OF ASPARTATE AMINOTRANSFERASE (SGOT) METHODS

Method description	Temperature (°C)	Unit system	Total no. of results	Mean	SD	CV	Lowest result	Highest result	Excluding those outside 2 × SD			
									No. of results	Mean	SD	CV
UV optimized	25°	IU/liter	22	111.9	35.7	31.9	70	254	21	105.1	16.8	16.0
	30°	IU/liter	2	166	—	—	164	168	—	—	—	—
	35°	IU/liter	7	197.4	—	—	120	240	—	—	—	—
	37°	IU/liter	73	208.3	53.2	25.5	62	343	67	216.6	35.2	16.2
	25°	Karmen	3	205.3	—	—	165	231	—	—	—	—
	37°	Karmen	1	229	—	—	—	—	—	—	—	—
	37°	Reitman–Frankel	1	255	—	—	—	—	—	—	—	—
UV nonoptimized	25°	IU/liter	24	87.8	24.3	27.6	47	175	23	84.0	16.0	19.1
	30°	IU/liter	3	131.3	—	—	94	153	—	—	—	—
	35°	IU/liter	11	158.4	13.9	8.7	142	182	11	158.4	13.9	8.7
	37°	IU/liter	40	194.5	48.1	24.7	89	315	37	196.9	38.8	19.7
	25°	Karmen	8	187.2	—	—	127	230	—	—	—	—
	37°	Reitman–Frankel	2	183.5	—	—	181	186	—	—	—	—
	37°	Reitman–Frankel	3	161.7	—	—	91	210	—	—	—	—
Manual colorimetric, two point	25°	IU/liter	6	112.4	—	—	72	210	—	—	—	—
	37°	IU/liter	18	131.9	83.2	63.1	48	350	17	119.1	64.9	54.5
	37°	Reitman–Frankel	11	217.9	151.9	69.7	95	650	10	174.8	53.4	30.5
	37°	Karmen	3	113.3	—	—	105	126	—	—	—	—
	Sigma kit	Sigma–Frankel	10	144.1	47.8	33.1	50	222	10	144.1	47.8	33.1
AutoAnalyzer, two point	25°	IU/liter	2	130	—	—	110	150	—	—	—	—
	37°	IU/liter	7	271.7	—	—	160	375	—	—	—	—
	45°	IU/liter	6	229.1	—	—	132	365	—	—	—	—
	37°	Reitman–Frankel	3	216.3	—	—	179	263	—	—	—	—
	37°	Karmen	4	284	—	—	210	345	—	—	—	—
SMA 12/60 UV	37°	IU/liter	3	219.3	—	—	135	340	—	—	—	—
Colorimetric	40°	IU/liter	1	300	—	—	—	—	—	—	—	—
Colorimetric	45°	IU/liter	1	365	—	—	—	—	—	—	—	—
Colorimetric	37°	Reitman–Frankel	1	170	—	—	—	—	—	—	—	—

Accuracy

Analytical method

Assigned value

Carry-over

Control material

External quality control

Internal quality control

Random

Reference value

Result

Sample

Specifically

Specimen

Standard

True value

The author has added five new terms that he has found to be important in quality control:

Random mistake

Variance

Correct value

Optimal conditions variance

Routine conditions variance

2.1. Random Mistake

This term is used in compliance with the colloquial use of the word *mistake,* and the term random means haphazard and unpredictable. The ability to detect such mistakes by quality control techniques is limited because they will, by their very nature, occur in a haphazard and unpredictable manner. Examples include: the misreading of instruments, haphazard errors in calculation, transcription errors, incorrect patient identity, incorrect specimen identity.

The term random mistake may be defined as an incorrect value that has occurred in an unpredictable and haphazard manner; note that it is concerned with a single value.

2.2. Variance

The IFCC Expert Panel obviously had considerable difficulty in defining the terms accuracy and precision and eventually decided that the terms were better expressed as inaccuracy and imprecision so that the definitions could be expressed in quantitative terms. The definitions proposed by the Panel are as follows:

Inaccuracy: Numerical difference between the mean of a set of results and the true value. This difference (positive or negative) may be expressed in the units in which a quantity is measured or as a percentage of the true value.

Imprecision: Standard deviation or coefficient of variation of the results in a set of replicate measurements. The mean value and number of replicates must be stated and the design used must be described in such a way that other workers can repeat it. This is particularly important whenever a specific term is used to denote a particular type of imprecision, such as between laboratory within-day or between-day.

The emphasis in the Panel's recommendations that precision and accuracy, or in their terms, imprecision and inaccuracy, can only be assessed in *sets* of results is a point frequently missed by many authors. Accuracy and precision cannot be assessed for an individual result; they can be assessed only in relation to a set of results on the same material. However, the Panel, in stating that imprecision and inaccuracy can be expressed in quantitative terms, have ignored an extremely important point. One of these attributes can be correctly assessed only if the other is constant. Thus imprecision of a set of results can be calculated, but if accuracy alters during the observation of the set of results, then the calculation of imprecision is meaningless. Equally, calculation of the inaccuracy of a set of results may be invalidated if the precision does not remain constant during the set of observations. This problem is referred to later.

When faced with discord and discrepancy of a set of results, there is often difficulty in deciding which of the three sources of discrepancy—accuracy, precision, or random mistakes—is responsible. A term is needed, and the use of the word *variance* is advocated. It means discord and discrepancy in the results of measuring the same quantity on the same material. Statisticians use the same word to describe the square of the standard deviation; this is the waste of a good English word on a statistic that is rarely communicated. The author's use of the word variance will be illustrated in later sections of this chapter.

2.3. CORRECT VALUE

A third additional term found to be necessary is concerned with the definition of accuracy. The inclusion in the definition of accuracy of the term true value is academic if the true value is rarely known. This is often the situation in clinical chemistry.

Again using serum calcium as an example, it is now possible to determine calcium in serum by an absolute method of isotopic dilution. The mean value of results obtained by such a method is of considerable interest in comparison with the mean result obtained by other methods. However, for other methods a correct result should be available. For example, if the analysis is performed by a Technicon AutoAnalyzer method, the laboratory will want to know the correct result for that material by that method. It will almost certainly be different from the true result, but nevertheless correct in itself.

Correct value could be defined as the best estimate of a quantity for a particular material using a defined analytical method. Accuracy could then have a broader definition as the relationship of a set of results to the correct value. Sometimes the correct value will be the same as the true value.

3. Quality Control Techniques

Quality control in the clinical chemistry laboratory involves several related activities: (1) preventive measures adopted to minimize variance; (2) assessing the variance of an analytical technique by performing analyses on control material at the same time as on patients' material; (3) statistical analysis of patients' results; (4) taking part in interlaboratory surveys.

In many laboratories the occasional analysis of a particular control material and plotting the result on a conventional control chart is the limit of the quality control activity of the laboratory. Such repetitive activity carried out without understanding or thought may give false comfort and assurance rather than a truly objective assessment of the variance of results. Quality control techniques must truly assess the variance in the results of the analyses performed. When a particular analytical method has been shown to be yielding results with an unacceptably high variance, or there has been a deterioration in the variance of a method during its routine use, then solving the problem and incorporating the solution into the preventive measures is frequently very demanding in scientific skill.

Skill must stem from a sound scientific training in clinical chemistry, so that the basic chemical and physical techniques used are fully understood. It is of interest that this point was made in the first published papers on interlaboratory surveys by Belk and Sundermann (B2). Despite this, poorly trained personnel are used in too many laboratories, and poor results ensue. It is relatively easy to teach laboratory personnel how to analyze control material and plot the results on a Levey and Jennings (L1) type chart. It is much more difficult to teach laboratory workers how to reduce the variance of a method.

4. Preventive Measures in Quality Control

The precautions taken prior to the performance of an analysis are preventive measures; some are obvious and reflect the basic knowledge and correctness of approach of the laboratory worker. Rarely are the preventive measures complete when an analytical method is first used. Experience gained by analysis of control material will result in the addition of other preventive measures.

The sources of variance in analytical results that need to be the subject of preventive measures are frequently obvious to well-trained laboratory workers, but there are some measures that many laboratories ignore. For this reason they are worth emphasizing. The steps in many clinical chemistry analyses that contribute to the total variance may be conveniently grouped as follows: (1) specimen collection and preparation; (2) sampling of the specimen; (3) the analytical process (e.g., addition of reagents, mixing, temperature control, etc.); (4) measurement (e.g., colorimetric reading); (5) calculation of results. A further source of variance may be the transport variance due to the contamination of one sample by a previous sample (carry-over).

The standard deviation of the method could be calculated from the individual standard deviations of each step, provided that each step is independent of others. The S of the method is the square root of the sum of the squares of each individual stage:

$$S = (S_1^2 + S_2^2 + 5_3^2 \cdots S_n^2)^{1/2}$$

Knowledge of the possible contribution of each step of a technique to the total variance is important in using correct preventive measures.

4.1.   Specimen Collection and Preparation

The variances in results that can be introduced at this stage are considerable. They include changes that occur in a wide range of substances, and many are well documented. Such variance may far exceed the analytical variance unless correct specimen handling procedures are used. Space will not allow detailed consideration, but the following factors are frequently of importance.

a. Physiological state of the patient (e.g., time of day, diet, posture).

b. Method of collection (e.g., application of tourniquet).

c. Correct patient and specimen identification (e.g., the importance of unique identity).

d. Specimen containers: The materials in which biological fluids are collected and stored may have important effects on the final result. The false assumption that all plastics are inert has led to high variance in analysis.

e. Specimen transport (e.g., exposure to high or low ambient temperatures, sunlight, etc.). The effect of sunlight is not confined to changes in bilirubin; uric acid is light sensitive in serum.

f. Specimen handling in the laboratory (e.g., speedy separation of serum free from white cells, avoiding evaporation, exposure to sunlight, etc.).

4.2. SAMPLING

A sample is that portion of a specimen used in the analytical process. It is usually a measured portion, and the measurement will have a variance. Mouth pipetting is unwise in the clinical laboratory, and many semi-automatic pipettes are now available. They are reasonably priced; many have a precision of less than ±0.5% at serum volume of less than 25 μl.

4.3. ANALYTICAL PROCESS VARIANCE

Although the contributions of such activities as pipetting, colorimetric reading, and calculation are appreciated by many clinical chemists, there is increasing evidence that the role of the analytical process variance is severely underestimated. The term analytical process variance is not ideal. It is the variance of the chemical reaction, including variance produced by (a) failure to mix reactants effectively at any stage; (b) failure to maintain the reactants at a constant and correct temperature; (c) failure to time reactants correctly; (d) exposure of the reactant to light. In addition, variance produced by deterioration of reagents or standards is included in this variance.

For many colorimetric assays the magnitude of the variances of pipetting, colorimetric measurement, and calculation of result are common to several methods, yet the total variance of the analytical method is vastly different. Those determinations where there is difficulty in controlling the reaction, e.g., cholesterol determination by acetic anhydride/sulfuric acid reagent, have a high variance owing to difficulties in controlling the chemical reaction.

There is increasing evidence that a large part of the variance of enzyme determination is due to the high analytical process variance. The introduction of automatic methods of analysis has not necessarily increased the precision of pipetting and colorimetric reading, but it has improved the replication of analytical conditions under which reactions take place. It is for this reason that many automated methods of analysis are more precise than manual methods (W4).

4.4. MEASUREMENT

As stated previously the variance of such activities as spectrophotometry, flame photometry, etc., is reasonably well understood and documented. Extremely precise instruments are now available to many clinical chemistry laboratories.

4.5. CALCULATION

The variance introduced at the calculation stage of an analytical method is frequently underestimated. The plotting of a graph of concentration of calibration material against instrument reading and the drawing of a freehand calibration curve is a source of high variance unless particular care is taken. The process of reading off results from such a graph frequently has a subjective bias (W2).

4.6. ADDITIONAL PREVENTIVE MEASURES

Other areas in which important preventive measures are sometimes more nebulous than those listed above, but are equally important, are listed below:

a. Laboratory environment. This includes such factors as laboratory cleanliness and layout. Noise, lighting, temperature, and humidity also have obvious importance.

b. Apparatus. The availability of well-maintained apparatus the operation of which is clearly understood by the staff.

c. Qualification and training of staff. This has been discussed earlier.

d. Work load. A constant and inappropriately high work load can lead to poor staff morale. Too low a work load can be equally damaging and unstimulating.

e. Management–staff relationships.

f. Documentation. Passing of techniques from one laboratory worker to another without correct documentation is an important factor in poor analytical work.

5. The Techniques of Quality Control—Determining the Variance of a Method

The most commonly practised quality control technique in clinical chemistry is the analysis of control material at the same time as patients' material. If the same control material is used on each occasion, then a conventional quality control graph can be prepared where the observed value is recorded daily on a chart showing a "target" or mean value and the expected confidence limits based upon standard deviation calculations.

Since the introduction of such charts in clinical chemistry by Levey and Jennings (L1), their use has been described on many occasions by various authors. The limitations of such a technique have not been as clearly stated. Their use can lead to the situation described earlier, that of falsely assuring the laboratory worker regarding the variance.

When a technique is first introduced in a laboratory or when the quality control of an established technique is introduced, Levey-Jennings charts are essential. In the author's laboratory two such charts are prepared: one shows the results of assessing the optional conditions variance and the second the routine conditions variance.

5.1. OPTIMAL CONDITIONS VARIANCE (OCV)

It is usual, in the author's laboratory, to determine OCV by carrying out approximately twenty analyses for the same quantity on the same material. The objective is to try to repeat analyses with the conditions of analysis as ideal and stable as possible, hence the term "optimal conditions." All known appropriate preventive measures need to be rigidly applied.

The following is not a complete list of such measures, but a guide to the approach: (a) use the same apparatus for all determinations and make sure it is functioning correctly; (b) use freshly prepared and checked reagents; (c) prepare the analyses on stable, homogeneous material; (d) check instrument readings and calculations; (e) perform the analyses as close in time as possible; (f) carefully control those factors that may contribute to the analytical process variance described in an earlier section (e.g., time, temperature, mixing, etc.); (g) use experienced personnel.

The mean and standard deviation of the results are plotted on a control chart, as in Fig. 2. Drift of results during the course of performing the analyses and outlier results may be detected by using such charts.

The statistics of the OCV are an important basis for the method. If the variance is unacceptably high, it is usually easier to detect causes at this stage rather than in later procedures. The relationship of the OCV to other variances provides important information, as shown later. If a method in routine use develops a high variance and the cause cannot be detected, then a return to check whether the original OCV can be repeated is frequently useful.

5.2. ROUTINE CONDITIONS VARIANCE (RCV)

The material used to assess the OVC should be incorporated into sets of analyses and performed under the conditions normally met during analysis of patients' material. It is not possible to lay down rigid guide-

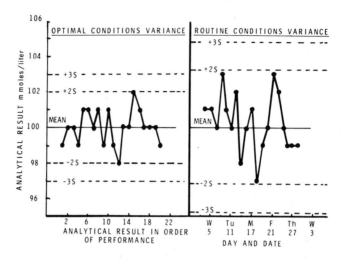

Fig. 2. An example of graphs of optimal conditions and routine conditions variance. S = standard deviation.

lines if the method has not yet been used in routine work, but the following illustrate the approach: (a) The analyses should be performed by the grade of staff who will be required to perform the test routinely. (b) The method should be communicated to such staff using the documentation that is to be used routinely and should particularly include all the known necessary preventive measures. (c) The analyses should be spanned over a period of time, say one a day for 20 days. (d) The analyses should be randomly placed in batches of patient material, not always in favored positions, such as close to standards.

The mean and standard deviation of the results are calculated, and the results plotted on a continuation of the OCV graph (Fig. 2). Note that the horizontal scale now includes day and date. These may have importance in investigating changes in variance.

The OVC and RCV mean value should be the same; if they are not, there has been a change in accuracy. Study the graph for alteration of precision and accuracy. Solving the problem and incorporating the solution into preventive measures is essential before proceeding further. The relationship between the variance of OCV and RCV is an important statistic. The standard deviation of the RCV results is rarely less than twice the RCV for common clinical chemistry determination. Particularly if the ratio of RCV to OCV is greater than two, the possible reasons for the increase of variance under routine conditions should be investigated.

5.3. LIMITATIONS OF OCV AND RCV ASSESSMENTS

As outlined, the suggested techniques check the variance at only one concentration of the substance under consideration. Variance may be different at other concentrations.

In addition, the operator will become familiar with the expected value, and if it is possible for the operator to bias the technique then bias will almost certainly occur. For this reason, when RCV is determined with the operator knowing the expected value, it is described as routine conditions variance-known values (RCVK). Many laboratories only use RCVK for assessment of their variance. This is why they obtain a variance that is comforting but does not accurately reflect the variance obtained on patients' material. Other methods of quality control are essential.

5.4. ROUTINE CONDITIONS VARIANCE—VALUES UNKNOWN TO OPERATOR (RCVU)

This method of assessment of the variance of a method checks the variance at various concentration levels. The range of values should approximate those likely to be met in routine practice.

To avoid bias, the concentration expected should not be known to the operator, and this implies the use of many different types of material. The variations of material may be increased by, say, occasionally reconstituting material in slightly less or more than the prescribed amount of distilled water, e.g., 10.5 ml or 9.5 ml instead of 10.0 ml. Obtaining adequate supplies of good quality control material with correctly assigned values is difficult, but increasingly such products are becoming available.

Plotting the results of RCVU studies is tedious if a separate chart is used for each of the individual materials analyzed. For this reason plotting percentage deviation from the assigned value is useful; several materials can then be incorporated on the same graph. Occasionally, assigned values will be incorrect, and detection of such inaccuracy for a particular material may be detected on such a graph (see the examples given in Fig. 3). The mean coefficient of variation for RCVU gives a reasonably accurate assessment of the variance of the results of patients' material.

5.5. GENERAL COMMENTS

The terms within batch and between batch, within series and between series, repeatability and reproducibility, all have meanings related to

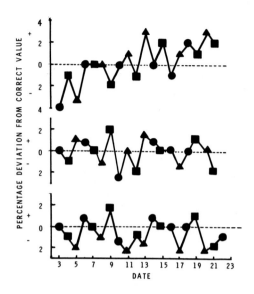

Fig. 3. Examples of routine conditions variance (unknown values) where the percentage variation from the assigned value is plotted. In example 1 (top) all values are drifting to higher values. Example 2 (middle) shows a satisfactory result. In example 3 (bottom), control serum A gives low results on each occasion. This could be because the method gives lower values for this serum or because the correct value for control serum A has not been properly assessed. ▲, control serum A; ●, control serum B; ■, control serum C.

OCV and RCV, but these later terms are preferred because they make clear the objective in making the measurement of variance.

The continuous use of Levey–Jennings type charts, once the OCV and RCV have been assessed, is essential before a technique has been stabilized. Alterations in the variance of a method can occur at any time, even after years of use, but stabilization is established when all the necessary preventive measures have been incorporated. After such stabilization, alteration in variance could occur, for example, as the result of a supply of faulty reagent or standards or a defect developing in a pipette or instrument.

After stabilization, standard deviation lines on the Levey–Jennings graph can indicate the true variance of the method in routine use; prior to this, other calculation of standard deviation may have been made only to be shown later to be too wide as preventive measures became effective. At this time, values occurring outside ±2SD on more than one occasion in twenty indicate unacceptable variance. If they consistently occur on one side of the mean, this indicates unacceptable alteration of accuracy.

If they occur randomly either side of the mean, this indicates poor precision.

6. Using Patients' Results in the Quality Control of Laboratory Results

There are sources of variance in the analysis of patients' material that cannot be monitored by the techniques outlined in previous sections of this chapter. These sources of variance include those introduced during collection of the specimen, transport from patient to laboratory, and specimen preparation (e.g., separation of serum). Control material is not usually subjected to such processes.

Consideration of patient's results and making calculations on them may, in some instances, be a most useful aid to controlling quality. The pioneer of the technique was Hoffman, who published papers advocating such techniques as early as 1955 (W1). Such techniques are usually associated with the calculation of the mean of patients' values for a particular period of time and comparison of the result with previous experience. The plotting of the mean results on a Levey–Jennings-type chart and visual examination of any alteration in the results is frequently useful.

It is important to realize that the technique measures not precision, but changes in the accuracy of results. Frequently the mean value has to be calculated on a truncated set of results to avoid extreme values having an effect on the mean value. The use of truncated values frequently results in the values used being within the reference interval ("normal range") for the method. It is thus really controlling accuracy at that level only. Truncation also reduces the sensitivity of the technique to changes in analytical accuracy of results as shown by Northam and Dixon (N1).

The use of patients' mean values in the quality control of a laboratory's results is often an extremely important additional measure, but each laboratory will have to make its own decision on their usefulness because patient populations are so different. Certain laboratories may have different patient populations on different days; hence, changes detected may be due to patient population changes, not to analytical changes. However, it is the author's experience that the technique has considerable potential and has already been proved to be an essential part of quality control in the author's laboratory (W2, W3, W5).

7. Developments in Handling Laboratory Quality Control Data

As stated previously, when a new analytical method has been introduced, the performance of OCV and RCV are essential. Plotting the results on Levey-Jennings-type charts is also essential. Alterations in precision and accuracy can be detected by eye, and their cause be sought and incorporated in preventive measures.

Later, when the method is apparently working satisfactorily in routine use, the production of such charts may lead to boredom on the part of laboratory staff and their production certainly involves a considerable amount of time if graphs are produced manually for several different control materials. In addition, and more important, there is a limit to the ability of the eye to detect changes in precision and accuracy by Levey–Jennings charts, and therefore the necessity of further preventive measures may not be detected.

The use of cumulative sum charts is a considerable help in the interpretation of control charts, and their use is illustrated in Fig. 4. The conventional control chart at the top of the Fig. 4 is a plot of the patient's daily mean value for blood urea in the author's laboratory during a period of 1965 when results were manually read from AutoAnalyzer control charts. A cumulative sum plot showed that the accuracy of the technique was varying throughout this period as different technicians (A, B, C, and D) were responsible for reading off results. Some technicians tended to read "high," others "low." The use of cumulative sum graphs is described by Woodward and Goldsmith (W8).

The cumulative sum plot has been shown to be particularly useful for

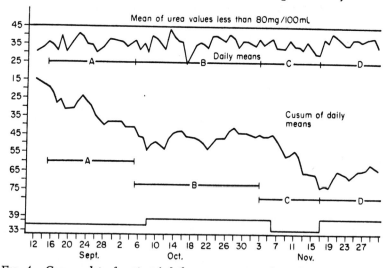

FIG. 4. Cusum plot of patients' daily mean urea results only using values below 80mg/100ml. The upper diagram shows a conventional plot of the mean value obtained each day. It is difficult to identify the changes in mean values that occurred when four different technicians (A, B, C, and D) read the AutoAnalyzer charts. This was due to subjective bias.

patient mean values; the tendency to a high variance in such calculations makes the interpretation of conventional control charts more difficult.

The preparation of cumulative sum plots is not without difficulty regarding the scale to use. Over long periods of study the values recorded may accumulate to large values, particularly if the correct value is unknown or has been incorrectly estimated. The index of accuracy technique described below is a useful alternative system. It is important to realize that cumulative plots indicate only changes in accuracy, not in precision.

7.1. ALTERNATIVES TO THE LEVEY–JENNINGS-TYPE CONTROL CHART

The following methods of calculating and plotting control material results are particularly useful in aiding interpretation of control charts in terms of both precision and accuracy. They may appear at first to imply the production of even more quality control data because one chart is replaced with two. Later in the chapter it will be shown how such a technique may considerably reduce data and yet, at the same time aid interpretation.

Both calculations are based upon results on the same control material, which has been incorporated in batches of patients' material. Ideally the correct result needs to be known; if not, a tentative value may be used for preliminary calculations.

7.1.1. *Index of Precision*

In this calculation, the observed value for a particular control material is subtracted from the previously obtained value, and the difference is expressed as a percentage of the correct value. This percentage variation is expressed as a percentage of the coefficient of variation of the method.

$$\text{Index of precision (PI)} = \frac{[(x_a - x_b)/a] \times 100}{c} \times 100$$

Where x_a and x_b are consecutive observed values, a is the correct value and c is the coefficient of variance of the method. The sign is ignored. The value of c should be that obtained in RCVU measurements. If this is not known, a tentative value may have to be used.

Example: Two consecutive measurements of a control material for glucose analysis were 5.1 and 5.0 mmoles/liter. The correct value was 5.0 mmoles/liter. The coefficient of variation was 2.5%. Then the PI for the second observation was

$$PI = \frac{[(5.1 - 5.0)/5.0] \times 100}{2.5} \times 100 = 80$$

The most convenient method of plotting such values is as a 10-day running mean value; when a value is added, then the most historical value is removed from the calculation. If the value of c is reasonably correct, then the daily value of PI usually lies between 0 and 200. The running daily mean value is theoretically correct at approximately 66. As with cumulative sum graphs, it is changes in PI that are important.

For illustrative purposes a simulated control chart is shown in Fig. 4, the running-mean PI calculation is shown in Table 3, and the graph of the results in Fig. 5. Obviously the running 10-day mean PI value cannot be calculated until the 11th observation is available. From that time it can be seen that the PI improves from the 18th to the 25th day and then deteriorates continuously until the 50th day. Such interpretation is very difficult by mere inspection of the conventional control chart.

7.1.2. *Accuracy Index*

A similar but slightly different approach can be used to assess changes in accuracy. In this calculation the correct value is subtracted from the observed value, and the sign is incorporated. The resultant figure is expressed as a percentage of the correct value. The accuracy index, either positive or negative, is calculated by dividing this percentage by the coefficient of variation c.

$$\text{Accuracy index (AI)} = \pm \frac{[(x_a - a)/a] \times 100}{c} \times 100$$

Thus for observation x_a for the glucose example given above, the AI would be

$$AI = \pm \frac{[(5.1 - 5.0)/5.0] \times 100}{2.5} = +80$$

The AI value for x_b would obviously be zero. The values of AI for the results in Table 3 are plotted in Fig. 5. The running 10-day mean value is plotted after 10 observations have been obtained. The value is reasonably correct from the 10th to the 20th day, but then increases until the 32nd day; there is then a fall in the observed value to give low values for approximately the last 10 days. Again this information is not easily obtained by visual inspection of the conventional control chart at the top of Fig. 4.

TABLE 3
TABLE OF PRECISION INDEX (PI) AND ACCURACY INDEX (AI)

Observation no.	Value x (mmoles/ liter)	$x_a - x_b$ (mmoles/ liter)	PI	Running mean PI, 10 day	$x - c$	AI	Running mean AI, 10 day
1	101				+1	+50	
2	101	0	0		+1	+50	
3	100	1	50		0	0	
4	98	2	100		−2	−100	
5	103	5	250		+3	+150	
6	101	2	100		+1	+150	
7	100	1	50		0	0	
8	101	1	50		+1	+50	
9	98	3	150		−2	−100	
10	100	2	100		0	0	+15
11	101	1	50	90	+1	+50	+15
12	99	2	100	100	−1	−50	+5
13	97	2	100	105	−3	−150	−10
14	100	3	150	110	0	0	0
15	103	3	150	100	+3	+150	0
16	102	1	100	95	+2	+100	+5
17	100	2	100	100	0	0	+5
18	99	1	50	100	−1	−50	−5
19	99	0	0	85	−1	−50	0
20	99	0	0	75	−1	−50	−5
21	99	0	0	70	−1	−50	−15
22	101	2	100	70	+1	+50	−5
23	101	0	0	60	+1	+50	+15
24	100	1	50	50	0	0	+15
25	101	1	50	40	+1	+50	+5
26	103	2	100	45	+3	+150	+10
27	99	4	200	55	−1	−50	+5
28	100	1	50	60	0	0	+10
29	101	1	50	60	+1	+50	+20
30	102	1	50	65	+2	+100	+35
31	100	2	100	75	0	0	+40
32	100	0	0	65	0	0	+35
33	102	2	100	75	+2	+100	+40
34	98	4	200	90	−2	−100	+30
35	100	2	100	95	0	0	+25
36	102	2	100	95	+2	+100	+20
37	98	4	200	95	−2	−100	+15
38	99	1	50	95	−1	−50	+10
39	100	1	50	95	0	0	+5
40	97	3	150	110	−3	−150	−10
41	99	2	100	115	−1	−50	−25
42	102	3	150	120	+2	+100	−15
43	99	3	150	125	−1	−50	−30
44	98	1	50	110	−2	−100	−30
45	103	5	250	125	+3	+150	−15
46	100	3	150	130	0	0	−25
47	97	3	150	125	−3	−150	−30
48	102	5	250	145	+2	+100	−25
49	96	6	300	170	−4	−200	−35
50	103	7	350	190	+3	+150	−5

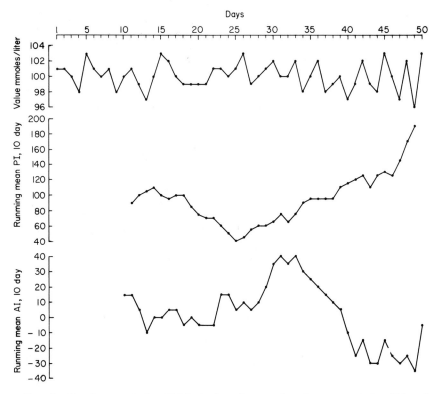

Fig. 5.   Results recorded in Table 3 plotted as graphs of precision index (PI) and accuracy index (AI). The upper graph shows observed values.

Obviously an ideal AI is 0. Setting limits on such a value is difficult; it is obvious that running mean values greater than ±50 indicate that on average the observed values are one standard deviation away from the mean, with a bias to the same side.

7.2.   DATA REDUCTION IN QUALITY CONTROL

There are considerable problems in handling quality control data in a laboratory, and the examples of accuracy and precision index plotting given above inevitably increase the amount of calculation, data recording, and graph plotting. It is the author's experience that the use of computers in clinical chemistry has considerably increased the ability of the laboratory worker to calculate, record, and graph the data, but there has been scant attention to techniques of data reduction or management of quality by exception techniques.

The precision index and accuracy index are useful basic calculations in such endeavors for the following reasons. First, they produce a figure that has the same magnitude in all determinations. One can record for the laboratory all values of PI falling outside 200 for an individual determination or, say, a running 10-day mean PI of greater than 100 or in addition any consistent changes in the values. Otherwise the data will be stored but not printed by the computer. Similarly with AI, exception values can be given. In addition PI and AI values for several control materials can be averaged. In the author's laboratory, the mean PI and AI of five control sera are averaged each day in operating the Technicon Sequential Multiple Analyzers (SMA) 12/60. This reduces five figures to two and considerably aids interpretation of results.

8. The Role of External Quality Control (EQC) Schemes

The technique of distributing portions of the same specimen of biological material to a number of laboratories, and comparing the results of analysis, started as an attempt merely to assess interlaboratory variance. Later it was adopted in some countries for licensing purposes. Only recently has the usefulness of such schemes been fully realized.

EQC is an essential stage in a laboratory's quality control techniques because it assesses the effectiveness of the internal quality control methods. If the internal systems are not accurately reflecting the performance of a laboratory and are designed to give false assurance, then this will be demonstrated by poor performance in external systems. The performance of the author's laboratory in external schemes is never as good as that shown by the internal techniques, but they are in reasonably close agreement.

Quantitative assessment of the performance of individual laboratories in EQC schemes is essential. Mere declaration of the percentage of laboratories with results within an arbitrarily decided acceptance limit is not sufficient information. Showing how well the best laboratories can perform is also an important demonstration of the "state of the art." Such quantitative information should assess the quality of the performance of laboratories over a wide range of quantities at different concentrations and also assess the changes of performance with time. Comparison of the performance of laboratories using different analytical methods is also an essential part of EQC. Inevitably such assessment requires a relatively complex organization with frequent distributions of material.

The United Kingdom National Quality Control Scheme (UKNQCS) is described to illustrate how these objectives may be achieved. The 420 laboratories taking part in the UKNQCS include virtually all laboratories in the United Kingdom which perform clinical chemical analyses. Distributions take place at approximately 14-day intervals, and the computer printout of results of all laboratories is received by the participants within 11 days of receipt of the specimen. The printout, previously described by Whitehead et al. (W7), includes various statistical calculations. The performance of each participant both overall and for particular substances is quantitatively assessed by calculation of the variance index.

8.1. Calculation of the Variance Index (VI)

The VI calculation is carried out on the results obtained from the participating laboratories for a particular determination. The mean value obtained by all those participating laboratories classified as using the same method is calculated. The types of analytical method used by participants for individual determinations have been classified, and those using the same or similar methods are grouped together for calculation of the method mean, with the participant's agreement. For some determinations, participants may use methods that are unclassified, and their results cannot be used in VI calculations, but more than 90% of the 420 participating laboratories use methods that can be used.

To avoid incorporating results that are random mistakes into the method mean calculation, the calculation uses only those values that fall within the mean ±3SD for all results returned by participants. The method mean ($\bar{x}_m$) is subtracted from the result of an individual laboratory (x), and the percentage variation from the method mean is calculated.

$$\% \text{ Variation} = V = [(x - \bar{x}_m)/\bar{x}_m] \times 100$$

The VI is calculated from this figure by dividing it by the chosen coefficient of variation (CCV) given in Table 4. To avoid decimal points, this figure is multiplied by 100.

$$VI = V/CCV \times 100$$

The lower the VI, the closer the result is to the method mean. The CCV values shown in Table 4 are the mean values for the particular determinations experienced over a period of several months early in the UKNQCS. They are kept constant so that improvements in the performance of laboratories can be detected. It is particularly important to avoid VI calculations on low mean values for serum determinations with a high variance, such as bilirubin, alkaline phosphatase, and iron, and therefore only mean values that fall within the limits shown in Table 5 are used for VI calculation.

A definition of variance index is as follows: the difference between the result obtained by a participant and calculated method mean expressed

TABLE 4

CHOSEN COEFFICIENT OF VARIATION (CCV) USED IN VARIANCE INDEX
(VI) CALCULATIONS

Determination	CCV (%)	Determination	CCV (%)
Sodium	1.6	Uric acid	7.7
Potassium	2.9	Creatinine	8.9
Chloride	2.2	Bilirubin	19.2
Urea	5.7	Total protein	3.9
Glucose	7.7	Albumin	7.5
Calcium	4.0	Alkaline phosphatase	19.6
Phosphorus	7.8	Cholesterol	7.6
Iron	15.0		

TABLE 5

RANGE OF VALUES USED IN THE VARIANCE INDEX CALCULATION

Determinations	Low	High	Units
Sodium	110	160	mmoles/liter
Potassium	1.5	8.0	mmoles/liter
Chloride	65	130	mmoles/liter
Urea	2.5	66.7	mmoles/liter
Glucose	0.8	22.2	mmoles/liter
Calcium	1.0	4.0	mmoles/liter
Phosphorus	0.6	3.9	mmoles/liter
Iron	3.6	53.6	μmoles/liter
Urate	179	893	μmoles/liter
Creatinine	62	1770	μmoles/liter
Bilirubin	9	342	μmoles/liter
Total protein	40	100	g/liter
Albumin	15	60	g/liter
Alkaline phosphatase	6.0	100.0	K.A. units[a]/100 ml
Cholesterol	1.3	12.9	mmoles/liter

[a] King–Armstrong units.

as a percentage of the mean, divided by a chosen coefficient of variation for that determination; the resultant figure is multiplied by 100.

The performance of an individual laboratory for several analyses of different material for the same substance may be expressed as the mean variance index. In the UKNQCS we use the term variance index score (VIS) because when a VI value for a particular result is less than 50 it contributes a nil score; this is to give encouragement to those laboratories whose results are closest to the mean. To avoid incorporating high VI values in the score, possibly due to a clerical error, VI values greater than 400 are treated as 400.

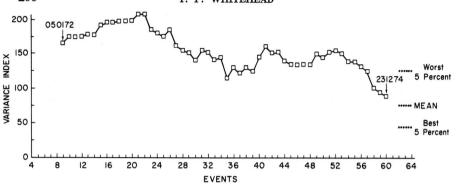

FIG. 6. Running VIS graph for a laboratory which, in general, has performed badly but has shown considerable improvement in the last few months of 1974.

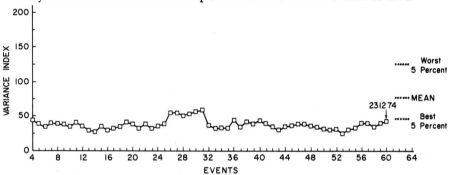

FIG. 7. Graph showing a good performance over a long period of time.

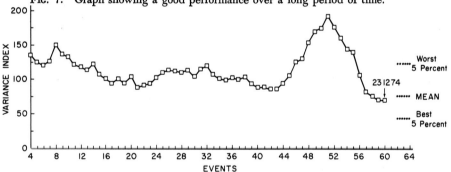

FIG. 8. Graph showing interesting changes in performance; the general trend is to improvement, but there was a period of poor performance early in 1974.

FIGS. 6–9. Examples of running variance index score (VIS). Graphs for four participating laboratories. A square (□) represents the running VIS for the most recent forty determinations after the distribution of a serum for eight or more different analyses. No line between the squares indicates that the laboratory did not return results for the particular distribution. The time span is approximately two years. To the right of the graph the mean variance index score and limits of 90% of results either side of the mean are shown. These graphs are prepared by computer graph plotter.

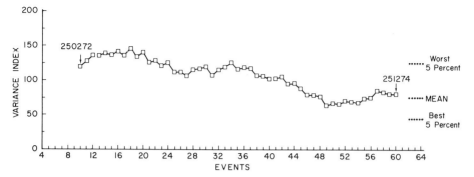

Fɪɢ. 9. Running VIS for a laboratory whose performance has gradually improved over a period of two years.

The mean VIS may be calculated for different determinations and several distributions; the resultant calculation is the overall VIS. In practice, it has been found useful to calculate the "running" overall VIS. In this, the overall VIS for the most recent 40 analyses is calculated. Where the scores for more recent results are added, the appropriate number of the earliest results are dropped out of the calculation.

At intervals, the running overall VIS over a period of the previous two years is prepared on the computer graph plotter. Examples are shown in Figs. 6–9. The mean running overall VIS and the range that includes 90% of all participants are shown in the graph. Thus, a laboratory can identify whether its performance is above or below average or whether it is included in the range associated with the best- or worst-performing laboratories. It does not indicate "acceptable" or "nonacceptable" performance.

Occasionally, the VIS for particular determinations are calculated, and the computer printout is distributed to participants. Along with the mean VIS for the individual laboratory, the mean VIS for all laboratories for that determination are reported (see Table 6). These statistics enable a laboratory to assess which determinations are making the most significant contribution to the overall variance index and whether their performance is above or below average. These calculations based on the VI have been accepted by the participating laboratories over a period of several years.

8.2   The Method Mean

In EQC schemes the correct value for a quantity is difficult to assess. Should laboratories be judged by their ability to obtain results close to the method mean? This was a question that was difficult to answer in the

TABLE 6

EXAMPLE OF RESULTS OF A PARTICIPATING LABORATORY SHOWING THE
VARIANCE INDEX SCORE (VIS) FOR INDIVIDUAL DETERMINATIONS
COMPARED WITH THE MEAN VIS FOR ALL PARTICIPATING
LABORATORIES

Determination	No. of possible results	No. of results returned	Mean VIS	Mean VIS for all laboratories
Sodium	34	34	46	86
Potassium	29	28	42	88
Chloride	20	11	61	80
Urea	34	34	21	79
Glucose	33	33	21	85
Calcium	34	34	45	78
Phosphate	34	32	33	75
Iron	20	19	90	77
Uric acid	33	33	28	79
Creatinine	32	32	51	98
Bilirubin	31	23	25	96
Total protein	33	31	47	75
Albumin	33	33	17	79
Alkaline phosphatase	28	26	38	79
Cholesterol	33	32	56	88

early days of the UKNQCS, but confidence in the use of such values has grown during the last 6 years. The evidence available is circumstantial, but, with the exception of enzyme activity, it is in favor of the correctness of such an approach, and for the following reasons:

1. Attempts to establish mean values from a group of reference laboratories have frequently resulted in values close to, or the same as, the method mean calculated for all laboratories.

2. Surveys have shown that the mean and mode for the determinations surveyed are virtually the same, indicating equal positive and negative effects on the mean value from the results of participating laboratories (W6).

3. Different analytical methods for determination of the same substance give virtually the same method mean value (W7).

The acceptance of the method mean value for the calculation of VI by participants in the UKNQCS over a period of 4 years is not necessarily a justification of the use of such statistics. However, none of the 420 participating laboratories have shown injustice in the use of such a value for assessing performance by VI calculations.

The VI and the associated statistical calculations are of particular use if the distribution of material is frequent and the return of the results to the participating laboratories is a matter of a few days. Too long a delay between analysis of the distributed material and the results of the survey being available in the participating laboratories means that the results will not be representative of current practice in the individual laboratories. In the UKNQCS there is an 11-day interval between receipt of material and the receipt of the computer printout with the statistical analysis on the results of all laboratories which participated. Material is distributed every 14 days, so that the distribution of material and statistical analysis of the results is completed for one distribution before the next distribution commences. The frequency of distribution of material is important. It may take several distributions to convince a laboratory that their performance in some or all methods is poor compared with that of other laboratories; it may then take some time while solutions are being sought, and then several more distributions to check that a correct solution has been found. The process could easily stretch over a year or more.

TABLE 7

THE NUMBER OF DISTRIBUTIONS OF MATERIAL MADE BY THE
UNITED KINGDOM NATIONAL QUALITY CONTROL SCHEME IN 1974

Determination	No. of distributions
Serum Sodium	11
Potassium	11
Chloride	11
Urea	11
Glucose	11
Calcium	11
Phosphate	11
Iron	11
Uric acid	10
Creatinine	10
Bilirubin	10
Total protein	10
Albumin	10
Alkaline phosphatase	10
Cholesterol	10
Blood lead	8
Serum pH	1
P_{CO_2}	1
Standard bicarbonate	1
Serum aspartate aminotransferase	2
Buffer solution for pH measurement	1
Total	172

The number of distributions and the determinations surveyed in 1974 are given in Table 7.

There are several advantages to be gained from using VI calculations in EQC schemes.

First, it is possible to identify laboratories which perform extremely well, as well as those which perform badly. The high-quality analytical performance that some laboratories can maintain over a period of many years has been illustrated by looking at the results from laboratories with a low overall VIS since the start of the scheme. Showing what other laboratories are capable of, and identifying the factors in those laboratories that are important in maintaining a low overall VIS, is an essential role of EQC schemes.

Second, the running VIS graph can show the level of performance over a wide range of determinations over a long period of time.

Third, the factors making for better performance can be assessed using the VIS. In a previous publication (W6) we have shown how the VIS can be used to illustrate that, in general, the laboratories with higher work loads have performed better in the scheme. It was also shown that, since the introduction of the VIS, the performance of the smaller laboratories had considerably improved.

Over the 7 years since the scheme commenced, methods with poor precision have been replaced by methods that have good precision. This is illustrated in Table 8 for serum cholesterol. In the 4 years 1971–1974, the participants using the AutoAnalyzer have increased from 16% to 45%. Those using various manual methods have decreased from 84% to 55%. The mean values of all methods have been shown to be very similar, but the precision of the alternative methods is much better by a factor of 0.6.

TABLE 8

Changes in the Methods Used for the Determination of Serum
Cholesterol 1971–1974[a]

| | AutoAnalyzer[b] | | Manual | Manual | |
Year	AAI	AAII	L. Burch	ZAK	Others
1971	43 (16%)		93 (34%)	49 (18%)	86 (32%)
1972	48 (17%)		98 (35%)	52 (18%)	86 (30%)
1973	87 (30%)	32 (11%)	80 (27%)	25 (9%)	68 (23%)
1974	94 (32%)	37 (13%)	76 (26%)	19 (7%)	66 (23%)

[a] Values are number and percentage of laboratories using various techniques.
[b] Technicon AutoAnalyzer I and II.

Similar alterations in methods used have been shown for other determinations. The role of EQC schemes in encouraging laboratories to change to better methods is of obvious importance.

REFERENCES

B1. Barnett, R. N., *Am. J. Clin. Pathol.* **50,** 671 (1968).
B2. Belk, W. P., and Sunderman, F. W., *Am. J. Clin. Pathol.* **17,** 853 (1947).
B3. Büttner, J., Borth, R., Boutwell, J. H., and Broughton, P. M. G., *Clin. Chim. Acta* **63,** F25 (1975).
C1. Cotlove, E., and Harris, E. K., and Williams, G. Z., *Clin. Chem.* **16,** 1028 (1970).
G1. Gilbert, R. K., "Survey Data 1974." College of American Pathologists, Illinois, 1975.
L1. Levey, S., and Jennings, E. R., *Am. J. Clin. Pathol.* **20,** 1059 (1950).
N1. Northam, B., and Dixon, K., *Clin. Chim. Acta* **30,** 433 (1970).
T1. Tonks, D., *Postgrad. Med.* **34,** 58 (1963).
W1. Waid, M. E., and Hoffman, R. G., *Am. Clin. Pathol.* **25,** 585 (1955).
W2. Whitehead, T. P., *in* "Progress in Medical Computing," p. 52. Blackwell, Oxford, 1965.
W3. Whitehead, T. P., *in* "A Question of Quality?" p. 99. Oxford Univ. Press, London and New York, 1976.
W4. Whitehead, T. P., "Quality Control of Clinical Chemical Analysis." Wiley, New York, 1976.
W5. Whitehead, T. P., and Morris, L. O., *Ann. Clin. Biochem.* **6,** 94 (1969).
W6. Whitehead, T. P., Browning, D. M., and Gregory, A., *J. Clin. Pathol.* **26,** 453 (1973).
W7. Whitehead, T. P., Browning, D. M., and Gregory, A., *in* "Quality Control in Clinical Chemistry" (G. Anido, E. J. van Kampers, S. B. Rosalki, and M. Rubin, eds.). de Gruyter, Berlin, 1975.
W8. Woodward, R. H., and Goldsmith, P. L., "Cumulative Sum Techniques," ICI Monogr. No. 3. Oliver & Boyd, Edinburgh, 1964.
W9. Wootton, I. D. P., and King, E. J., *Lancet* **1,** 470 (1953).

BIOCHEMICAL CONSEQUENCES OF INTRAVENOUS NUTRITION IN THE NEWBORN

Gordon Dale

Department of Clinical Biochemistry, University of Newcastle upon Tyne
and Royal Victoria Infirmary, Newcastle upon Tyne, England

1. Introduction

A major advance in the management of severe nutritional failure has been the development of intravenous infusions that provide not only sufficient calories for energy requirements, but also amino acids and other nutrients. These can be used to put a stop to the "draft on the body nitrogen bank, and, even though the patient cannot eat, to promote redeposit and resynthesis of muscle protein" (M8). The technique is known variously as intravenous nutrition, parenteral nutrition, intravenous hyperalimentation, parenteral feeding, and hyperalimentation (B10). It had not proved to be clinically satisfactory until the researches of Dudrick et al. (D12,

D13), who developed a procedure capable of supporting beagle puppies so that they could be kept alive for months, growing and developing normally. This work was quickly followed by use in the treatment of humans (D14), and it is now possible to provide long-term support for patients with total intestinal resection allowing at the same time a reasonable quality of life (B9, J4).

In its commonest application, intravenous nutrition is used as a temporary measure preventing malnutrition in patients with conditions from which recovery is possible, usually of the intestinal tract, and is employed with increasing frequency in pediatrics, where it can be a life-saving procedure.

The increasing use of intravenous nutrition has revealed a variety of complications (G12, W2); this has tempered enthusiasm with caution (F2). Many of the problems encountered are associated with the intravenous catheter itself, either its siting or bacterial colonization (P5), and the high sepsis rate is a major cause of concern (B8, N1). In addition, a number of metabolic complications have been reported (D11). The purpose of this review is to draw attention to these metabolic problems and to indicate the areas in which the pediatrician may expect the clinical chemist to provide a "responsive laboratory service essential to serial monitoring of relevant plasma and urine constituents" (H17).

2. Intravenous Nutrition and the Newborn Infant

The newborn infant, with its relatively high metabolic rate, its requirements for growth, and its limited calorie stores is particularly susceptible to the effects of starvation. Heird *et al.* (H17) have predicted that while an adult should have sufficient calorie reserve for almost 100 days of total starvation, a normal full-term baby might be expected to live only 32 days under such conditions. The low-birth-weight infant is particularly vulnerable. With a total energy reserve of perhaps little more than 200 cal/kg, the very small baby cannot be expected to survive more than 4 days of absolute starvation. The infusion of conventional amounts of 10% glucose will probably not prolong life for much more than 7 days.

In dealing with congenital anomalies of the gastrointestinal tract, the pediatric surgeon must consider not only the surgical difficulties, but also the effects of malnutrition on a vulnerable newborn infant with temporary, but total, intestinal malfunction. In many of these cases, intravenous nutrition has proved to be of considerable benefit (B11, C14, D5), permitting not merely survival, but also the prospect of normal mental and physical development when formerly the outlook was uniformly bad. The technique is also of value in the management of infants with chronic intractable diarrhea, when the loss of endogenous nitrogen produces a vicious cycle of protein depletion resulting in impaired synthesis of intestinal mucosa and digestive enzymes and consequent malabsorption (G6). A third major group that is particularly susceptible to the effects of malnutrition is that of the low-birth-weight infant. Studies of the application of total intravenous nutrition to the management of very small babies have given encouraging results (B4, D7) with a probable reduction in mortality and morbidity. In this situation, however, the procedure has not yet been firmly established as being of proven value in other than specialized centers (B13, W7).

Although details of the different regimes of intravenous nutrition vary considerably (B6, D14), the aim is to provide an adequate source both of calories and of amino acids. The first satisfactory amino acid solutions were obtained by hydrolysis of a suitable protein, such as casein or fibrin. Such preparations are still used extensively and have the advantage that they contain only L-amino acids with adequate amounts of most of the individual components and a high rate of essential to nonessential amino acids (E2). However, hydrolyzates tend to be of inconstant composition, with variable amounts of poorly metabolized peptides and excessive concentrations of sodium and ammonium, so that increasing use is made of synthetic L-amino acid preparations in which the composition can be better adjusted to nutritional requirements.

In addition to the provision of a nitrogen source for protein synthesis, sufficient calories are provided for growth and energy expenditure. The amount of amino acid utilized for protein synthesis is proportional to the calorie intake (C6). In the majority of cases a carbohydrate, such as glucose or fructose, is employed, although ethanol, sorbitol, or xylitol may also be used. Although safe and effective fat emulsions, such as those prepared from soybean oil, have been available and in use in Europe for several years, the toxic effects of some of the early fat preparations delayed the introduction into the United States of fat as a major calorie source in intravenous nutrition (W7).

Unlike normal oral feeding, intravenous infusion bypasses the liver so that the patient does not have the immediate benefit of hepatic regulation. If adequate nutrition is to be supplied by this means, the process may result in abnormally high concentrations of nutrients in the peripheral circulation, and consequent metabolic derangement, which may be further complicated by nutritional deficiencies (W2).

3. Effects of the Individual Nutrients

3.1. GLUCOSE

Glucose, the traditional energy-providing intravenous infusate, is the carbohydrate most frequently used in intravenous nutrition. The normal human adult can metabolize glucose at rates up to 1.2 g/kg per hour (G3). The problem, particularly in schemes of intravenous nutrition that do not provide energy-rich fat emulsion as an additional caloric source, is to supply sufficient glucose for metabolic needs without producing hyperglycemia, glycosuria, osmotic diuresis, and hyperosmolar nonketotic dehydration and coma (D11).

In the newborn, there is a considerable range of metabolic response to the use of hypertonic glucose. The normal-birth-weight infant is more likely to tolerate high initial rates of glucose infusion than the infant of low birth weight. During long-term intravenous nutrition, mature infants may be able to tolerate glucose infusions in excess of 1 g/kg per hour without producing hyperglycemia (D5, F4, K1). The degree of glycosuria is often greater than might be expected from the peripheral blood glucose level and may well be related to the unusually high solute load delivered to the renal artery as a result of infusion into a systemic vein (G5).

The optimal rate of glucose infusion may be more difficult to determine in the low-birth-weight newborn. Decreased hepatic glycogen stores, defective gluconeogenesis (H9), hypoxemia from birth asphyxia (H7), and relatively high basal levels of plasma insulin may all act to increase the incidence of neonatal hypoglycemia. In the low-birth-weight infant, there is a pressing requirement for calories in order to prevent the damaging effects of hypoglycemia and to reduce the negative nitrogen balance caused by protein catabolism (A10). Unfortunately, glucose metabolism in this group of babies is very fragile; they readily become hyperglycemic (B13, B15, D8, D16, H11, H19, P3) and may require the administration of insulin. Despite the urgent need for calories, babies in this group can tolerate only low initial rates of glucose infusion, perhaps 0.4 g/kg per hour increasing gradually to 1.1–1.2 g/kg per hour, which is usually tolerated by day 11 of intravenous nutrition (D8, P3). The use of a computer has been advocated to adjust the composition of the infusate in order to reduce the incidence of metabolic complications, such as hyperglycemia (B2).

Surgical operation, hypothermia, and sepsis may all affect the stability of glucose metabolism in the newborn (D16, F2). The postsurgical newborn is particularly prone to develop hyperglycemia (E9), and care is needed in determining the optimal infusion rate. Reactive hypoglycemia, which may be a problem whenever hypertonic glucose infusions are terminated abruptly, is especially dangerous during surgical operation, when the clinical status of the anesthetized patient is more difficult to assess (D11).

The clinical chemist bears a considerable responsibility in providing a blood glucose monitoring service for the newborn receiving intravenous nutrition. Care should be taken to ensure that reports not only of abnormally low concentrations of glucose but also high levels are not misinterpreted. Blood glucose concentrations may be very high indeed, and a result reported as greater than 250 mg/100 ml, without repeating at a higher dilution, can be misinterpreted, and gross, perhaps fatal, hyperosmolality be unrecognized or inadequately treated (C5).

3.2. FRUCTOSE

Fructose is commonly used in regimes of intravenous nutrition. It is a stable sugar, and its use has been advocated on the grounds that it is relatively, but not totally, independent of the action of insulin; it is antiketogenic and rapidly metabolized particularly by the liver to form glycogen. In addition, it is said to be less thrombogenic than glucose, although Harries (H5) suggests that there is no good published evidence to support this view. Compared with glucose, intravenous fructose appears to improve nitrogen retention (E7) and produces lower urinary losses, and consequently less diuretic effects (A7), although osmotic diuresis and dehydration can still be a problem (D2). Fructose-loading in newborn infants stimulates plasma insulin release to a lesser degree than glucose (P8).

The phosphorylation of fructose is mediated either by hexokinase to form fructose 6-phosphate or by fructose kinase forming fructose 1-phosphate, the major pathway in the liver. Fructose 1-phosphate is split by the enzyme fructose 1-phosphate aldolase producing dihydroxyacetone phosphate, a metabolite of the glycolytic pathway, and glyceraldehyde, which is converted to glyceraldehyde 3-phosphate by the enzyme triose kinase. The conversion of a molecule of fructose into these triose phosphates is associated with the loss of 2 molecules of ATP and the production of two molecules of ADP (M10) (Fig. 1). The formation of fructose 1-phosphate from fructose is rapid and probably accounts for the fact that its removal from the circulation is faster than that of glucose. This feature of fructose metabolism has been advanced as one of the factors in favor of the use of this sugar as a calorie source in intravenous nutrition; however, it may have an important drawback, since it seems that, in some patients at least, the aldolase reaction cleaving the fructose 1-phosphate is slower, with consequent accumulation of the potentially toxic fructose 1-phosphate in liver and kidney (D2) producing a situation analogous to hereditary fructose intolerance. This accumulation of fructose 1-phosphate may interfere with gluconeogenesis, which, coupled with a defect in glycogenolysis (perhaps due to a shortage of the ATP essential for activation of phosphorylase b), may account for the hypoglycemia seen in some newborn infants receiving fructose infusion.

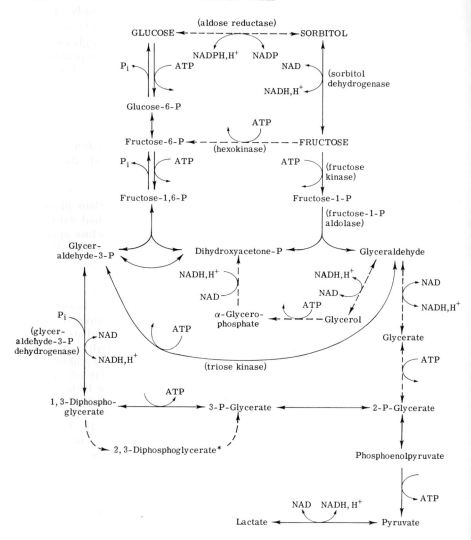

FIG. 1. Metabolism of glucose, fructose, and sorbitol, showing NADH, H⁺, ATP production and formation of lactate. Minor pathways are indicated by dashed lines. *: Formed in the red cell; Pi, inorganic phosphate.

The work of Mäenpää et al. (M2) shows that, in rats at least, intravenous fructose may have other unwanted side effects. The incorporation of [¹⁴C] leucine into liver protein is inhibited, suggesting that intracellular ATP is preferentially used to produce fructose 1-phosphate rather than to facilitate protein synthesis.

3.2.1.   Fructose Intolerance

Danks *et al.* (D2) have drawn attention to the dangers of the use of fructose in pediatric patients. They reported a fatality due to hereditary fructose intolerance, a disorder in which deficiency of the enzyme fructose-1-phosphate aldolase produces toxic accumulation of fructose 1-phosphate. This condition should be borne in mind whenever there is a history, or a family history, of intolerance to or abhorrence of sweet foods or when unexplained hypoglycemia follows the use of fructose. These workers also described a severe reaction to fructose in three infants, two of them new-born, in whom the diagnosis of hereditary fructose intolerance was un-likely. These babies were all very ill before treatment was started, but infusion of fructose was followed by bile-stained vomiting, metabolic acidosis, hypoglycemia, osmotic diuresis, and dehydration. The authors urged that fructose be avoided in patients with severe liver disease and in newborn infants with hypoglycemia.

3.2.2.   Lactic Acidosis

Both infants and older children may develop a metabolic acidosis when supported by regimes of intravenous nutrition which include fructose. A similar clinical picture is sometimes seen when ethanol or the polyols are used. The etiology of this acidosis is by no means clear and because of the complicated nature of most intravenous solutions cannot always be attributed solely to fructose. In many cases, the description of "lactic acidosis" is based upon circumstantial evidence. However, the infusion of fructose into healthy adults (S1) and newborns (P8) has been shown to produce a raise in blood lactate that may be accompanied by a fall in plasma bicarbonate. It is probable that the metabolic acidosis following fructose infusion in some children (A5) and infants (H6) is substantially due to the accumulation of lactic acid.

The mechanism of lactic acid production is not certain but appears to be dose-dependant and may be exaggerated if ethanol is used. A large proportion of a fructose load is rapidly metabolized to lactate by the liver, especially under anaerobic conditions (W13), and the presence of tissue anoxia may result in greater conversion to lactate (W11). Hypoxia, perhaps coupled with impaired liver function reducing the capacity of the liver to remove lactate, may lead to increasing lactic acidosis. Perheentupa and Raivio (P6) suggested that the hepatic generation of lactic acid might be due to a block in the gluconeogenetic pathway caused by inhibition of glucose phosphate isomerase by fructose 1-phos-phate—a block that might also be expected to aggravate hypoglycemia.

3.2.3. *Fructose-Induced Hyperuricemia*

Perheentupa and Raivio (P6) have reported fructose-induced increases in the plasma uric acid and uric acid excretion in both normal children and children with hereditary fructose intolerance. These changes were not seen in an adult with essential fructosuria. It was suggested that these changes in plasma and urine uric acid concentrations were not due to increased purine synthesis, but probably originated from the preexisting purine pool. The metabolism of fructose, with consequent accumulation of fructose 1-phosphate, reduces the net available ATP and inorganic phosphate in liver (M2). Depletion of adenine nucleotides in human liver has also been noted in fructose infusion (B7). Reduced hepatic ATP and inorganic phosphorus levels may increase the activity of both AMP deaminase (which is inhibited by both inorganic phosphorus and ATP) (N2) and 5'-nucleotidase (inhibited by ATP) (B1). The action of these two enzymes is to increase the breakdown of AMP to IMP (B1, W12) and adenosine, eventually producing uric acid (Fig. 2). Woods and Alberti (W11) suggested this as a mechanism for the uricemia, perhaps aggra-

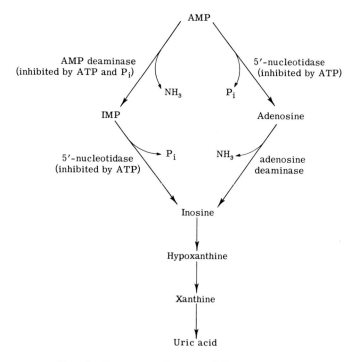

FIG. 2. Formation of uric acid from AMP (W12).

vated by the inhibitory effect of lactate of urinary uric acid excretion (G7).

It is clear that fructose may not be without its complications as a calorie source. Although thousands of fructose-based infusions have been used over the past decade or so without serious consequence, it would seem to be wise to recommend amino acid–glucose solutions rather than amino acid–fructose (P2). In the perinatal period in healthy newborns, the use of fructose offers no clear advantage (P8) and the increasing incidence of metabolic disturbances has led to a more cautious attitude to its use (D2, E1, P2, W11). Certainly, fructose should not be used in the presence of lactic acidosis, and probably at least 50% of the carbohydrate should be given as glucose to counteract possible hypoglycemia in the newborn (B10, H5).

3.2.4. Heat-Induced Changes in Carbohydrate-Containing Nutrient Solutions

Unwanted, and potentially toxic, products may be formed during the process of preparation of intravenous nutrients. These changes are frequently the result of heating the solutions as part of the sterilization process and usually affect the carbohydrate moiety, either alone, or by reaction with amino acids.

Jellum et al. (J5) investigated two severely ill babies found to be excreting in their urine non-glucose reducing substances identified as furan derivatives. These infants had been receiving intravenous nutrition with heat-sterilized mixtures containing glucose, fructose, amino acids, electrolytes, and vitamins. The fructose-containing solutions were found to contain large amounts of 5-hydroxymethyl-2-furfural, 2-(2-hydroxyacetyl)-furan, levulinic acid, and 2-keto-3-deoxyglucose as impurities. The two first-named compounds are potentially toxic and inevitably formed whenever fructose-containing solutions with pH lower than 3.5–4.0 are heated to 110°–130°C.

A major problem affecting the stability and nutritional value of infusates containing mixtures of amino acids and sugars is the so-called "Maillard reaction" or "browning reaction." In this reaction, amino acids or peptides combine with the glycosidic center of sugars. This is followed by other more complex changes, depending upon the nature of the amino acid involved and on the conditions, resulting eventually in the formation of brown polymeric pigments (E6).

Christensen et al. (C10) found that the presence of glucose and fructose in commercially available protein hydrolyzate solutions increased the urinary losses of amino acids. This did not seem to be the result of higher plasma amino acid levels and did not occur if glucose was added immediately before infusion but reappeared if this mixture was then autoclaved. This wastage of amino acids occurred particularly in the presence of high concentrations of glucose, although fructose had a similar effect, but to a lesser extent. It seems, therefore, that the Maillard reaction reduces the nutritional value of amino acids and is likely to occur in preparations sterilized by autoclaving. The compounds produced may increase urinary losses of trace elements, particularly zinc (see Section 7.1.).

3.3. ALCOHOLS

Alcohols, either polyols or ethanol, have been used as energy sources in regimes of intravenous nutrition. They have an advantage over hexoses in that they are less likely to undergo the heat-induced Maillard reaction with amino acids and such mixtures can be more easily sterilized by autoclaving. The polyols most commonly employed are sorbitol and xylitol; the metabolism of these compounds is closely related to that of sugars. Diols, such as 1,3-butanediol and 1,2-propanediol, have been investigated experimentally and advantages have been claimed for them (H8, K8), but they have not been generally adopted for intravenous nutrition in humans.

3.3.1. *Sorbitol*

The intravenous infusion of sorbitol has been found to give satisfactory results in animal studies (M3) and is rapidly metabolized in man (A2). Although some sorbitol may be converted directly to glucose by the NADP-requiring enzyme aldose reductase, the main pathway is to fructose (Fig. 1); this latter reaction is effected by sorbitol dehydrogenase, found largely in liver and kidney.

In view of its metabolic fate, sorbitol appears to have no particular advantage over fructose and retains the disadvantages of that sugar. In combination with amino acids and ethanol, sorbitol may be especially liable to produce hyperlactatemia during the intravenous nutrition of children (A11)—not surprising, perhaps, considering the increased formation of NADH occasioned by the metabolism of both ethanol and sorbitol.

When infused rapidly, sorbitol has quite a marked diuretic effect, and acute reactions, such as severe epigastric pain, tachycardia, nausea, and weakness, have been observed in adult volunteers (L2). In view of the increased urinary losses of sorbitol and the suggestion of a reduced rate of metabolism, this polyol should be used with caution in patients with liver diseases (L2).

There is at present little evidence to suggest that sorbitol offers any particular advantage in the intravenous nutrition of infants.

3.3.2. Xylitol

Xylitol, a pentahydroxy alcohol, is a normal constituent of the glucuronic acid–xylulose pathway (Fig. 3), being converted into D-xylulose by the NAD-linked xylitol dehydrogenase. D-Xylulose is phosphorylated to xylulose 5-phosphate, which is metabolized via the pentose phosphate pathway. The conversion of xylitol to D-xylulose is associated with an increase in the NADH:NAD ratio. Gluconeogenesis from lactate is inhibited by xylitol, probably by a mechanism involving decreased flux through pyruvate carboxylase caused by diminished substrate concentration and decreased acetyl-CoA activation (J2).

Xylitol is metabolized readily by newborn infants (E8), its uptake by the cells being independent of the action of insulin. It is an effective energy source when used either alone or in combination with other carbohydrates (B3). Metabolic complications of its use have, however, been described; most of the severe complications have been reported in adults, who on the whole, tend to have much higher blood levels than babies, have greater urinary losses (E8), and are more likely to experience osmotic diuresis.

Metabolic disorders following the intravenous administration of xylitol include osmotic diuresis, lactic acidosis, and increases in serum uric acid,

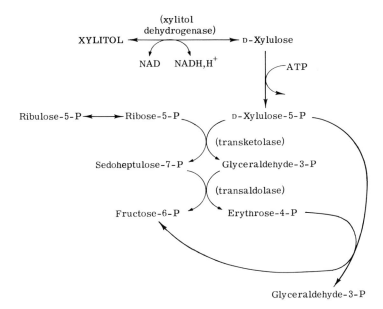

Fig. 3.   Metabolism of xylitol.

bilirubin, and alkaline phosphatase (F10, S4, T2, T3). Thomas *et al.* (T2) described a syndrome ·of diuresis, acidosis, oliguria, and azotemia with liver and cerebral disturbances, elevated serum uric acid levels, and calcium oxalate crystal deposition in kidney and brain. While lactic acidosis and uricacidemia may occur as complications of the use of other nutrients, particularly fructose, the deposition of oxalate crystals, if they are indeed related to this therapy rather than to a preexisting renal disorder, is unusual. Thomas *et al.* (T2) speculated that the oxalate precursor, glycolaldehyde, may be generated during the metabolism of xylitol. Transketolase, a thiamine-dependent enzyme, produces as a transient intermediate a glycolaldehyde–enzyme complex. Usually this two-carbon fragment is accepted by ribulose 5-phosphate to form sedoheptulose 7-phosphate. Failure of transfer may cause release of the glycolaldehyde and subsequent metabolism to oxalic acid. These workers commented that the occurrence in some patients of disturbed liver function with histological evidence of centrilobular hepatic cell necrosis is reminiscent of ethylene glycol poisoning (in which oxalate precipitates in the renal tubules and renal failure is also observed).

The clinical and biochemical complications of the use of xylitol as a calorific source suggest that this particular nutrient should be used with caution (S4).

3.3.3. *Ethanol*

The nitrogen-sparing effect of ethanol has been known for some considerable time (A9). Ethanol has some attractive features as a nutrient. It has a high calorie value (7.1 cal/g), it imposes little or no osmotic load, and a very small proportion of it is excreted in the urine or expired air. A mild euphoria produced by its use has been considered to be advantageous (C11); however, because of the well-known toxic effect it is never used as the sole source of calories but always in combination, usually with carbohydrate. At least in adults, ethanol has been used successfully in medium- and long-term intravenous nutrition, supplying 25–33% of the calorie needs without adverse reaction (C11).

Over 90% of the oxidation of ethanol occurs in the liver, so that blood levels give an indication of hepatic oxidation (R4). Ethanol is oxidized by liver alcohol dehydrogenase to acetaldehyde, which is further oxidized to acetate by the ubiquitous aldehyde dehydrogenases; more than 60% is probably metabolized extrahepatically. The rate-limiting step in the oxidation of ethanol is the first one (Fig. 4). The equilibrium of the alcohol dehydrogenase reaction lies far to the left, and the oxidation of ethanol proceeds because acetaldehyde is continuously removed by the irreversible aldehyde dehydrogenase step.

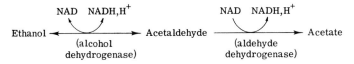

FIG. 4.   Metabolism of ethanol.

Although ethanol has been used frequently in the intravenous nutrition of adults, pediatricians have been more cautious. Heird and co-workers (H17) noted that the provision of additional calories as ethanol contributed to impressive improvement in the children treated. Although they infused alcohol at quite a high rate (3–4 g/kg per day), they encountered no obvious toxicity, sedation was minimal, liver function results remained normal, and diuresis secondary to suppression of antidiuretic hormone was not troublesome. However, these workers were worried by the possibility of hepatic and central nervous system toxicity as well as the difficulty in maintaining long-term infusions by peripheral vein, and they discontinued the use of alcohol. Peden *et al.* (P4) investigated plasma ethanol levels in 13 newborn premature infants receiving total intravenous nutrition. They found elevated plasma alcohol levels ranging from 39 mg/100 ml to 183 mg/100 ml in four; in each case, unusual lethargy was noted. Two of these infants had edema that was refractory to treatment with salt-poor albumin —a paradoxical finding considering the known effect of ethanol diminishing the release of antidiuretic hormone. It may have been that, in these particular premature infants, there was an immaturity of the liver alcohol dehyrogenase system. The state of nutrition may also be important since it has been shown, at least in experimental animals (V3), that the fasting state reduces the ability to oxidize alcohol.

Ethanol should be used with great caution in the intravenous nutrition of infants, especially those of low birth weight. Its use requires careful monitoring of plasma alcohol levels regardless of the rate of infusion. It is not advisable to discontinue abruptly, not only because of the risk of hypoglycemia but also because of the possibility of withdrawal symptoms resembling delirium tremens (P4).

The nature of the combination with other energy-providing nutrients may have a considerable influence on metabolism. Ethanol/fructose mixtures appear to be particularly liable to produce lactic acidosis (W11). The excessive production of NADH coupled with the inhibition of gluconeogenesis from lactate (K7) leads to a striking rise in lactate. The ratio of NAD:NADH in liver is especially adverse when a combination of ethanol and sorbitol is used, and this combination has been noted to give a lactic acidosis in infants and children (A11).

Although hypoglycemia attributable to ethanol in intravenous nutrition has not been reported, the occurrence as a consequence of accidental ingestion is well known (H12, M1). Depletion of glycogen stores and inhibition of gluconeogenesis by alcohol (K7) may be important.

3.4. Fat Emulsions

Some early fat preparations used for intravenous feeding were found to be unsatisfactory, either because of instability of the emulsion or because of toxic reactions (A3, H1, S3) caused by the emulsifying agent. Although safe and effective fat infusions have been used for some considerable time in Europe, these have not until recently been generally available in the United States, where hypertonic glucose solutions have been rather more extensively employed (E2).

The use of fat emulsions has a number of attractions. These preparations can provide a major source of calories (B12, G13) in a relatively small volume [an advantage in the management of small infants (C15, W15)] and may reduce the sepsis rate (E3) by decreasing reliance on hypertonic glucose solutions which predispose to bacterial and fungal infection (B14). They may be administered through a peripheral vein without causing phlebitis and can be useful in preventing essential fatty acid deficiency (see Section 6).

The emulsions presently available contain a vegetable oil, either cottonseed oil or soybean oil, together with stabilizing emulsifiers, which may be either egg-yolk phospholipids, soybean lecithin, or soybean phospholipids. The infusate is made isotonic by the addition of a polyol, such as sorbitol, xylitol, or glycerol. Details of the composition of commercially available fat emulsions have been outlined by Wretlind (W14) and Coran (C15).

Because of considerable differences among fat preparations, it is not possible to generalize upon their metabolism or effects (C15, W15). Intralipid, an emulsion of soybean oil, is probably the most frequently used preparation; it has physical characteristics similar to those of natural chylomicrons (W15), being eliminated from the circulation in much the same way (H1, H2, W15). Intravenously administered fat is associated with a rise in the levels of plasma free fatty acid (C16). Forget et al. (F9) demonstrated, in an 8-year-old girl receiving treatment for anorexia nervosa, that over a period of 4 weeks the Intralipid elimination constant increased more than 3-fold, and the postheparin liproprotein lipase activity 6-fold, enabling the dose of infused fat to be increased progressively without raising plasma triglyceride levels. It is possible that such adaptation can occur in the newborn (B10). Small amounts of heparin, by increasing the lipolytic activity of lipoprotein lipase, can facilitate the disappearance of fat from the blood (B12, V2).

Other plasma lipids may be altered by infused fat. An initial fall in serum cholesterol levels is sometimes noticed; this has been attributed (B5) to the cholesterol-lowering effect of the high linoleic acid content of soybean oil.

Even with Intralipid, currently the most intensively investigated of the fat emulsions, there is still much to be learned about its metabolism in the newborn period, especially of low-birth-weight infants. Small-for-date and preterm appropriate-for-date newborns appear to respond differently to a single injection of 0.5 g of Intralipid per kilogram (G13, V2). In the light-for-dates group, a lower disappearance rate of lipid particles and a reduced rate of triglyceride clearance was reported. During the 2 hours after the injection, the appearance of pre-β-lipoprotein was found to be absent or slight in the preterms, but pronounced in the small-for-date infants. The explanation for these differences in the latter group is not apparent, but is probably independent of the action of insulin (G13) and may be related to an inefficient lipoprotein lipase response, to a reduced number of fat cells (impairing fatty acid uptake), and to inadequate formation by the adipose tissue of α-glycerophosphate for esterification of fatty acids.

A study of the endocrine effects of intravenous nutrition of infants during the first 3 months of life (A6) showed that a regime including Intralipid, combined with 12% glucose and a nitrogen source, produced higher glucagon and lower growth hormone and insulin levels than the fat-free procedures. It was suggested that the reduction in growth hormone was probably due to the inhibitory effect of high concentrations of free fatty acids and that the significantly higher carbohydrate load in the fat-free regimens accounted for the lower glucagon and high insulin concentrations in that group.

Complications of the use of the recently developed intravenous fat emulsions, particularly 10% Intralipid, are surprisingly few (H1, V2). Although incriminating evidence is lacking, the rise in free fatty acids, particularly after heparin injection (V2) carries with it theoretical dangers. Glucose metabolism may be impeded and growth hormone depressed. Of particular concern is the possibility of displacement of albumin-bound bilirubin by plasma free fatty acids, which may compete with bilirubin for free albumin binding sites (H16), increasing the risk of kernicterus.

The uptake of Intralipid into the endothelial cells of the lung vessels has been reported to occur shortly after infusion (G8). Pulmonary gas exchange has been found to be reversibly impaired after brief infusion of massive doses of Intralipid. Greene (G11) studied pulmonary function in 10 normal adult males during the 48 hours following infusion of 500 ml of 10% Intralipid over a 4-hour period. There was a decrease in membrane diffusing capacity in 6 of the 10 subjects. Greene injected an equivalent amount of Intralipid into rabbits and showed that during the early phase of the infusion more lipid was retained in the lung than in the liver. However, at no time was there any lipid deposition in the capillary endothelium or alveolar epithelium. On such evidence, it is difficult to draw firm conclusions on the pulmonary effects in the newborn infant. In the very ill baby with respiratory distress syndrome, tolerance to Intralipid may be reduced. In this situation, a decrease in membrane diffusing capacity could have a deleterious effect and measurement of triglyceride levels could be helpful in preventing dangerous overloading.

In view of the variability of handling infused fat emulsions it should not be automatically assumed that low-birth-weight infants are capable of metabolizing large quantities of fat (H16). Lipoprotein lipase is saturated at levels of about 100 mg/100 ml. Severely ill patients receiving modest amounts of Intralipid may have plasma triglyceride concentrations in excess of 400–500 mg/100 ml. By monitoring the total serum triglyceride concentration, it is possible to modify the rate of Intralipid infusion in order to prevent the plasma level from exceeding 200 mg/100 ml. Nothing is to be gained by infusing at a rate greater than that which can be metabolized. In the laboratory, the turbidity of the plasma produced by excessive fat infusion can interfere with routine biochemical analyses.

3.5. Amino Acids

The provision of a solution containing amino acids is the one common factor essential to all regimes of total intravenous nutrition. This nitrogen source may be obtained either as beef fibrin or casein hydrolyzates or as the more recently introduced totally synthetic solutions of crystalline amino acids. The process of hydrolysis, either acid- or enzyme-catalyzed, tends to destroy some of the amino acids, and this deficit, especially of the essential amino acids, is corrected by addition of the pure substances. A disturbing feature of these amino acid solutions, particularly the protein hydrolyzates, is the inconsistency in composition and the discrepancies between the claimed and the actual composition (D4, G5, S12). Just how much of the peptide content of hydrolyzates is utilized is in doubt; certainly peptiduria can be produced (C8, C9), but it would appear that at least a portion of the peptide content can be metabolized (H17). An important factor affecting the losses of peptide in the urine may be related to the effects of heat sterilization; although the amount of material modified by the Maillard reaction is minute compared with the peptide wastage, it may be that the urinary losses are the consequence of trace amounts of antagonistic, and presumably toxic, material (C7).

Even moderate heat may cause glutamine to be converted either to glutamate and ammonium or to cyclic compound, pyrrolidone-5-carboxylate and ammonium. In consequent of such reactions, the ammonium content of hydrolyzates solutions is usually considerably higher than that of synthetic amino acid mixtures. There is no evidence that pyrrolidone carboxylate is harmful, and, in rat at least, it is rapidly metabolized (R3).

Although relatively cheap to produce, protein hydrolyzates have the major disadvantage of variability and inflexibility of composition and may contain random collections of peptides with unknown, and possibly undesirable, effects (C7). Solutions of crystalline amino acids are considerably more expensive than the hydrolyzates but offer the potential benefits of consistency of composition and adaptability to meet the nutritional and metabolic needs of the patient.

Few of the commercially available solutions have been specifically formulated with the newborn in mind, although some are better than others (B11). Unfortunately, it cannot be assumed that the infant's metabolic requirements with respect to amino acids are similar to those of the adult. For most of the amino acids, the per kilogram requirement of the newborn infant may be almost an order of magnitude greater than that of the adult (H3, M9). Considerable individual differences in the metabolism of amino acids are seen among infants. In this respect, the maturity of the newborn plays an important part. Small-for-gestational-age infants may present metabolic problems seen less frequently in normal full-term newborns.

Compared with normal full-term infants, low-birth-weight infants tend to have lower total plasma amino acid concentration (R5) with lower levels of glutamine, glycine, histidine (A1, R5), serine, methionine, isoleucine (R5), alanine, and ornithine (A1).

Although low-birth-weight infants can be induced to gain weight when infused with solutions that contain amino acids, the factors determining the ability of these infants to metabolize amino acids are incompletely understood. This group of newborns is particularly prone to develop hyperaminoacidemias when fed intravenously, and the possible deleterious effects of such disturbances is a cause of concern (A1).

An "immaturity" of some pathways of amino acid metabolism may hinder proper utilization producing elevated, and possibly toxic, concentration of amino acids and their metabolites. Increased levels of methionine and low concentrations of cystine have been noted in infants receiving intravenous nutrition (B16, P7, W10); this is almost certainly related to a block in the pathway synthesizing cystine from methionine. Cystathionase is known to be absent in human fetal liver and premature infants (R2, S15). This may be further complicated by low levels in the liver of the methionine-activating enzyme (R2). The consequences of such a block are elevation of methionine, low rate of synthesis of cystine, and possibly high levels of cystathionine, similar to those reported by Valman and colleagues (V1) in 4 out of 5 low-birth-weight infants on high-protein feeds. Considerable changes in the metabolism of sulfur-containing amino acids occur in the newborn period; taurine, which is excreted in very large amounts by the normal newborn, is less prominent in the urine of infants aged between 1 and 12 months (S7).

Tyrosinemia is a frequent problem in low-birth-weight infants, especially those receiving intravenous amino acids (A1). This appears to be due to an effective deficiency of the enzyme p-hydroxyphenylpyruvic acid oxidase in the premature infant and to substrate inhibition of the enzyme in the presence of inadequate amounts of ascorbic acid; supplementation with vitamin C may correct the defect.

Although the hepatic phenylalanine hydroxylase system is usually well developed in the full-term infant, so that there is usually no difficulty in the conversion of phenylalanine to tyrosine, a metabolic block may occur at this level in low-birth-weight infants, with consequent hyperphenylalaninemia and impaired synthesis of tyrosine (D4, R2).

Although many of the currently available solutions are largely devoid of cystine and contain low concentrations of tyrosine (S12), even from the incomplete evidence presently available, it would seem that these amino acids, especially cystine, may be essential in some newborn infants, and, indeed, even in some adults receiving intravenous nutrition (D6). Histidine, which may be a nutritionally essential amino acid in some infants (S8), may also be deficient in some regimes and result in low plasma concentrations (W10).

The ability of the low-birth-weight infant to convert amino acid into glucose may be impaired. In the adult, alanine stimulates glucagon secretion, increasing gluconeogenesis (W9). In the healthy full-term newborn infant, alanine administered either intravenously (S10), or orally (F6) also raises plasma glucagon and glucose levels, indicating that in the normally nourished infant alanine, the major gluconeogenic amino acid, enhances hepatic glucose output. Although some infants of gestational age as low as 31 weeks appear to be able to utilize amino acid for gluconeogenesis (B16), in some small-for-gestational-age infants the plasma concentrations of potentially gluconeogenic amino acids normally metabolized through pyruvate (alanine, aspartate, serine, glycine, and methionine) may be significantly higher than in normal full-term infants, and the concentration of alanine may remain persistently elevated at 24 hours (H9). Oral administration of alanine to small-for-gestational-age infants may be associated with a significantly lower rise in both plasma glucose and insulin concentrations than in healthy newborns (W6). It is apparent, therefore, that in the malnourished infant (small-for-gestational-age) gluconeogenesis may be ineffective and gluconeogenic amino acids, such as alanine, cannot be relied upon as energy sources.

As a consequence of undernutrition and metabolic immaturity, the low-birth-weight infant may not easily handle infused amino acids. In this situation, monitoring of amino acid metabolism should play an important part. At this time, this presents considerable technical difficulties. It is not feasible to measure tissue incorporation or even amino acid concentrations and, in view of the expense incurred in equipment and materials, and the time taken to perform plasma aminograms on relatively large samples of blood, it is perhaps not surprising that plasma levels of amino acids are rarely determined routinely. Thin-layer chromatography of plasma amino acids can be used to give useful information (B15). There is, however, a dearth of data concerning the effects of intravenous nutrition upon tissue amino acid pools (S11). Because of the very nature of the regimes, in particular the amino acid concentration, the rate of infusion, the degree of maturity of the infant, and the circumstances of its illness, generalizations are difficult to make. Gross excesses of amino acid concentration in plasma and also deficiencies are observed (G6). In general, the plasma amino acid profile tends to be considerably influenced by the composition of the preparation and its rate of infusion (J3, S11, S12); high rates of infusion tend to be associated with hyperaminoacidemia (D1, J3). With reasonably balanced solutions, 300–350 mg of N per kilogram per day can be infused without producing gross hyperaminoacidemia in most infants, with plasma levels usually within two standard deviations of the normal plasma mean (D1).

Olney et al. (O1) have questioned the safety of protein hydrolyzates in the total intravenous nutrition of the human infant. They found that hydrolyzate solutions containing glutamate, aspartate, and cysteic acid, when injected into mice, were capable of producing hypothalamic damage, which did not occur after the injection of control solutions from which these amino acids have been excluded. On the available data, Filer and Stegink (F3) considered that it was unwarranted to impugn the safety of protein hydrolyzates as nitrogen sources in the total intravenous nutrition of the human infant. However, high rates of infusion may produce isosmolar coma (T4), and in the absence of adequate data, it would not seem to be wise to produce gross elevations of the plasma concentrations of these, and other, amino acids, particularly as the intake of disproportionate amounts may result not only in toxicity but also antagonisms and imbalances (H3, H4, M6, W1).

3.5.1. *Hyperammonemia*

Elevated plasma ammonium concentrations have been reported in infants receiving intravenous nutrition. The degree of hyperammonemia appears to be related to the rate of infusion of the amino acid solution (J6); at low rates of infusion, this complication is not seen (S11). It has been suggested (G5, J6) that hyperammonemia may be the result of infusion with protein hydrolyzates solutions that have high ammonium concentrations (F5, M7). However, the finding of high blood levels of ammonium in infants receiving mixtures of synthetic L-amino acids (H18) with low ammonium concentrations (M7), suggests that the etiology is probably more complex and depends on such factors as imbalance of the amino acid mixture, high rates of infusion of the amino acid preparation, and an inability to handle endogenous and/or exogenous ammonium.

Arginine, a component of the ammonium-removing urea cycle, is known to play a protective role with respect to the toxic effects of some amino acids (M6). Plasma arginine levels in infants receiving intravenous nutrition are rarely raised and, indeed, may be low; the administration of arginine to some infants with hyperammonemia appears to be associated with a reduction in the plasma ammonium level (B11, H18).

The observations of Stephen and Waterlow (S14) suggested that, in a state of malnutrition, the infant liver may have depressed activity of argininosuccinase. It is likely that many of the infants receiving intravenous nutrition will have experienced pre- and postnatal malnutrition, and it is possible that, in the cases with hyperammonemia, there is a block in the urea cycle. The low-birth-weight infant with immaturity of the liver enzyme systems, or with overt liver disease, is likely to be more susceptible to hyperammonemia. In their study, Ghadimi and co-workers (G5) recorded abnormal levels of plasma aminotransferases in two of their infants. Ghadimi (G4) has suggested that the clinical entity described by Silvis and Paragas (S5) as "fatal hyperalimentation syndrome" may be explained by hyperammonemia.

Clinically, infants with this condition develop lethargy, unresponsiveness, and twitching movements of eyes and limbs followed by fits. Heird *et al.* (H17) suggest that all infants receiving total intravenous nutrition should have careful monitoring of plasma ammonium levels. In view of uncertainty over the incidence of this complication and the limitation upon the number of different investigations possible imposed by the small blood volume of many of the infants involved, this is, perhaps, a counsel of perfection difficult in practice to achieve.

4. Disorders of Hydrogen Ion Regulation

Alterations in hydrogen ion regulation may be encountered in infants receiving total intravenous nutrition. Helmuth *et al.* (H19), describing metabolic changes occurring in four low-birth-weight infants receiving a protein hydrolyzate–monosaccharide (fructose/glucose) regime, noted a rapid fall in arterial blood pH associated with commencement of this infusion. In some cases, severe metabolic acidosis may occur, especially in small infants (C3, C4, H6, H14), although not in all cases (F11, P3), and in some low-birth-weight infants, the fall in pH may be due to chronic respiratory acidosis with increased plasma P_{CO_2} values (D8).

The etiology of this metabolic acidosis is almost certainly multifactorial and may be further complicated by the fact that infused nutrients bypass that major regulator of hydrogen ion concentration, the gastrointestinal tract, which by secreting acid through the gastric and jejunal mucosa and base from the pancreas and colon considerably modifies the acid-base effects of ingested food (K4).

Heird *et al.* (H14) investigated the possible cause of hyperchloremic metabolic acidosis in 11 infants receiving total intravenous nutrition for functional impairment of the gastrointestinal tract. They concluded that endogenous causes resulting in excessive loss of base were unlikely to account for the complication. Using the undetermined anion (i.e., Na + K + 2 Ca + 2 Mg − Cl − 1.8 total P) as an index of bicarbonate and organic bases, they found that there was no appreciable difference between the excretion of base in patients receiving either the synthetic amino acid mixture or fibrin hydrolyzate. Indeed, in both groups, the loss of base was less than that of normal milk-fed infants and considerably less than that of infants with diarrhea. Infants who became acidotic during intravenous nutrition with the synthetic amino acid mixture were found to have normal, or even high, values for the daily urinary excretion of net acid (urinary titratable acidity + NH_4 − HCO_3). It therefore seemed very unlikely that the hyperchloremic acidosis was the result of excessive urinary excretion of base.

Metabolic acidosis associated with intravenous nutrition has been attributed to a variety of causes.

4.1. Hyperosmolar Acidosis

An increase in urine and plasma osmolality may be encountered, particularly in low-birth-weight infants receiving hypertonic monosaccharide–amino acid infusions (B13, G5, H11); this may be associated with a fall in arterial pH (H19).

Studies in animals have revealed that experimentally induced hypertonicity of body fluids results in the formation and release of large quantities of hydrogen ion and the development of a severe extracellular metabolic acidosis, which improves with restoration of normal osmolality (S9, W8). The magnitude of fall in plasma bicarbonate concentration can be largely accounted for by shift of water from the intracellular to the extracellular space, reducing the bicarbonate concentration by dilution (W8). Such a mechanism should increase the intracellular pH, since the bicarbonate concentration within the cells would increase as a result of the transfer of water. Some support for this view was gained by examination of the cerebrospinal fluid (CSF) (in which there is rapid equilibration of water and carbon dioxide, but not of bicarbonate). It was found that the pH of cerebrospinal fluid rose while that of the blood fell, the change being apparently due to increased concentrations of bicarbonate in the CSF (W8). Since the solutions used in total intravenous nutrition are, in the main, appreciably hypertonic, this mechanism may be a cause of metabolic acidosis, although direct evidence is at present lacking.

4.2. LACTIC ACIDOSIS

Lactic acidosis, with a concomitant increase in NADH:NAD ratio, may be seen in intravenous nutrition particularly when fructose, ethanol, or polyols are used (A11, H6). This is discussed in Section 3.2.1.

4.3. AMINO ACIDS IN RELATION TO HYDROGEN ION REGULATION

A relationship between the nature and rate of infusion of the amino acid solution to the development of acid-base disorders is well established. Some synthetic mixtures of L-amino acids are more likely to produce metabolic acidosis than are protein hydrolyzates (C4, H13).

The amino acid solutions used in intravenous nutrition are usually acidic, with pII in the range of 5.5 5.8, and have appreciable titratable acidity and ammonium concentrations. It is probable, however, that this direct infusion of acid is not the most important factor leading to metabolic acidosis since the fibrin hydrolyzates have a much greater titratable acidity and a higher ammonium concentration than the synthetic amino acid mixtures, while the latter may be more liable to produce acidosis (H13, H14).

Chan (C3) found that the infusion of amino acid solutions into 4 premature infants and a 10-year-old child was associated with a 4- to 14-fold increase in sulfuric acid production. Although the rate of organic acid production in patients receiving casein hydrolyzate was about twice that when synthetic amino acid solutions were infused, the sulfuric acid production was the more important, so that the total amount of acid produced as a consequence of the synthetic amino acid infusion was greater than that associated with the use of casein hydrolyzate. This work suggested that the increased production of sulfuric acid associated with the use of synthetic infusates was likely to be related to the high concentrations of sulfur-containing amino acids, especially methionine.

Although there is no doubt that sulfuric acid is produced by the metabolism of sulfur-containing amino acids, this may not be the major source of acid production (H15). Heird *et al.* (H14) suggested that the increased acidogenic properties of the synthetic amino acid mixtures which they used (Neoaminosol and Freamine) is due to the higher concentrations of the cationic amino acids, arginine, lysine, and histidine. These, especially arginine and lysine, are effectively acidic at physiological pH. In Neoaminosol, the cation gap (inorganic anion in excess of inorganic cation) can be accounted for by the concentrations of these metabolizable cationic amino acids. Protein hydrolyzates have a small *anion* gap, probably due to the presence of the negatively charged amino acids (glutamate and aspartate) and negatively charged peptides. The catabolism of cationic amino acids releases hydrogen ion whereas that of the anionic amino acids is associated with the removal of hydrogen ions. The relative proportions of lysine and arginine on the one hand and glutamate and aspartate on the other are probably important in the genesis of acid–base disturbances.

If totally catabolized, the acidogenic effects of lysine and arginine are neutralized by roughly similar concentrations of glutamate and aspartate. It is, however, difficult to determine an ideal ratio between these two groups of amino acids since most proteins contain more glutamate and asparatate than arginine and lysine, so that, during protein synthesis, additional glutamate and aspartate are required (C7). The hydrogen ion status is therefore dependent not only on the absolute amounts of these amino acids, but also upon the relationship between anabolism and catabolism (C7).

In view of the frequency with which potentially dangerous acid-base disorders are associated with intravenous nutrition of the newborn, the provision of an adequate laboratory service for the monitoring of hydrogen ion parameters is of the utmost importance.

5. Hypophosphatemia

Hypophosphatemia may occur as a complication of intravenous nutrition both in adult patients (L3, M4, S2, S6, T7) and in children (F12, R6).

This complication occurs particularly in regimes not supplemented by phosphate, especially when the amino acid solution used is either a synthetic mixture of crystalline amino acids or a fibrin hydrolyzate. Hypophosphatemia occurs less frequently with casein hydrolyzates or the soybean emulsion Intralipid, since both contain appreciable amounts of organic phosphorus; however, the use of these infusates should not lead to complacency since this phosphorus may not readily be utilized. In infants and children, there may be an associated hypercalcemia (D8, U1). The clinical features include hypotonia, areflexia, lethargy, tremor, and polypnea (R6) paresthesia, muscular weakness, and coma (P9, S2). The intravenous administration of potassium phosphate will correct the hypophosphatemia but may not always affect the neurological symptoms (S2).

Silvis and Paragas (S5) described a "fatal hyperalimentation syndrome" in which high rates of infusion of fibrin hydrolyzate and glucose into starved animals produced a profound fall in serum inorganic phosphate; correction of the hypophosphatemia did not give protection.

The fall in plasma inorganic phosphorus levels is related to the reduced intake, and 2 mmoles/kg/per day of inorganic phosphate is usually sufficient to maintain a positive phosphorus balance and normal plasma inorganic phosphorus concentration (H17). However, other mechanisms appear to play a part. In children, there may be a transient, inappropriate, hyperphosphaturia as the hypophosphatemia develops, and negative phosphorus balances have been observed (R6). This phosphaturia may be due to inhibition of tubular phosphate reabsorption by amino acids, especially alanine (D9). The excessive excretion of phosphates is a feature of the postoperative period in the newborn, paralleling the urinary excretion of potassium (K5). Once hypophosphatemia is established it is usually associated with a simultaneous fall of urinary phosphorus excretion, both in children (R6) and in adults (T7). There may be associated hypercalciuria (R6).

Urinary losses of phosphate, combined with a reduced intake, cannot entirely account for the degree of hypophosphatemia. The plasma inorganic phosphorus level rapidly returns to normal when intravenous nutrition is ended, suggesting massive shifts in body inorganic phosphate (L4). In the adult case reported by Silvis and Paragas (S6), death coincided with a marked increase in calorie intake. They observed that the fall in serum inorganic phosphorus in response to a calorie load resembled that seen in the glucose tolerance test, and it may be that the clinical features and the hypophosphatemia are related to abrupt changes in glucose utilization.

In their study of the relationship between intravenous nutrition, hy-

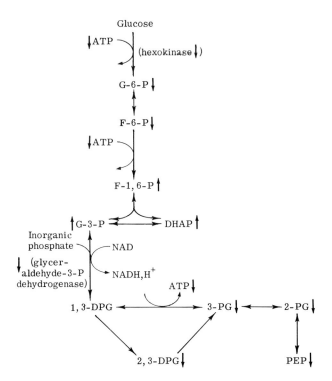

Fig. 5.   Effects of hypophosphatemia on red-cell glycolysis, postulated by Travis *et al.* (T7). Abbreviations correspond to metabolites named in Fig. 1.

pophosphatemia, and red cell metabolism, Travis *et al.* (T7) noted that of 8 hypophosphatemic patients the 3 with paresthesias, mental obtundity, and hyperventilation had the lowest p_{50} values. This was attributable to decreased levels of erythrocyte 2,3-diphosphoglycerate (2,3-DPG) and ATP causing a "shift to the left" of the oxygen–hemoglobin dissociation curve, with increased affinity for oxygen and consequent decreased tissue oxygenation. Their data suggest that the glycolytic pathway is regulated by inorganic phosphorus at the glyceraldehyde-3-phosphate dehydrogenase step, so that hypophosphatemia results in decreases in erythrocyte 2,3-DPG and ATP and increases in the triose phosphates. The decreased ATP reduces the hexokinase activity and, by virtue of reduction in allosteric inhibition, increases phosphofructokinase activity, adding further to the accumulation of triose phosphates while reducing the amounts of glucose 6-phosphate and fructose 6-phosphate. Phosphate repletion, either by intravenous phosphate infusion or by cessation of intravenous feeding, restores the erythrocyte concentrations of ATP and

2,3-DPG only rather slowly over a period of several days, with rise in 2,3-DPG favored over that of ATP. A lag period of 1–3 weeks occurs before restoration to normal of erythrocyte ATP levels (L4). It seems likely, therefore, that the clinical features associated with hypophosphatemia depend to a large extent on decreased oxygen delivery to the tissues rather than on the concentrations of tissue organic phosphates as such.

The red cell content of ATP appears to affect its membrane deformability and consequently its life-span (L1). Although low concentrations of erythrocyte ATP, resulting from hypophosphatemia, appear to increase the rigidity of the cell membrane, Travis *et al.* (T7) showed no change in osmotic fragility in one patient investigated during the entire period of hypophosphatemia.

Although it is clear that hypophosphatemia has considerable effects upon the metabolism of the red cell, evidence of a similar dependence of the nonerythroid cells upon plasma inorganic phosphorus metabolism is not so well documented. It may be that such cells become the beneficiaries of the accumulation of phosphate which accompanies glucose and amino acid entry (L3). In patients receiving intravenous nutrition, low plasma inorganic phosphorus concentrations have been shown to be associated with a reduction in leukocyte ATP (C17). This was found to be associated with a depression of chemotactic, phagocytic, and bactericidal actions of granulocytes. While this may have some relevance to the problem of infection in patients receiving intravenous nutrition, the mechanism is still not clear, since correction of the subnormal concentrations of ATP with phosphate supplements do not completely restore the chemotactic response.

6. Essential Fatty Acid Deficiency

Intravenous feeding with glucose-amino acid regimes may affect the lipid profile producing a fall to low levels of plasma free fatty acids (D5, W4), free glycerol, and triglycerides (D5), and a rise in ester cholesterol (W4). Concern has been expressed over the lack of dietary essential fatty acids in infants receiving fat-free regimes (W4). Essential fatty acids, which are prostaglandin precursors and are found in phospholipids, may play an important role in maintaining the structural integrity of cell membranes. Deficiencies are likely to occur in linoleic acid, the precursor of the $\omega6$ family of fatty acids and in linolenic acid, the source of the $\omega3$ series.

Essential fatty acid deficiency is now established as a human disease (C2). Since the newborn infant has a serum pattern of polyunsaturated acids resembling that of marginal essential fatty acid deficiency (H21), it is possible for infants to develop evidence of deficiency when fed on some infant formula diets. Fat emulsions, especially the soybean preparations, contain considerable amounts of both linoleic and linolenic acid. Fat-free intravenous feeding may induce a deficiency of essential fatty acids, both in adults (J4) and in infants (C1, P1). It seems likely that the deficiency will occur more regularly with some regimes than with others (D10).

Essential fatty acid deficiency is characterized by the development of a dry scaly dermatitis, which may be associated with impaired wound healing, susceptibility to sepsis, and thrombocytopenia. These clinical findings are accompanied by the characteristic changes in serum fatty acid composition—decreased amounts of $18:2\omega6$ (linoleic acid), $20:4\omega6$ (arachidonic acid), and $22:6\omega3$ with elevated concentrations of $20:3\omega9$ (eicosatrienoic acid) (H21, P1, W3). There is a rise in the trienoic/tetranoic fatty acid ratio—a useful indicator of the intensity of essential fatty acid deficiency. Although the changes in fatty acid levels are seen within the first week, with little additional change during the subsequent weeks, the clinical features of essential fatty acid deficiency may not be apparent until some considerable time after the institution of fat-free intravenous feeding. The fatty acid changes may be accompanied by elevation of the plasma cholesterol ester, but not of free cholesterol, and higher mean plasma levels of total lipid and triglyceride with little change in the phospholipid concentration (W4).

The rise in the plasma concentration of eicosatrienoic acid associated with a fall in both linoleic and linolenic acids is presumably due to the increased conversion of oleic acid to the 20-carbon acid. Although linoleic acid cannot be synthesized, it can be elongated and converted to arachidonic acid, so that the decrease in the latter parallels that of the former. The decline in arachidonic acid is not always observed. Jeejeebhoy et al. (J4) reported essential fatty acid deficiency in an adult receiving intravenous nutrition for 23 months and noted that during the period of fat-free infusion there was evidence of essential fatty acid deficiency together with a reduction in linoleic acid and a slight rise, rather than the anticipated decline, in arachidonic acid; this was associated with higher concentrations of eicosatrienoic acid than found in normal plasma. Jeejeebhoy et al. noted that their patient developed a fatty liver while on a fat-free diet; this histological finding reverted to normal when Intralipid was added to the regime—supporting the view that lipid emulsions can play an important part in long-term intravenous feeding (although not proving that the effects were due to the essential fatty acid content of the product.)

At least in rats, essential fatty acid deficiency may be associated with increased skin permeability to water, abnormalities of mitochondria (H22) and of fatty acid composition of brain lipids affecting the developing central nervous system (G1, G2).

Patients with cystic fibrosis have low levels of some essential fatty acids. These changes have been reviewed by Rivers and Hassam (R7), who suggest that patients with cystic fibrosis have increased requirements of linoleic acid, and possibly of its desaturation products. Regular infusion of Intralipid administered to an infant with cystic fibrosis was associated with a decline in sweat sodium concentration, relief of pancreatic achylia, and improvement in general health, with weight gain progressing from the third percentile to the fiftieth percentile (E5). Although it is too early to draw firm conclusions, these data suggest that Intralipid may have some value in the treatment of cystic fibrosis.

7. Trace Element Deficiencies

The use of prolonged total intravenous nutrition is likely to produce deficiencies of minor dietary components, such as the trace elements, including manganese, zinc, copper, and cobalt (W14). Although some groups of workers have included in their regimes regular plasma infusions, hoping thereby to prevent trace element deficiencies, it is unlikely that such attempts at replacement therapy are effective. Solutions providing what appear to be adequate amounts of these elements have been regularly added to the infusate without obvious toxic effects and with maintenance of the measured zinc and copper levels (J4).

To date, little is known of the incidence or effects of trace element deficiency in man, and even less in patients receiving intravenous nutrition. What little information is available is largely restricted to zinc and copper.

7.1. ZINC

Zinc is involved in many important metabolic processes (M5); it provides the metal constituent of a number of metalloenzymes, including carbonic anhydrase, carboxypeptidase, alkaline phosphatase, and dehydrogenases, including alcohol dehydrogenase, glutamate dehydrogenase, glyceraldehyde-3-phosphate dehydrogenase, lactate dehydrogenase, and malate dehydrogenase. In addition, it activates many hydrolytic enzymes. DNA synthesis, RNA polymerase, ribonuclease, and thymidine kinase are zinc-dependent. The element plays an important part in protein anabolism (H20), and it appears to participate in the synthesis of collagen.

In man, the metabolism and consequent importance, of zinc has been the subject of much investigation and speculation (E4, W5). Zinc deficiency resulting from inadequate nutrition, appears to be associated with growth failure, hypogonadism, idiopathic hypogeusia, and impaired wound healing.

Under normal circumstances, dietary sources are adequate and zinc deficiency does not occur. Tissue catabolism, especially of skeletal muscle, may be associated with increased urinary zinc excretion (F1), and there is evidence that hyperactivity of the hypothalamic–pituitary–adrenal axis is associated with an increased mobilization of body stores, raised urinary excretion, and a decrease in serum zinc concentration (F8, H20). The cachectic patient with gastrointestinal disorder receiving intravenous nutrition, with consequent deficient intake combined with increased excretion, is especially liable to become zinc deficient (K3).

In some circumstances, intravenous nutrition may increase the urinary zinc losses. Freeman et al. (F13) investigated the effect of intravenous nutrition on urinary zinc excretion in groups of postsurgical adult patients and healthy volunteers. They found a 4-fold increase in urinary zinc losses when the solution used was a protein hydrolyzate previously autoclaved with glucose. No such increase was noted in subjects receiving solutions in which the amino acid source had not been previously heated with glucose. This work suggests that the sugar-amine compounds produced by the "browning reaction" (see Section 3.2.4.) chelate zinc, and that tubular reabsorption of the filtered complex does not occur. Amino acid binding of zinc does not appear to be a significant factor, since the urinary free amino acid excretion was similar in patients receiving both kinds of solution.

The introduction of more sensitive methods of analysis has greatly facilitated the estimation of zinc in biological fluids (M5). Unfortunately, in man the concentration of zinc in serum may not accurately reflect total body stores (H20). Normal levels may be found in states of depletion and low serum levels may be encountered in the presence of acute or chronic infection, anemia, liver disease, and malignancy without associated zinc deficiency. The measurement of urinary zinc excretion is probably a better indicator of zinc deficiency, particularly when the intake of the element is known, as is usually the case in patients receiving intravenous nutrition.

When providing a monitoring service, the clinical chemist should be aware of the possibility of contamination of blood samples by zinc, which may be in high concentration in the rubber end-cap of the piston of some disposable plastic syringes (T1).

7.2. COPPER

Copper depletion is not uncommon in severely malnourished infants with chronic diarrhea (A4, G10). Clinical features associated with copper deficiency include sideroblastic anemia, neutropenia, hypoproteinemia, hypoferremia, scorbutic-like bone changes in the presence of ascorbic acid intake, depigmentation of skin and hair, hypotonia, psychomotor retardation, and difficulties with vision (A4, A8, G9). Low-birth-weight infants appear to be particularly susceptible; although such infants have correspondingly small livers, the copper content is not usually decreased, and the development of the deficiency is dependent not only on a poor copper intake but probably also on gastrointestinal losses (G9).

The clinical and biochemical features of copper deficiency occurring during long-term intravenous nutrition have been described in infants (A8, K2) and in adults (D15). In each case, the condition developed in patients receiving prolonged courses of intravenous nutrition following gastrointestinal surgery, and the signs of copper deficiency responded promptly to copper supplementation. The work of Dunlap et al. (D15) suggests that the duodenum is a major site of copper absorption, since oral administration to their patients, both of whom had the duodenum anastomosed to the transverse colon, corrected the deficiency. In each of these patients, the serum copper and ceruloplasmin concentrations were depressed to about 10% of their normal value. The renal and gastrointestinal losses of copper were not measured. Similar clinical findings have been noted in Menkes' "kinky-hair" syndrome, an X-lined recessive inherited condition in which copper deficiency appears to be related to a defect in intestinal absorption (D3).

The nature of the biochemical lesions produced by copper deficiency is unknown. Cytochrome oxidase is an important copper-containing enzyme whose activity is markedly decreased in the presence of copper depletion (W5), possibly accounting for the neurological and metabolic disturbance. Copper is an important component of other oxidases, including monoamine oxidase, concerned with the oxidation of lysine to provide cross-links between elastin polypeptides. The scorbutic-like bone changes may be explained by the copper requirement of ascorbic acid oxidase.

8. Intravenous Nutrition and the Liver

Hepatic disorders may be encountered in association with intravenous nutrition. The incidence of liver dysfunction varies considerably in pediatric patients, with reports as low as one in 118 (H17) to three of 18 (T6) and even 15 out of 17 (C13). The factors influencing such a wide spectrum of incidence include the age of the patient (and, in the case of newborn infants, the developmental maturity), the nature and duration of the infusion, and the means of detecting liver dysfunction. Biochemical tests of liver function are relatively infrequently used in the particularly vulnerable low-birth-weight newborn (R1). Three types of structural liver changes have been described: fatty liver, intrahepatic cholestasis, and hepatic deposition of "lipid pigment."

8.1. Fatty Liver

The development of fatty liver as a result of dietary deficiencies is well documented (F7). Steiger *et al.* (S13) showed that the treatment of protein-depleted rats with intravenous glucose solutions produced a deleterious change in liver morphology, with an associated fall in serum albumin level, reversed by the addition to the regime of an amino acid mixture. Jeejeebhoy *et al.* (J4), in their study of prolonged intravenous feeding, found that extensive fatty change occurred when intravenous lipid emulsion was removed from the protocol: subsequent biopsies showed rapid resolution to normal after the reintroduction of Intralipid in adequate amounts. This work strongly suggested that lipid infusions may be effective in preventing the development of fatty liver. In their patient, elevated serum glutamic–oxaloacetic transaminase occurred both during lipid-containing and lipid-free periods; this rise did not appear to be correlated with obvious liver disease other than mild triaditis. The serum alkaline phosphatase changes paralleled those of the transaminase, and the plasma albumin rose to normal values during intravenous nutrition and appeared to be unaffected by therapy with Intralipid.

8.2. Intrahepatic Cholestasis Associated with Long-Term Intravenous Nutrition

Peden *et al.* (P5) first drew attention to the problem of cholestasis. Their patient, a 1-kg infant, had developed well-marked hepatosplenomegaly by day 48 of total parenteral nutrition with a 20% glucose/3.3% protein hydrolyzate solution into a central vein. The patient died at the age of 71 days, and at postmortem examination was found to have early cirrhosis with prominent bile duct reduplication and centrilobular cholestasis. No clear relationship between liver disease and therapy was established. Touloukian and Downing (T6) subsequently reported obstructive jaundice in three newborn infants, two of whom died, receiving a similar regime for periods in excess of 50 days. In each, there were parallel elevations of total and direct bilirubin with relatively normal levels of serum alkaline phosphatase and transaminase and, in the two examined histologically, there was an unusual form of hepatitis with parenchymal cholestasis. In the surviving child, jaundice cleared when the intravenous feeding was stopped. The two patients with unremitting jaundice shonwed no sign of hepatic insufficiency. Similar cholestatic jaundice with rising serum transaminases and alkaline phosphatase have been reported in older children (C12).

Increasing serum transaminases after 2 months of intravenous nutrition have been observed in an adult receiving crystalline amino acids, glucose, and Intralipid for over 7 months (B5). These changes normalized when the fat infusion was replaced by hypertonic glucose with a transitory increase when fat was reintroduced. In this case, the serum alkaline phosphatase activity was in the high-normal range for the first 2 months and subsequently varied between 2 and 4 times the upper normal value, being parallel to the changes in transaminases. The serum bilirubin levels were never excessive. Serum triglycerides, cholesterol, and phospholipids increased in concentration during therapy but remained largely within the normal range.

The mechanism of this form of jaundice is not clear. Experimental studies with guinea pig liver explants (C12) suggest that glycine, leucine, threonine, and isoleucine (and possibly cysteine and arginine) produced considerable increases in transaminase activity in the explant medium.

Cholestasis, at least in the premature infant, may be related not so much to the nature of the intravenous nutrient as to the poor state of general nutrition and the lack of oral feeding. Failure to feed has been suggested as a factor acting by reducing the normal increase in bile flow and bile salt excretion found after oral feeding (R1). Perhaps some disorder of amino acid metabolism impairs normal bile salt formation (T6).

8.3. HEPATIC "INTRAVENOUS FAT PIGMENT"

A feature of intravenous nutrition with regimes including Intralipid is the inclusion in the liver of yellow-brown, PAS-positive, diastase-resistant acid-fast pigment—so-called "intravenous fat pigment" (J1). A retrospective examination of postmortem material from 23 infants and children receiving intravenous lipid emulsion before death revealed that in 14 patients pigment was demonstrable in the hepatic cells, and in 22 patients it was present in the reticuloendothelial cells (K6). It appears that the amount of hepatic cell pigment is related directly to the rate of lipid infusion whereas that in the reticuloendothelial cell bears no relationship to age, diagnosis, rate, or total dose of fat emulsion. This accumulation does not appear to signify liver damage (B5). The pigment probably persists for a considerable time (H10) so that long-standing harmful effects cannot be excluded (T5).

REFERENCES

A1. Abitbol, C. L., Feldman, D. B., Ahmann, P., and Rudman, D., Plasma amino acid patterns during supplemental nutrition of low-birth-weight infants. *J. Pediatr.* **86,** 766–772 (1975).

A2. Adcock, L. H., and Gray, C. H., The metabolism of sorbitol in the human subject. *Biochem. J.* **65**, 554–560 (1957).

A3. Allen, P. C., Biochemical principles in parenteral nutrition. *In* "A Clinical Guide to Intravenous Nutrition" (P. C. Allen and H. A. Lee, eds.), pp. 5–25. Blackwell, Oxford, 1969.

A4. Al-Rashid, R. A., and Spangler, J., Neonatal copper deficiency. *N. Engl. J. Med.* **285**, 841–843 (1971).

A5. Andersson, G., Brohult, J., and Sterner, G., Increasing metabolic acidosis following fructose infusion in two children. *Acta Pediatr. Scand.* **58**, 301–304 (1969).

A6. Asch, M. J., Sperling, M., Fiser, R., Leake, R., Moore, T. C., and Oh W., Metabolic and hormonal studies comparing three parenteral nutrition regimens in infants. *Ann. Surg.* **182**, 62–65 (1975).

A7. Ashare, R., Moore, R., and Ellison, E. H., Utilization of glucose, fructose and invert sugar. *Arch. Surg. (Chicago)* **70**, 428–435 (1955).

A8. Ashkenazi, A., Levin, S., Djaldetti, M., Fishel, E., and Benvenisti, D., The syndrome of neonatal copper deficiency. *Pediatrics* **52**, 525–533 (1973).

A9. Atwater, W. O., and Benedict, F. C., An experimental inquiry regarding the nutritive value of alcohol. *Mem. Natl. Acad. Sci.* **8**, 235 (1897).

A10. Auld, P. A. M., Bhangananda, P., and Mehta, S., The influence of an early calorie intake with I.V. glucose on catabolism of premature infants. *Pediatrics* **37**, 592–596 (1966).

A11. Aynsley-Green, A., Baum, J. D., Alberti, K. G. M. M., and Woods, H. F., Hyperlactataemia during intravenous feeding in childhood. *Arch. Dis. Child.* **49**, 647–653 (1974).

B1. Baer, H. P., Drummond, G. I., and Duncan, E. L., Formation and deamination of adenosine by cardiac muscle enzymes. *Mol. Pharmacol.* **2**, 67–76 (1966).

B2. Baker, J. A., Kirkman, H., Woodley, C., and Eckel, F. M., Computer-assisted pediatric hyperalimentation. *Am. J. Hosp. Pharm.* **31**, 752–758 (1974).

B3. Bässler, K. H., and Bickel, H., The use of carbohydrates alone and in combination in parenteral nutrition. *In* "Parenteral Nutrition" (A. W. Wilkinson, ed.), pp. 99–104. Churchill Livingstone, Edinburgh and London, 1972.

B4. Benda, G. I. M., and Babson, S. G., Peripheral intravenous alimentation of the small premature infant. *J. Pediatr.* **79**, 494–498 (1971).

B5. Bergström, K., Blomstrand, R., and Jacobson, S., Long-term complete intravenous nutrition in man. *Nutr. Metab.* **14**, Suppl., 118–149 (1972).

B6. Blackburn, G. L., Flatt, J. P., Clowes, G. H. A., and O'Donnell, T. E., Peripheral intravenous feeding with isotonic amino acid solutions. *Am. J. Surg.* **125**, 447–454 (1973).

B7. Bode, C., Schumacher, H., Goebell, H., Zelder, O., and Pelzel, H., Fructose induced depletion of liver adenine nucleotides in man. *Horm. Metab. Res.* **3**, 289–290 (1971).

B8. Boeckman, C. R., and Krill, C. E., Bacterial and fungal infections complicating parenteral alimentation in infants and children. *J. Pediatr. Surg.* **5**, 117–126 (1970).

B9. Bordos, D. C., and Cameron, J. L., Successful long-term intravenous hyperalimentation in the hospital and at home. *Arch. Surg. (Chicago)* **110**, 439–441 (1975).

B10. Børresen, H. C., Clinical applications in paediatric surgery and paediatrics. *In* "Parenteral Nutrition in Acute Metabolic Illness" (H. A. Lee, ed.), pp. 221–272. Academic Press, New York, 1974.

B11. Børresen, H. C., Bjordal, R., and Knutrud, O., Total balanced intravenous feeding by peripheral veins in paediatric surgery. *Ann. Chir. Gynaecol. Fenn.* **62**, 319–327 (1973).

B12. Børresen, H. C., Coran, A. G., and Knutrud, O., Metabolic results of parenteral feeding in neonatal surgery: A balanced program based on a synthetic L-amino acid solution and a commercial fat emulsion. *Ann. Surg.* **172**, 291–301 (1970).

B13. Brans, Y. W., Sumners, J. E., Dweck, H. S., and Cassady, G., Feeding the low birth weight infant: orally or parenterally? Preliminary results of a comparative study. *Pediatrics* **54**, 15–21 (1974).

B14. Brennan, M. F., Goldman, M. H., O'Connell, R. C., Kundsin, R. B., and Moore, F. D., Prolonged parenteral alimentation: *Candida* growth and the prevention of candidemia by Amphotericin installation. *Ann. Surg.* **176**, 265–269 (1972).

B15. Bryan, M. H., Wei, P., Hamilton, J. R., and Chance, G. W., Supplemental intravenous alimentation in low-birth-weight infants. *J. Pediatr.* **82**, 940–944 (1973).

B16. Bryan, M. H., Anderson, G. H., Roy, R. N., and Jeejeebhoy, K. N., Effect of gestational age on the utilization of intravenous amino acids in the first week of life. *Pediatr. Res.* **8**, 379/105 (1974).

C1. Caldwell, M. D., Jonsson, H. T., and Othersen, H. B., Essential fatty acid deficiency in an infant receiving prolonged parenteral alimentation. *J. Pediatr.* **81**, 894–898 (1972).

C2. Caldwell, M. D., Meng, H. C., and Jonsson, H. T., Essential fatty acid deficiency (EFAD)—now a human disease. *Fed. Proc., Fed. Am. Soc. Exp. Biol.* **32**, 915 (1973).

C3. Chan, J. C. M., The influence of synthetic amino acid and casein hydrolysate on the endogenous production and urinary excretion of acid in total intravenous alimentation. *Pediatr. Res.* **6**, 789–796 (1972).

C4. Chan, J. C. M., Asch, M. J., Lin, S., and Hays, D. M., Hyperalimentation with amino acid and casein hydrolysate solutions. Mechanism of acidosis. *J. Am. Med. Assoc.* **220**, 1700–1705 (1972).

C5. Chance, G. W., Results in very low birth weight infants ($<$ 1300 gm birth weight). *In* "Intravenous Nutrition in the High Risk Infant" (R. W. Winters and E. G. Hasselmeyer, eds.), pp. 39–50. Wiley, New York.

C6. Chen, W.-J., Ohashi, E., and Kasai, M., Amino acid metabolism in parenteral nutrition: with special reference to the calorie:nitrogen ratio and the blood urea nitrogen level. *Metab., Clin. Exp.* **23**, 1117–1123 (1974).

C7. Christensen, H. N., Factors that should be considered for the improvement of amino acid solutions for intravenous nutrition. *In* "Intravenous Nutrition in the High Risk Infant" (R. W. Winters and E. G. Hasselmeyer, eds.), pp. 237–244. Wiley, New York, 1975.

C8. Christensen, H. N., Lynch, E. L., and Powers, J. H., The conjugated, non-protein, amino acids of plasma. III. Peptidemia and hyperpeptiduria as a result of the intravenous administration of partially hydrolyzed casein (Amigen). *J. Biol. Chem.* **166**, 649–652 (1946).

C9. Christensen, H. N., Lynch, E. L., Decker, D. G., and Powers, J. H., The conjugated, non-protein, amino acids of plasma. IV. A difference in the utilization of the peptides of hydrolysates of fibrin and casein. *J. Clin. Invest.* **26**, 849–852 (1947).

C10. Christensen, H. N., Wilber, P. B., Coyne, B. A., and Fisher, J. H., Effects of simultaneous or prior infusion of sugars on the fate of protein hydrolysates. *J. Clin. Invest.* **34**, 86–93 (1955).

C11. Coats, D. A., The place of ethanol in parenteral nutrition. *In* "Parenteral Nutrition" (A. W. Wilkinson, ed.), pp. 152–159. Churchill Livingstone, Edinburgh, and London, 1972.

C12. Cohen, M. I., Changes in hepatic function. *In* "Intravenous Nutrition in the High Risk Infant" (R. W. Winters and E. G. Hasselmeyer, eds.), pp. 293–305. Wiley, New York, 1975.

C13. Cohen, M. I., Litt, I. F., Schonberg, S. K., Daum, F., and Spigland, I., Hepatic dysfunction associated with parenteral alimentation: Clinical and experimental studies. *Pediatr. Res.* **7**, 334/106 (1973).

C14. Coran, A. G., The long-term total intravenous feeding of infants using peripheral veins. *J. Pediatr. Surg.* **8**, 801–807 (1973).

C15. Coran, A. G., Intravenous use of fat for the total parenteral nutrition of the infant. *In* "Intravenous Nutrition in the High Risk Infant" (R. W. Winters and E. G. Hasselmeyer, eds.), pp. 343–355. Wiley, New York, 1975.

C16. Coran, A. G., and Nesbakken, R., The metabolism of intravenously administered fat in adult and newborn dogs. *Surgery* **66**, 922–928 (1969).

C17. Craddock, P. R., Yawata, Y., VanSanten, L., Gilberstadt, S., Silvis, S., and Jacob, H. S., Acquired phagocyte dysfunction. A complication of the hypophosphatemia of parenteral hyperalimentation. *N. Engl. J. Med.* **290**, 1403–1407 (1974).

D1. Dale, G., Panter-Brick, M., Wagget, J., and Young, G., Plasma amino acid changes in the postsurgical newborn during intravenous nutrition with a synthetic amino acid solution. *J. Pediatr. Surg.* **11**, 17–22 (1976).

D2. Danks, D. M., Connellan, J. M., and Solomon, J. R., Hereditary fructose intolerance: Report of a case and comments on the hazards of fructose infusion. *Aust. Paediatr. J.* **8**, 282–286 (1972).

D3. Danks, D. M., Stevens, B. J., Campbell, P. E., Gillespie, J. M., Walker-Smith, J., Bloomfield, J., and Turner, B., Menkes' kinky-hair syndrome. *Lancet* **1**, 1100–1102 (1972).

D4. Das, J. B., and Filler, R. M., Amino acid utilization during total parenteral nutrition in the surgical neonate. *J. Pediatr. Surg.* **8**, 793–799 (1973).

D5. Das, J. B., Filler, R. M., Rubin, V. G., and Eraklis, A. J., Intravenous dextrose-amino acid feeding: The metabolic response in the surgical neonate. *J. Pediatr. Surg.* **5**, 127–135 (1970).

D6. Den Besten, L., and Stegink, L. D., Effect of parenteral alimentation mixtures on plasma amino acid levels in adult subjects: Comparison of the route of administration. *Fed. Proc., Fed. Am. Soc. Exp. Biol.* **31**, 732 (1972).

D7. Dolanski, E. A., Stahlman, M. T., and Meng, H. C., Parenteral Alimentation of premature infants under 1,200 grams. *South. Med. J.* **66**, 41–46 (1973).

D8. Driscoll, J. M., Heird, W. C., Schullinger, J. N., Gongaware, R. D., and Winters, R. W., Total intravenous alimentation in low-birth-weight infants. A preliminary report. *J. Pediatr.* **81**, 145–153 (1972).

D9. Drummond, K. N., and Michael, A. F., Specificity of the inhibition of tubular phosphate reabsorption by certain amino acids. *Nature (London)* **201**, 1333–1334 (1964).

D10. Dudrick, S. J., Essential fatty acids. *In* "Intravenous Nutrition in the High Risk Infant" (R. W. Winters and E. G. Hasselmeyer, eds.), pp. 285–289. Wiley, New York, 1975.

D11. Dudrick, S. J., MacFadyen, B. V., Van Buren, C. T., Ruberg, R. L., and Maynard, A. T., Parenteral hyperalimentation:metabolic problems and solutions. *Ann. Surg.* **176**, 259–264 (1972).

D12. Dudrick, S. J., Vars, H. M., Rawnsley, H. M., and Rhoads, J. E., Total intravenous feeding and growth in puppies. *Fed. Proc., Fed. Am. Soc. Exp. Biol.* **25**, 481 (1966).

D13. Dudrick, S. J., Wilmore, D. W., Vars, H. M., and Rhoads, J. E., Long-term total parenteral nutrition with growth, development and positive nitrogen balance. *Surgery* **64**, 134–142 (1968).

D14. Dudrick, S. J., Wilmore, D. W., Vars, H. M., and Rhoads, J. E., Can intravenous feeding as the sole means of nutrition support growth in the child and restore weight loss in an adult? An affirmative answer. *Ann. Surg.* **169**, 974–984 (1969).

D15. Dunlap, W. M., James, G. W., and Hume, D. M., Anemia and neutropenia caused by copper deficiency. *Ann. Intern. Med.* **80**, 470–476 (1974).

D16. Dweck, H. S., and Cassady, G., Glucose intolerance in infants of very low birth weight. I. Incidence of hyperglycemia in infants of birthweights 1,100 grams or less. *Pediatrics* **53**, 189–195 (1974).

E1. Editorial, Fructose infusion hazards. *Can. Med. Assoc. J.* **108**, 1208 (1973).

E2. Editorial, Intravenous feeding. *Lancet* **2**, 1179–1180 (1973).

E3. Editorial, Postoperative feeding and metabolism. *Lancet* **2**, 263–264 (1975).

E4. Editorial, Zinc in human medicine. *Lancet* **2**, 351–352 (1975).

E5. Elliott, R. B., and Robinson, P. G., Unusual clinical course in a child with cystic fibrosis treated with fat emulsion. *Arch. Dis. Child.* **50**, 76–78 (1975).

E6. Ellis, G. P., The Maillard reaction. *Adv. Carbohydr. Chem.* **14**, 63–134 (1959).

E7. Elman, R., Pareira, M. D., Conrad, E. J., Weichselbaum, T. E., Moncrief, J. A., and Wren, C., The metabolism of fructose as related to the utilization of amino acids when both are given by intravenous infusion. *Ann. Surg.* **136**, 635–642 (1952).

E8. Elphick, M. C., Dougall, A. J., and Wilkinson, A. W., The utilisation of solutions of glucose and xylitol administered by intravenous infusion to neonatal surgical patients. *In* "Parenteral Nutrition" (A. W. Wilkinson, ed.), pp. 138–147. Churchill Livingstone, Edinburgh and London, 1972.

E9. Elphick, M. C., and Wilkinson, A. W., Glucose intolerance in newborn infants undergoing surgery for alimentary-tract anomalies. *Lancet* **2**, 539–541 (1968).

F1. Fell, G. S., Fleck, A., Cuthbertson, D. P., Queen, K., Morrison, C., Bessent, R. G., and Husain, S. L., Urinary zinc levels as an indication of muscle catabolism. *Lancet* **1**, 280–282 (1973).

F2. Filer, L. J., Barness, L. A., Goldbloom, R. B., Holliday, M. A., Miller, R. W., O'Brien, D., Pearson, H. A., Scriver, C. R., Weil, W. B., Whitten, C. F., Cravioto, J., and Kline, O. L., Parenteral feeding—a note of caution. *Pediatrics* **49**, 776–779 (1972).

F3. Filer, L. J., and Stegink, L. D., Safety of hydrolysates in parenteral nutrition. *N. Engl. J. Med.* **289**, 426–427 (1973).

F4. Filler, R. M., Eraklis, A. J., Rubin, V. G., and Das, J. B., Long-term total parenteral nutrition in infants. *N. Engl. J. Med.* **281**, 589–594 (1969).

F5. Finkbiner, R. B., Arcos, M., and Ahmed, S. Z., Arterial and venous ammonia response to intravenous protein hydrolysate administration. *Metab., Clin. Exp.* **11**, 1077–1086 (1962).

F6. Fiser, R. H., Williams, P. R., Fisher, D. A., DeLameter, P. V., Sperling, M. A., and Oh, W., The effect of oral alanine on blood glucose and glucagon in the human newborn infant. *Pediatrics* **56**, 78–81 (1975).

F7. Flores, H., Seakins, A., and Mönckeberg, F., Mechanism of fatty liver in infantile malnutrition. *In* "Dietary Lipids and Postnatal Development" (C. Galli, G. Jacini, and A. Pecile, eds.), pp. 115–125. Raven, New York, 1973.

F8. Flynn, A., Pories, W. J., Strain, W. H., Hill, O. A., and Fratianne, R. B., Rapid zinc depletion associated with corticosteroid therapy. *Lancet* **2**, 1169–1171 (1971).

F9. Forget, P. P. F. X., Fernandes, J., and Haverkamp Begemann, P., Enhancement of fat elimination during intravenous feeding. *Acta Paediatr. Scand.* **63**, 750–752 (1974).

F10. Förster, H., Meyer, E., and Ziege, M., Erhöhung von Serumharnsäure und Serumbilirubin nach hochdosierten Infusion von Sorbit, Xylit und Fructose. *Klin. Wochenschr.* **48**, 878–879 (1970).

F11. Fox, H. A., and Krasna, I. H., Total intravenous nutrition by peripheral vein in neonatal surgical patients. *Pediatrics* **52**, 14–20 (1973).

F12. Frédérich, A., Guibaud, P., Marcon, G., and Larbre, F., Le risque de déplétion phosphorée dans l'alimentation parentérale prolongée du nourrisson. *Pediatrie* **28**, 453–454 (1973).

F13. Freeman, J. B., Steglink, L. D., Meyer, P. D., Fry, L. K., and DenBesten, L., Excessive urinary zinc losses during parenteral alimentation. *J. Surg. Res.* **18**, 463–469 (1975).

G1. Galli, C., Dietary lipids and brain development. *In* "Dietary Lipids and Postnatal Development" (C. Galli, G. Jacini, and A. Pecile, eds.), pp. 191–202. Raven, New York, 1973.

G2. Galli, C., White, H. B., and Paoletti, R., Brain lipid modifications induced by essential fatty acid deficiency in growing male and female rats. *J. Neurochem.* **17**, 347–355 (1970).

G3. Geyer, R. P., Parenteral nutrition. *Physiol. Rev.* **40**, 150–186 (1960).

G4. Ghadimi, H., A review: Current status of parenteral amino acid therapy. *Pediatr. Res.* **7**, 169–173 (1973).

G5. Ghadimi, H., Abaci, F., Kumar, S., and Rathi, M., Biochemical aspects of intravenous alimentation. *Pediatrics* **48**, 955–965 (1971).

G6. Ghadimi, H., Kumar, S., and Abaci, F., Endogenous amino acid loss and its significance in infantile diarrhea. *Pediatr. Res.* **7**, 161–168 (1973).

G7. Gibson, H. V., and Doisy, E. A., A note on the effect of some organic acids upon the uric acid excretion of man. *J. Biol. Chem.* **55**, 605–610 (1923).

G8. Gigon, J. P., Enderlein, F., and Scheidegger, S., Über das Schicksal infundierter Fettemulsionen in der menschlichen Lunge. *Schweiz. Med. Wochenschr.* **96**, 71–75 (1966).

G9. Graham, G. G., Human copper deficiency. *N. Engl. J. Med.* **285**, 857–858 (1971).

G10. Graham, G. G., and Cordano, A., Copper depletion and deficiency in the malnourished infant. *Johns Hopkins Med. J.* **124**, 139–150 (1969).

G11. Greene, H. L., Effects of intralipid on the lung. *In* "Intravenous Nutrition in the High Risk Infant" (R. W. Winter and E. G. Hasselmeyer, eds.), pp. 369–375. Wiley, New York, 1975.

G12. Groff, D. B., Complications of intravenous hyperalimentation in newborns and infants. *J. Pediatr. Surg.* **4**, 460–464 (1969).

G13. Gustafson, A., Kjellmer, I., Olegård, R., and Victorin, L., Nutrition in low-birth-weight infants. *Acta Paediatr. Scand.* **61**, 149–158 (1972).

H1. Hallberg, D., Holm, I., Obel, A. L., Schuberth, O., and Wretlind, A., Fat emulsions for complete intravenous nutrition. *Postgrad. Med. J.* **43**, 307–316 (1967).

H2. Hallberg, D., Schuberth, O., and Wretlind, A., Experimental and clinical studies with fat emulsion for intravenous nutrition. *Nutr. Dieta* **8**, 245–281 (1966).

H3. Harper, A. E., Amino acid imbalance. *In* "Intravenous Nutrition in the High Risk Infant" (R. W. Winters and E. G. Hasselmeyer, eds.), pp. 215–228. Wiley, New York, 1975.

H4. Harper, A. E., Benevenga, N. J., and Wohlhueter, R. M., Effects of ingestion of disproportionate amounts of amino acids. *Physiol. Rev.* **50**, 428–550 (1970).

H5. Harries, J. T., Intravenous feeding in infants. *Arch. Dis. Child.* **46**, 855–863 (1971).

H6. Harries, J. T., Metabolic acidosis during intravenous feeding of infants. *In* "Parenteral Nutrition" (A. W. Wilkinson, ed.), pp. 266–274. Churchill, London, 1972.

H7. Harris, R. J., Plasma nonesterified fatty acid and blood glucose levels in healthy and hypoxemic newborn infants. *J. Pediatr.* **84**, 578–584 (1974).

H8. Harris, R. L., Mehlman, M. A., and Veech, R. L., Effect of chronic feeding of 1,3-butanediol and ethanol on brain redox states and metabolite levels. *Fed. Proc., Fed. Am. Soc. Exp. Biol.* **31**, 670 (1972).

H9. Haymond, M. W., Karl, I. E., and Pagliara, A. S., Increased gluconeogenic substrates in the small-for-gestational-age infants. *N. Engl. J. Med.* **291**, 322–328 (1974).

H10. Hays, D. M., in discussion of "Hepatic 'intravenous fat pigment' in infants and children receiving lipid emulsion," by Y. Koga, V. L. Swanson, and D. M. Hays. *J. Pediatr. Surg.* **10**, 641–648 (1975).

H11. Hays, D. M., Kaplan, M. S., Mahour, G. H., Strauss, J., and Huxtable, R. F., High-calorie infusion therapy following surgery in low-birth-weight infants: Metabolic problems encountered. *Surgery* **71**, 834–841 (1972).

H12. Heggarty, H. J., Acute alcoholic hypoglycaemia in two 4-year-olds. *Br. Med. J.* **1**, 280 (1970).

H13. Heird, W. C., Disorders of acid-base metabolism. *In* "Intravenous Nutrition in the High Risk Infant" (R. W. Winters and E. G. Hasselmeyer, eds.), pp. 257–262. Wiley, New York, 1975.

H14. Heird, W. C., Dell, R. B., Driscoll, J. M., Grebin, B., and Winters, R. W., Metabolic acidosis resulting from intravenous alimentation mixtures containing synthetic amino acids. *N. Engl. J. Med.* **287**, 943–948 (1972).

H15. Heird, W. C., Dell, R. B., and Winters, R. W., Acid-base problems after intravenous amino acids. *N. Engl. J. Med.* **288**, 421 (1973).

H16. Heird, W. C., and Driscoll, J. M., Use of intravenously administered lipid in neonates. *Pediatrics* **56**, 5–7 (1975).

H17. Heird, W. C., Driscoll, J. M., Schullinger, J. N., Grebin, B., and Winters, R. W., Intravenous alimentation in pediatric patients. *J. Pediatr.* **80**, 351–372 (1972).

H18. Heird, W. C., Nicholson, J. F., Driscoll, J. M., Schullinger, J. N., and Winters, R. W., Hyperammonemia resulting from intravenous alimentation using a mixture of synthetic L-amino acids: A preliminary report. *J. Pediatr.* **81**, 162–165 (1972).

H19. Helmuth, W. V., Adam, P. A. J., and Sweet, A. Y., The effects of protein hydrolysate-monosaccharide infusion on low-birth-weight infants. *J. Pediatr.* **81**, 129–136 (1972).

H20. Henkin, R. I., Zinc in wound healing. *N. Engl. J. Med.* **291**, 675–676 (1974).

H21. Holman, R. T., Essential fatty acid deficiency in humans. *In* "Dietary Lipids and Postnatal Development" (C. Galli, G. Jacini, and A. Pecile, eds.), pp. 127–143. Raven, New York, 1973.

H22. Houtsmuller, U. M. T., Differentiation in the biological activity of polyunsaturated fatty acids. In "Dietary Lipids and Postnatal Development" (C. Galli, G. Jacini, and A. Pecile, eds.), pp. 145–155. Raven, New York, 1973.

J1. Jacobson, S., Ericsson, J. L. E., and Obel, A.-L., Histopathological and ultrastructural changes in the human liver during complete intravenous nutrition for seven months. Acta Chir. Scand. 137, 335–349 (1971).

J2. Jakob, A., Williamson, J. R., and Asakura, T., Xylitol metabolism in perfused rat liver. Interactions with gluconeogenesis and ketogenesis. J. Biol. Chem. 246, 7623–7631 (1971).

J3. Jean, R., Castel, J., Rieu, D., Montoya, F., Alquier, J., Belay, J. M., and Dubar, J., Acides amines plasmatiques au cours de l'alimentation parentérale par l'"Aminosol Vitrum." Rev. Pediatr. 9, 641–652 (1973).

J4. Jeejeebhoy, K. N., Zohrab, W. J., Langer, B., Phillips, M. J., Kuksis, A., and Anderson, G. H., Total parenteral nutrition at home for 23 months, without complication, and with good rehabilitation. Gastroenterology 65, 811–820 (1973).

J5. Jellum, E., Børresen, H. C., and Eldjarn, L., The presence of furan derivatives in patients receiving fructose-containing solutions intravenously. Clin. Chim. Acta 47, 191–201 (1973).

J6. Johnson, J. D., Albritton, W. L., and Sunshine, P., Hyperammonemia accompanying parenteral nutrition in newborn infants. J. Pediatr. 81, 154–161 (1972).

K1. Kaplan, M. S., Mares, A., Quintana, P., Strauss, J., Huxtable, R. F., Brennan, P., and Hays, D. M., High caloric glucose-nitrogen infusions: Postoperative management of neonatal infants. Arch. Surg. (Chicago) 99, 567–571 (1969).

K2. Karpel, J. T., and Peden, V. H., Copper deficiency in long-term parenteral nutrition. J. Pediatr. 80, 32–36 (1972).

K3. Kay, R. G., and Tasman-Jones, C., Zinc deficiency and intravenous feeding. Lancet 2, 605–606 (1975).

K4. Kildeberg, P., Engel, K., and Winters, R. W., Balance of net acid in growing infants. Endogenous and transintestinal aspects. Acta Paediatr. Scand. 58, 321–329 (1969).

K5. Knutrud, O., Postoperative homeostasis in the neonatal period. Acta Chir. Scand., Suppl. 357, 138–141 (1966)

K6. Koga, Y., Swanson, V. L., and Hays, D. M., Hepatic "intravenous fat pigment" in infants and children receiving lipid emulsion. J. Pediatr. Surg. 10, 641–648 (1975).

K7. Krebs, H. A., Freedland, R. A., Hems, R., and Stubbs, M., Inhibition of hepatic gluconeogenesis by ethanol. Biochem. J. 112, 117–124 (1969).

K8. Kremer, J. N., Vitolinia, S. P., Frank, E. L., Baumann, V. R., and Schmidt, A. A., The utilization of diols as an energy source in parenteral nutrition. In "Advances in Parenteral Nutrition" (G. Berg, ed.), p. 170. Thieme, Stuttgart, 1969.

L1. LaCelle, P. L., Alteration of membrane deformability in hemolytic anemias. Semin. Hematol. 7, 355–371 (1970).

L2. Lee, H. A., Morgan, A. G., Waldram, R., and Bennett, J., Sorbitol: Some aspects of its metabolism and role as an intravenous nutrient. In "Parenteral Nutrition" (A. W. Wilkinson, ed.), pp. 121–137. Churchill Livingstone, Edinburgh and London, 1972.

L3. Lichtman, M. A., Hypoalimentation during hyperalimentation. N. Engl. J. Med. 290, 1432–1433 (1974).

L4. Lichtman, M. A., Miller, D. R., Cohen, J., and Waterhouse, C., Reduced red cell glycolysis, 2,3-diphosphoglycerate and adenosine triphosphate concentration, and increased hemoglobin-oxygen affinity caused by hypophosphatemia. *Ann. Intern. Med.* **74**, 562–568 (1971).

M1. MacLaren, N. K., Valman, H. B., and Levin, B., Alcohol-induced hypoglycaemia in childhood. *Br. Med. J.* **1**, 278–280 (1970).

M2. Mäenpää, P. H., Raivio, K. O., Kekomäki, M. P., Liver adenine nucleotides. Fructose-induced depletion and its effect on protein synthesis. *Science* **161**, 1253–1254 (1968).

M3. Meng, H. C., and Anderson, G. E., The use of sorbitol in parenteral nutrition. *Fed. Proc., Fed. Am. Soc. Exp. Biol.* **31**, 670 (1972).

M4. Metzger, R., Burke, P., Thompson, A., Lordon, R., and Frimpter, G. W., Hypophosphatemia and hypouricemia during parenteral hyperalimentation with an amino acid-glucose preparation. *J. Clin. Invest.* **50**, 65a–66a (1971).

M5. Mikac-Dević, D., Methodology of zinc determinations and the role of zinc in biochemical processes. *Adv. Clin. Chem.* **13**, 271–333 (1970).

M6. Milne, M. D., Pharmacology of amino acids. *Clin. Pharmacol. Ther.* **9**, 484–516 (1968).

M7. Monnens, L., Trijbels, F., Van Galen, M., Henrichs, Y., and Baars, P., Complications of intravenous feeding. *Lancet* **1**, 1116–1117 (1973).

M8. Moore, F. D., and Brennan, M. R., Intravenous aminoacids. *N. Engl. J. Med.* **293**, 194–195 (1975).

M9. Munro, H. N., Amino acid requirements and metabolism and their relevance to parenteral nutrition. *In* "Parenteral Nutrition" (A. W. Wilkinson, ed.), pp. 34–67. Churchill Livingstone, Edinburgh and London, 1972.

M10. Muntz, J. A., and Vanko, M., The metabolism of intraportally injected fructose in rat liver *in vivo. J. Biol. Chem.* **237**, 3582–3587 (1962).

N1. Nelson, R., Minimizing systemic infection during complete parenteral alimentation of small infants. *Arch. Dis. Child.* **49**, 16–20 (1974).

N2. Nikiforuk, G., and Colowick, S. P., The purification and properties of 5-adenylic acid deaminase from muscle. *J. Biol. Chem.* **219**, 119–129 (1956).

O1. Olney, J. W., Ho, O. L., and Rhee, V., Brain-damaging potential of protein hydrolysates. *N. Engl. J. Med.* **289**, 391–395 (1973).

P1. Paulsrud, J. R., Pensler, L., Whitten, C. F., Stewart, S., and Holman, R. T., Essential fatty acid deficiency in infants induced by fat-free intravenous feeding. *Am. J. Clin. Nutr.* **25**, 897–704 (1972).

P2. Peaston, M. J. T., Dangers of Intravenous fructose. *Lancet* **1**, 266 (1973).

P3. Peden, V. H., and Karpel, J. T., Total parenteral nutrition in premature infants. *J. Pediatr.* **81**, 137–144 (1972).

P4. Peden, V. H., Sammon, T. J., and Downey, D. A., Intravenously induced infantile intoxication with ethanol. *J. Pediatr.* **83**, 490–493 (1973).

P5. Peden, V. H., Witzleben, C. L., and Skelton, M. A., Total parenteral nutrition. *J. Pediatr.* **78**, 180–181 (1971).

P6. Perheentupa, J., and Raivio, K., Fructose-induced hyperuricaemia. *Lancet* **2**, 528–531 (1967).

P7. Pildes, R. S., Ramamurthy, R. S., Cordero, G. V., and Wong, P. W. K., Intravenous supplementation of L-amino acids and dextrose in low-birth-weight infants. *J. Pediatr.* **82**, 945–950 (1973).

P8. Pr̆ibylová, H., Kimlová, I., and Štroufová, A., The effect of intravenous fructose and glucose on metabolism and plasma insulin levels in newborn infants. *Biol. Neonate* **23**, 205–213 (1973).

P9. Prins, J. G., Schrijver, H., and Staghouwer, J. H., Hyperalimentation, hypophosphataemia, and coma. *Lancet* 1, 1253–1254 (1973).

R1. Ragcr, R., and Finegold, M. J., Cholestasis in immature newborn infants: Is parenteral alimentation responsible? *J. Pediatr.* 86, 264–269 (1975).

R2. Räihä, N. C. R., Biochemical basis for nutritional management of preterm infants. *Pediatrics* 53, 147–156 (1974).

R3. Ramakrishna, M., Krishnaswamy, P. R., and Rao, D. R., Metabolism of pyrrolidonecarboxylic acid in the rat. *Biochem. J.* 118, 895–897 (1970).

R4. Raskin,, N. H., Alcoholism or acetaldehydism? *N. Engl. J. Med.* 293, 422–423 (1975).

R5. Reisner, S. H., Aranda, J. V., Colle, E., Papageorgiou, A., Schiff, D., Scriver, C. R., and Stern, L., The effect of intravenous glucagon on plasma amino acids in the newborn. *Pediatr. Res.* 7, 184–191 (1973).

R6. Ricour, C., Millot, M., and Balsan, S., Phosphorus depletion in children on long-term total parenteral nutrition. *Acta Paediatr. Scand.* 64, 385–392 (1975).

R7. Rivers, J. P. W., and Hassam, A. G., Defective essential-fatty-acid metabolism in cystic fibrosis. *Lancet* 2, 642–643 (1975).

S1. Sahebjami, H., and Scalettar, R., Effects of fructose infusion on lactate and uric acid metabolism. *Lancet* 1, 366–369 (1971).

S2. Sand, D. W., and Pastore, R. A., Paresthesias and hypophosphatemia occurring with parenteral alimentation. *Am. J. Dig. Dis.* 18, 709–713 (1973).

S3. Schuberth, O., and Wretlind, A., Intravenous infusion of fat emulsions, phosphatides and emulsifying agents. *Acta Chir. Scand., Suppl.* 278, 1–21 (1961).

S4. Schumer, W., Adverse effects of xylitol in parenteral alimentation. *Metab., Clin. Exp.* 20, 345–347 (1971).

S5. Silvis, S. E., and Paragas, P. V., Fatal hyperalimentation syndrome. Animal studies. *J. Lab. Clin. Med.* 78, 918–930 (1971).

S6. Silvis, S. E., and Paragas, P. D., Paresthesias, weakness, seizures and hypophosphatemia in patients receiving hyperalimentation. *Gastroenterology* 62, 513–520 (1972).

S7. Snyderman, S. E., Metabolism of amino acids. A review. *Pediatrics* 21, 117–142 (1958).

S8. Snyderman, S. E., Boyer, A., Roitman, E., Holt, L. E., and Prose, P. H., The histidine requirement of the infant. *Pediatrics* 31, 786–801 (1963).

S9. Sotos, J. F., Dodge, P. R., and Talbot, N. B., Studies in experimental hypertonicity. II. Hypertonicity of body fluids as a cause of acidosis. *Pediatrics* 30, 180–193 (1962).

S10. Sperling, M. A., DeLamater, P. V., Phelps, D., Fiser, R. H., Oh, W., and Fisher, D. A., Spontaneous and amino acid-stimulated glucagon secretion in the immediate postnatal period: Relation to glucose and insulin. *J. Clin. Invest.* 53, 1159–1166 (1974).

S11. Stegink, L. D., Amino acid metabolism. *In* "Intravenous Nutrition in the High Risk Infant" (R. W. Winters and E. G. Hasselmeyer, eds.), pp. 181–203. Wiley, New York, 1975.

S12. Stegink, L. D., and Baker, G. L., Infusion of protein hydrolysates in the newborn infant: Plasma amino acid concentrations. *J. Pediatr.* 78, 595–602 (1971).

S13. Steiger, E., Daly, J. M., Allen, T. R., Dudrick, S. J., and Vars, H. M., Postoperative intravenous nutrition: Effects on body weight, protein regeneration, wound healing, and liver morphology. *Surgery* 73, 686–691 (1973).

S14. Stephen, J. M. L., and Waterlow, J. C., Effect of malnutrition on activity of two enzymes concerned with amino acid metabolism in human liver. *Lancet* **1**, 118–119 (1968).

S15. Sturman, J. A., Gaul, G., and Räihä, N. C. R., Absence of cystathionase in human fetal liver: Is cystine essential? *Science* **169**, 74–75 (1970).

T1. Taylor, A., and Marks, V., Contamination from syringes and blood container pots in trace element analysis. *Ann. Clin. Biochem.* **10**, 42–46 (1973).

T2. Thomas, D. W., Edwards, J. B., Gilligan, J. E., Lawrence, J. R., and Edwards, R. G., Complications following intravenous administration of solutions containing xylitol. *Med. J. Aust.* **1**, 1238–1246 (1972).

T3. Thomas, D. W., Gilligan, J. E., Edwards, J. B., and Edwards, R. G., Lactic acidosis and osmotic diuresis produced by xylitol infusion. *Med. J. Aust.* **1**, 1246–1248 (1972).

T4. Touloukian, R. J., Isomolar coma during parenteral alimentation with protein hydrolysate in excess of 4gm/kg/day. *J. Pediatr.* **86**, 270–273 (1975).

T5. Touloukian, R., in discussion of "Hepatic 'intravenous fat pigment' in infants and children receiving lipid emulsion," by Y. Koga, V. L. Swanson, and D. M. Hays. *J. Pediatr. Surg.* **10**, 641–648 (1975).

T6. Touloukian, R. J., and Downing, S. E., Cholestasis associated with long-term parenteral hyperalimentation. *Arch. Surg. (Chicago)* **106**, 58–62 (1973).

T7. Travis, S. F., Sugerman, H. J., Ruberg, R. L., Dudrick, S. J., Delivoria-Papadopoulos, M., Miller, L. D., and Oski, F. A., Alterations of red-cell glycolytic intermediates and oxygen transport as a consequence of hypophosphatemia in patients receiving intravenous hyperalimentation. *N. Engl. J. Med.* **285**, 763–768 (1971).

U1. Ulstrom, R. A., and Brown, D. M., Hypercalcemia as a complication of parenteral alimentation. *J. Pediatr.* **81**, 419–420 (1972).

V1. Valman, H. B., Brown, R. J. K., Palmer, T., Oberholzer, V. G., and Levin, B., Protein intake and plasma amino-acids of infants of low birth weight. *Br. Med. J.* **4**, 789–791 (1971).

V2. Victorin, L. H., Intralipid metabolism in low birth weight infants. *In* "Intravenous Nutrition in the High Risk Infant" (R. W. Winters and E. G. Hasselmeyer, eds.), pp. 357–367. Wiley, New York, 1975.

V3. Vitale, J. J., DiGiorgio, J., McGrath, H., May, J., and Hegsted, D. M., Alcohol oxidation in relation to alcohol dosage and the effect of fasting. *J. Biol. Chem.* **204**, 257–264 (1953).

W1. Wannemacher, R. W., Cooper, W. K. C., and Muramatsu, K., Effect of amino acid levels on a cell-free system for protein synthesis. *Proc. Soc. Exp. Biol. Med.* **135**, 180–183 (1970).

W2. Wardrop, C. A. J., Heatley, R. V., Tennant, G. B., and Hughes, L. E., Acute folate deficiency in surgical patients on aminoacid/ethanol intravenous nutrition. *Lancet* **2**, 640–642 (1975).

W3. Wene, J. D., Connor, W. E., and DenBesten, L., The development of essential fatty acid deficiency in healthy men fed fat-free diets intravenously and orally. *J. Clin. Invest.* **56**, 127–134 (1975).

W4. White, H. B., Turner, M. D., Turner, M. S., and Miller, R. C., Blood lipid alterations in infants receiving intravenous fat-free alimentation. *J. Pediatr.* **83**, 305–313 (1973).

W5. "World Health Organization" Expert Committee, Trace elements in human nutrition. *W.H.O., Tech. Rep. Ser.* **532**, 9–19 (1973).

W6. Williams, P. R., Fiser, R. H., Sperling, M. A., and Oh, W., Effects of oral alanine feeding on blood glucose, plasma glucagon and insulin concentrations in small-for-gestational-age infants. *N. Engl. J. Med.* **292**, 612–614 (1975).

W7. Winters, R. W., Total parenteral nutrition in pediatrics: The Borden Award Address. *Pediatrics* **56**, 17–23 (1975).

W8. Winters, R. W., Scaglione, P. R., Nahas, G. G., and Verosky, M., The mechanism of acidosis produced by hyperosmotic infusions. *J. Clin. Invest.* **43**, 647–657 (1964).

W9. Wise, J. K., Hendler, R., and Felig, P., Evaluation of alpha-cell function by infusion of alanine in normal, diabetic and obese subjects. *N. Engl. J. Med.* **288**, 487–490 (1973).

W10. Wolf, H., Melichar, V., von Berg, W., and Kerstan, J., Intravenous alimentation with a mixture of fat, carbohydrates and amino acids in small newborn infants. *Infusionstherapie* **1**, 479–481 (1973).

W11. Woods, H. F., and Alberti, K. G. M. M., Dangers of intravenous fructose. *Lancet* **2**, 1354–1357 (1972).

W12. Woods, H. F., Eggleston, L. V., and Krebs, H. A., The cause of hepatic accumulation of fructose-1-phosphate on fructose loading. *Biochem. J.* **119**, 501–510 (1970).

W13. Woods, H. F., and Krebs, H. A., Lactate production in the perfused rat liver. *Biochem. J.* **125**, 129–139 (1971).

W14. Wretlind, A., Complete intravenous nutrition. Theoretical and experimental background. *Nutr. Metab.* **14**, Suppl., 1–57 (1972).

W15. Wretlind, A., Modern principles of the use of fat emulsions in parenteral nutrition. *Z. Ernaehrungswiss., Suppl.* **13**, 16–27 (1972).

SUBJECT INDEX

A

Advances in quality control, 175–205
 data handling, 191–192
 external schemes, 197–205
 preventive measures, 183–186
 techniques, 183
 terminology, 179–183
 use of patients' results, 191
 variance determinations, 186–191
Analogs of 1,25-(OH)$_2$D$_3$, 148–154
 biological activity requires fully
  extended side chain, 154
 3-deoxy-1-hydroxylated vitamin D's,
  151–152
 dihydrotachysterol, 149–150
  treatment of hypocalcemic diseases,
   149
  vitamin D-resistant rickets, 150
 epi-25-OH-D$_2$, 153
 3-epi-1,25-(OH)$_2$D$_3$, 153
 25-hydroxydihydrotachysterol, 150
 hydroxyl functions all related to
  biological activity, 154
 3-hydroxyl, biological significance,
  152
 24-hydroxylation, significance of, 152
 hydroxytachysterols and nephrectomized vitamin D-deficient
  animals, 150
 1α-hydroxyvitamin D$_2$, 151
 1α-hydroxyvitamin D$_3$, 151
  conversion to 1,25-(OH)$_2$D$_3$, 151
 isolated target-organ systems, in
  biological activity studies, 153
 length of side chain and biological
  activity, 153
 NMR studies, ring A, 154
 1,25-(OH)$_2$D$_2$, 153
 2α,25-(OH)$_2$D$_3$, 153
 organ-culture experiments, 153
 plants containing 1,25-(OH)$_2$D$_3$ and
  1,25-(OH)$_2$D$_2$, 154
 1,24R, 25-(OH)$_3$D$_3$, 153

24S- and 24R-hydroxy derivatives,
  152
 side chain derivatives, 153
 5,6-trans isomers, 150
 X-ray crystallography, 25-OH-D, 154
Analytical performance, quality of,
  176–179
 calcium determinations, hyperparathyroidism, 176
 evidence concerning quality, 176
 improvement, techniques and equipment, 176
 interlaboratory surveys, 176
  United Kingdom, 176, 177
  United States, 176
 introduction of automation, 176
 quality control techniques, 176
 radioimmunoassay, 178
 reference interval, 177
 serum albumin determination, 177
 serum calcium determination, 176
 UK National Quality Control Scheme,
  177
Antibodies to hormone receptors, 110–
  115
 acetylcholine receptor, 113–114
 insulin-receptor antibodies, 113
 other receptors, 114–115
 thyrotropin receptor antibodies, 110–
  113
Assigned value, 181
Automatic enzyme analyzers, 1–56
 continuous-monitoring assays, 10–23
  Abbott Laboratories ABA 100, 19
  amplifier characteristics, 17
  Beckman Instruments, Inc. System
   TR, 21
  data processing, 19–23
  enzyme activation or inactivation,
   16
  Gilford Instrument Laboratories
   Inc. 3500, 19
  I.F.C.C. recommended temperature,
   14
  inefficient mixing, 13

CONTENTS OF PREVIOUS VOLUMES

A
B
C
D
E
F
G
H
I
J